TARGETING NEW PATHWAYS AND CELL DEATH IN BREAST CANCER

Edited by **Rebecca L. Aft**

Targeting New Pathways and Cell Death in Breast Cancer
Edited by Rebecca L. Aft

Published by InTech
Janeza Trdine 9, 51000 Rijeka, Croatia

Publishing Process Manager Silvia Vlase

Technical Editor Teodora Smiljanic

Cover Designer InTech Design Team

Additional hard copies can be obtained from orders@intechopen.com

Targeting New Pathways and Cell Death in Breast Cancer, Edited by Rebecca L. Aft
p. cm.
ISBN 978-953-51-0145-1

For EU product safety concerns:
IN TECH d.o.o., Prolaz Marije Krucifikse Kozulić 3, 51000 Rijeka, Croatia,
info@intechopen.com or visit our website at intechopen.com.

Meet the editor

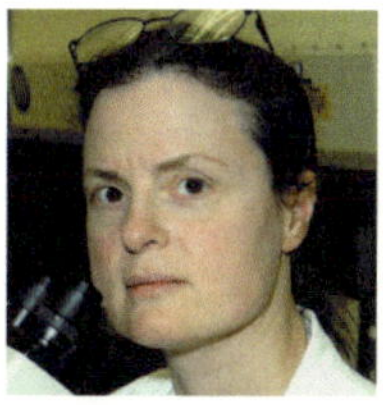

Dr Rebecca L. Aft is a Professor of Surgery, Washington University School of Medicine, in St. Louis. She received her PhD from the McArdle Laboratory for cancer Research at the University of Wisconsin-Madison and attended medical school at Washington University in St. Louis. Dr Aft has been the PI on multiple extramural and intramural grants as well as have been the PI on several clinic trials. Dr Aft's main research interest is characterizing disseminated tumor cells. These cells are intermediaries in the development of metastases. Specifically, her work focuses on molecularly characterizing these cells in order to develop new predictive detection modalities and new therapeutic interventions.

Contents

Preface

In this book we present manuscripts focusing on mechanisms of breast cancer cell death and new targets for therapeutic intervention by an accomplished group of international investigators. We have divided the book into 2 sections based on these topics. In the first section cell death by autophagy, estrogen induced apoptosis and by immunotherapy will be discussed. In the second section, there is an overview of the DNA damage response and discussion of new targets for intervention. Each of the experts contributing to this book discusses their topic thoughtfully and provides new insight into the topic leading to a new appreciation for these areas of investigation.

Dr. Rebecca L. Aft
Washington University School of Medicine
Department of Surgery
Saint Louis, Missouri
USA

Part 1

Breast Cancer Cell Death

1

Estrogen-Induced Apoptosis in Breast Cancer Cells: Translation to Clinical Relevance

Philipp Y. Maximov and Craig V. Jordan
Department of Oncology, Lombardi Comprehensive Cancer Center, Georgetown, University Medical Center, Washington, D.C., USA

1. Introduction

The first example of hormonal dependency of breast cancer can be dated back as far as 1896, when Dr. G.T. Beatson observed and described the reduction of breast cancer progression in a premenopausal patient after bilateral oophorectomy (Beatson 1896). It was an indication that the ovaries produced something in a woman's body that fueled breast cancer growth. This phenomenon was reconfirmed in a collected series of patients with advanced breast cancer following oophorectomy (Boyd 1900), however there was only a 30% percent response. In 1916 Lathrop and Loeb demonstrated in mice, that ovarian function has an influence on the growth of mammary glands and tumorigenesis, and that castration of immature female mice has delayed the evolution of mammary tumors (Lathrop 1916). However, the chemical control mechanisms of breast cancer progression and the relevance of ovarian function remained uncertain, until the first animal models were introduced to test the effects of oophorectomy and estrogenic properties of different chemical compounds under precise laboratory conditions (Allen 1923). This model allowed the indentification the ovarian hormone, which induced estrus in oophorectomized mice, estrogen.

In subsequent years during the 1930s and 1940s many other compounds, including diethylstilbestrol, and triphenylethylene derivatives would be identified as estrogens utilizing the ovariectomized mouse model (Robson 1937; Dodds 1938). The connection between the beneficial effects of oophorectomy as a treatment for advanced breast cancer provoked questions about the actual role of estrogen and other estrogenic compounds in breast cancer growth. High dose estrogen therapy was the first chemical therapy ("chemotherapy") to treat any cancer successfully. In 1944 Haddow (Haddow 1944) published the results of his clinical trial with the synthetic estrogens triphenylchlorethylene, triphenylmethylethylene, and diethylstilbestrol. He found that 10 out of 22 post-menopausal patients with advanced mammary carcinomas, who were treated with triphenylchlorethylene, had significant regression of tumor growth. Five patients out of 14 who were treated with high dose stilbestrol produced similar responses. The finding that high doses of synthetic estrogens induced regression of tumor growth in some, but not all postmenopausal patients with breast cancer (30% of patients responded to therapy favorably) was similar to the random responsiveness of oophorectomy in premenopausal patients with metastatic breast cancer (Boyd 1900). However, Haddow (Haddow 1944) noted that the first successful use of a chemical therapy to treat breast and prostate cancers was affiliated with significant systemic side effects, such as nausea, areola pigmentation, uterine bleeding, and edema of the lower extremities. At approximately same time Walpole was investigating the role of diethylstilbestrol and dienestrol in breast cancer (Walpole 1948). He confirmed the results obtained by Haddow that estrogens are effective in the treatment of breast cancer and can be of benefit for patients, but also noticed that older women, and women who received higher doses of estrogens had a better response to hormonal therapy (Walpole 1948; Haddow 1950). However, the mechanisms were again undefined.

The first successful attempt to decipher the biochemistry of estrogens in mammals occurred a decade later. Tritium-labeled hexestrol was found to accumulate in reproductive organs, including mammary glands, in female goats and sheep (Glascock and Hoekstra 1959). This finding was a crucial observation to understand the role of estrogens in processes involving target tissues, such as the mammary gland. Subsequently this research was translated to the clinic with the finding that tritium-labeled hexestrol accumulated at a higher rate in patients that favorably respond to adrenalectomy and oophorectomy, comparing to patients that do not (Folca et al. 1961). This indicated that patients who would accumulate estrogens better in target breast tissue would respond better to surgical castration. However, this technical approach was not pursued further.

During the 1950's Kennedy (Kennedy and Nathanson 1953) systematically investigated the efficacy of synthetic estrogens for the treatment of advanced breast cancer. Kennedy examined a variety of different estrogens, however he found no significant differences and diethylstilbestrol became the standard drug. However, side effects still remained a concern and responses lasted for only about a year in the majority of patients. By the 1960's, the standards for the hormonal treatment of breast cancer were established. Premenopausal women were to be treated with ovarian irradiation therapy or bilateral oophorectomy. However, based on data from the clinical trials, postmenopausal patients with advanced breast cancer were to be treated with high dose of the most potent synthetic estrogenic compound diethylstilboestrol (Kennedy 1965). Overall, one could anticipate that 36 % of patients would respond favorably to high dose estrogen therapy (Kennedy 1965). However, the molecular mechanisms of the anticancer action of estrogen remained elusive. In 1970 Haddow (Haddow 1970) was not enthusiastic about the overall prospects of chemical therapy of breast cancer, he felt that it was important that safer less toxic "estrogens" were developed that might extend therapeutic use. There were clues that deciphering the mysteries of endocrine therapy, such as unknown mechanisms of tumor regression after high-dose estrogen therapy, which could be of major benefit for patient's treatment. Haddow stated: "In spite of the extremely limited practicality of such measure [high dose estrogen], the extraordinary extent of tumor regression observed in perhaps 1% of post-menopausal cases has always been regarded as of major theoretical importance, and it is a matter of some disappointment that so much of the underlying mechanisms continues to elude us". However, as noted previously, high dose estrogen therapy was more successful as a treatment for breast cancer the farther the woman was from the menopause. Estrogen withdrawal somehow played a role in sensitizing tumors to the antitumor actions of estrogen, but this fact was not appreciated at that time. We will return to this concept.

Elwood Jensen predicted the existence of estrogen receptor (ER) in 1962 (Jensen 1962), and the isolation and identification of the ER protein by Toft and Gorski occurred in 1966 (Toft and Gorski 1966). The mediating role of the ER in the estrogen responsiveness of breast cancer was established, and eventually the ER became the molecular target for targeted therapy and prevention of ER-positive breast cancer (Jensen and Jordan 2003). It was suggested (Lacassagne 1936) in 1936 that a therapeutic agent to block estrogen action would be useful in breast cancer prevention, but there were no clues. Potential candidate antiestrogens were only discovered 20 years later in the late 1950s, but these agents were identified and screened as contraceptive drugs in laboratory animals. MER25 (Lerner et al. 1958), which was first reported as a non-steroidal antiestrogen and subsequently found to be a post-coital contraceptive in animals (Lerner and Jordan 1990). But the drug was too toxic. The first clinically useful compound MRL41 or clomiphene was tested in women; however, it was not a contraceptive, but actually induced ovulation. Nevertheless, clinical trials of clomiphene in the early 1960's did move forward to evaluate its activity in the treatment of breast cancer, but were terminated because of concerns about the drug's potential to cause cataracts (Jordan 2003). In parallel studies stimulated by the initial reports of the non-steroidal antiestrogens, ICI 46,474, the pure trans-isomer of a substituted triphenylethylene, was discovered at Imperial Chemicals Industry (ICI) Pharmaceuticals (now Astra Zeneca) and was described as a postcoital contraceptive in the rat (Harper and Walpole 1967). The Head of the Fertility Control program, Arthur Walpole, earlier in his career was interested in why only some postmenopausal women with metastatic breast cancer respond favorably to high dose estrogen therapy (Walpole 1948). Later Walpole ensured that ICI 46,474 was tested in the clinic and placed on the market as an orphan drug while ICI invested in the scientific research by others in academia to conduct a systematic study of the anticancer actions of tamoxifen and its metabolites (Jordan 2008). This investment reinvented tamoxifen as the first anticancer agent specifically targeted to the ER in the tumor and created the scientific principles to ultimately establish tamoxifen as the "gold standard" for the adjuvant therapy of breast cancer and as the first chemopreventative agent that reduces the incidence of breast cancer in women with elevated risk (Fisher et al. 1999; EBCTCG 2005).

2. Development and clinical application of antihormonal therapy

Since the clinical application of the laboratory principle of targeting the ER with long-term antihormonal therapy (Jordan 2008) to treat breast cancer has become the standard of care, two different approaches to adjuvant antihormonal therapy have been developed in the past 30 years: first, is the blockade of estrogen-stimulated growth (Jensen and Jordan 2003) at the tumor ERs with antiestrogens, and the second one, is the use of aromatase inhibitors to block estrogen biosynthesis in postmenopausal patients (Jordan and Brodie 2007). Tamoxifen was originally referred to as a non-steroidal antiestrogen (Harper and Walpole 1967). However, as more has become known about its molecular pharmacology (Jordan 2001) it has become the pioneering Selective Estrogen Receptor Modulator (SERM). The concept of SERM action was defined by four main pieces of laboratory evidence: 1) ER-positive breast cancer cells inoculated into athymic mice grew into tumors in response to estradiol, but not to tamoxifen (antiestrogenic action), however both estradiol and tamoxifen induced uterine weight increase in mice (estrogen action) (Jordan and Robinson 1987); 2) raloxifene (another non-steroidal antiestrogen), which is less estrogenic in rat uterus, maintained the bone density in ovariectomized rats (estrogen action), as did tamoxifen (Jordan et al. 1987), and prevented mammary carcinogenesis (antiestrogenic action) (Gottardis and Jordan 1987); 3) tamoxifen blocked estradiol-induced growth of ER-positive breast cancer cells in athymic mice (antiestrogenic action), but induced rapid growth of ER-positive endometrial carcinomas (estrogenic action) (Gottardis et al. 1988); 4) raloxifene was less effective in promoting endometrial cancer growth than tamoxifen (less estrogenic action in uterine tissue) (Gottardis et al. 1990). These laboratory results all translated into clinical practice where it was shown that tamoxifen effectively can reduce the incidence of breast cancer in high-risk pre- and postmenopausal women, however increases the incidence of blood clots and endometrial cancer, which is linked to estrogen-like actions of tamoxifen in these tissues in postmenopausal women, who have a low-estrogen environment (Fisher et al. 1998).

Aromatase inhibitors have an advantage in the therapy of postmenopausal patients over tamoxifen, firstly, because there are fewer side effects, such as blood clots or endometrial cancer, and aromatase inhibitors have a small, but still significant efficacy in increasing disease free survival (Howell et al. 2005). However, most postmenopausal patients worldwide continue treatment with tamoxifen, either for economic reasons or because they were hysterectomized and also have a low risk of developing blood clots (low body mass index and are athletically active). In premenopausal women, long term tamoxifen is the antihormonal therapy of choice for the treatment of ductal carcinoma in situ (DCIS) (Fisher et al. 1999), ER-positive breast cancer treatment (EBCTCG 2005) and the reduction of breast cancer incidence in those premenopausal women at elevated risk (Fisher et al. 1998). It is important to stress that premenopausal women treated with tamoxifen do not have elevations in endometrial cancer and blood clots, thus risk: benefit ratio is in favor of tamoxifen treatment (Gail et al. 1999).

The development of raloxifene from a laboratory concept (Jordan 2007) to a clinically effective drug to prevent both osteoporosis and breast cancer (Cummings et al. 1999; Vogel et al. 2006) has created new opportunities for clinical applications of SERMs. Raloxifene is the result. However, the biggest advantage of raloxifene is that it does not increase the incidence of endometrial cancer (Vogel et al. 2006), which was noted in postmenopausal women taking tamoxifen (Fisher et al. 1998). Raloxifene is used primarily for the prevention of osteoporosis and for the prevention of breast cancer in high risk postmenopausal women. The current clinical trend for the use of antihormonal therapy for the treatment and prevention of breast cancer is to employ long-term treatment durations. Currently aromatase inhibitors are used for a full 5 years after 5years of tamoxifen (Goss et al. 2005). Though, the clinical application of the SERM concept has proven itself to be successful for the prevention of osteoporosis and 50% of breast cancers (Vogel et al. 2006; Vogel et al. 2010), drug resistance remains an important issue arising from long-term SERM treatment. Studies have shown that after long-term SERM treatment, the pharmacology of the SERMs changes from an inhibitory antiestrogenic state to a stimulatory estrogen-like response (Gottardis and Jordan 1988).

3. Evolution of SERM resistance as deciphered by the laboratory models

Clinical and laboratory studies have identified possible mechanisms for the acquired resistance to SERMs, and tamoxifen. Acquired resistance to SERMs is unique as the tumors are SERM stimulated for growth (Howell et al. 1992). The first laboratory model (Gottardis and Jordan 1988; Gottardis et al. 1988; Gottardis et al. 1990) of transplantable tamoxifen resistant cells demonstrated that 1) tamoxifen or estrogen can cause tumors to grow, 2) tumors require a liganded receptor to grow, 3) an aromatase inhibitors (estrogen deprivation) or a pure antiestrogen that causes ER degradation would be useful second line agents, 4) there was cross resistance with other SERMs (O'Regan et al. 2002). Currently, numerous model systems exist to study SERM resistance. Some are engineered to increase the likelihood of resistance (Osborne et al. 2003) and others are engineered by transfection of the aromatase gene to study resistance to aromatase inhibitors and compare them with tamoxifen (Brodie et al. 2003). In contrast, others have chosen to develop models naturally through selective pressure either *in vivo* or *in vitro*. The natural selection approach is to either continuously transplant the resulting SERM resistant breast cancer into SERM-treated athymic animals (Wolf and Jordan 1993; Lee et al. 2000) or to employ strategies *in vitro* that use continuous SERM treatment (Herman and Katzenellenbogen 1996; Liu et al. 2003; Park et al. 2005) or long term estrogen deprivation in culture (Song et al. 2001; Lewis et al. 2005). Distinct phases of resistance were elucidated with the use of unique models of tamoxifen-resistant breast cancer developed *in vivo*, in order to better understand the biological consequences of extended antiestrogen treatment on the survival of breast cancer. The model for the treatment phase was developed by injecting ERα-positive MCF-7 cells into athymic mice and supplementing them with post-menopausal doses of estradiol (E2) (86–93 pg/ml) (Robinson and Jordan 1989), which were estradiol-stimulated and tamoxifen (TAM)-inhibited (Figure 1).

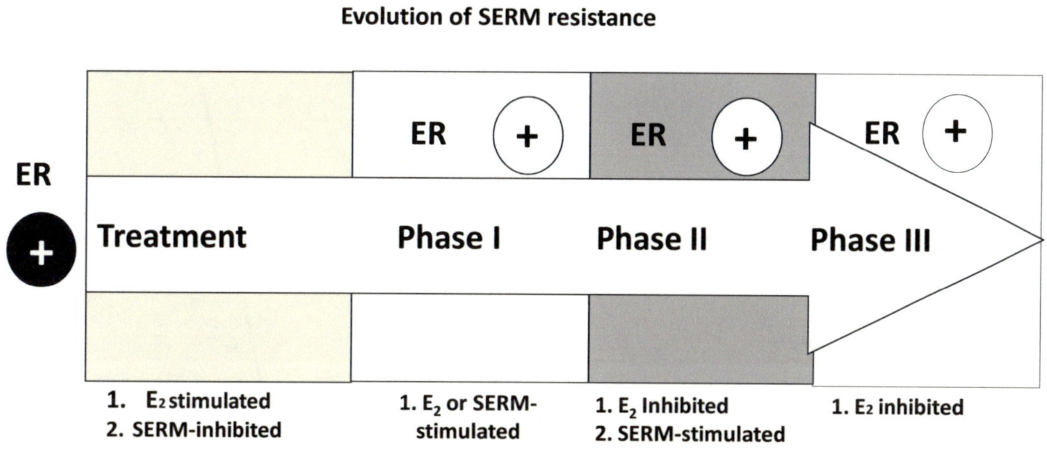

Fig. 1. Evolution of SERM resistance as observed in animal models.

With short term treatment (<2 years) with tamoxifen Phase I TAM-resistant breast tumors developed, which were stimulated to grow by both E2 and tamoxifen (Figure 1) (Gottardis and Jordan 1988; Osborne et al. 1991). The novel model of Phase II resistance to tamoxifen was developed by long-term treatment (>5 years) of breast tumors with tamoxifen (MCF-7TAMLT). These MCF-7TAMLT tumors were stimulated to grow with tamoxifen, but paradoxically were inhibited by estradiol (Figure 1) (Wolf and Jordan 1993; Yao et al. 2000; Osipo et al. 2003). The phase when all known therapies fail and only E2-inhibit the growth is referred to as phase III resistance (Figure 1) (Jordan 2004). Interestingly, during the progression from the treatment phase to Phase III resistance, a cyclic phenomenon was observed where initially estradiol-inhibited growth of Phase II TAM-resistant tumors followed by re-sensitization to estradiol as a growth stimulant (Yao et al. 2000). These new estradiol-stimulated MCF-7 tumors from Phase II tamoxifen-resistant tumors were inhibited by treatment with either TAM or fulvestrant demonstrating complete reversal of drug resistance to tamoxifen (Yao et al. 2000). A similar phenomenon was observed with raloxifen-resistance (Balaburski et al. 2010). In addition to SERM-resistant tumors, estradiol, at physiologic concentrations, has also been shown to induce apoptosis in long term estrogen deprived (LTED) breast cancer cells *in vitro* and *in vivo*. We noted previously, that in the past, pharmacologic estrogen was employed in therapy of advanced breast cancer that resulted in favorable responses with regression of disease (Haddow 1944). Estrogen therapy yields as high as 40% response rate as first-line treatment in patients with hormonally sensitive breast cancer with metastatic disease (Ingle et al. 1981) and approximately 31% in patients heavily pre-treated with previous endocrine therapies (Lonning et al. 2001). The unique aspect of current laboratory findings is that physiologic estrogen can induce tumor regression in long-term anti-hormone drug resistance (Wolf and Jordan 1993; Yao et al. 2000; Song et al. 2001; Jordan and Ford 2011). But what are the mechanisms?

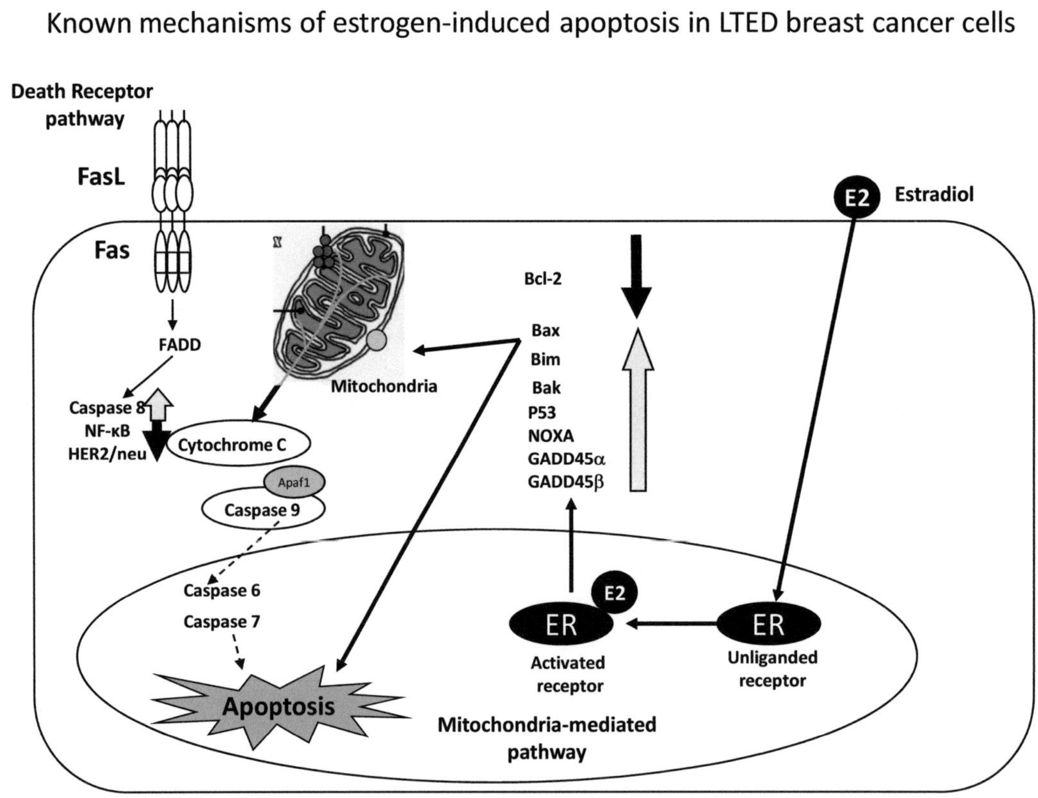

Fig. 2. Mechanisms of estrogen-induced apoptosis in Long-Term Estrogen Deprived (LTED) breast cancer cells. Both FasR/FasL death-signaling and mitochondrial pathways are involved.

4. Mechanism of estrogen-induced apoptosis

To investigate the mechnisms of estradiol-induced apoptosis SERM-stimulated models (Liu et al. 2003; Osipo et al. 2003) or long-term estrogen deprived MCF-7 breast cancer cell lines (Song et al. 2001; Lewis et al. 2005; Lewis et al. 2005) have been interrogated. A link between estradiol-induced apoptosis and activation of the FasR/FasL death-signaling pathway was demonstrated in tamoxifen-stimulated breast cancer tumors by inducing the death receptor

Fas with physiologic levels of estradiol and suppressing the antiapoptotic/prosurvival factors NF-κB and HER2/neu (Osipo et al. 2003; Lewis et al. 2005). A similar finding was reported (Liu et al. 2003) for raloxifene-resistant tumor cells where the growth of raloxifene-resistant MCF-7/Ral cells *in vitro* and *in vivo* was repressed by estradiol via mechanism involving increased Fas expression and decreased NF-κB activity. Furthermore, MCF-7 cells deprived of estrogen for up to 24 months (MCF-7LTED) *in vitro* expressed high levels of Fas compared to the parental MCF-7 cells, which do not express Fas and treatment of the MCF-7/LTED cells with estradiol resulted in a marked increase in Fas ligand (FasL) in these cells (Song et al. 2001). It was also noted that mitochondrial pathway could play a role in mediating estrogen induced apoptosis as the basal expression levels of Bcl-2 were higher in these cells than in the parental MCF-7 cells. Estradiol induced apoptosis occurs in a LTED breast cancer cell line named MCF-7:5C by neutralization of the Bcl-2/Bcl-XL proteins, and upregulation of proapoptotic proteins such as Bax, Bak and Bim, which proves the role of intrinsic mitochondrial pathway (Lewis et al. 2005) (Figure 2).

In MCF-7:5C cells the expression of several pro-apoptotic proteins—including Bax, Bak, Bim, Noxa, Puma, and p53—are markedly increased with estradiol treatment and blockade of Bax and Bim expression using siRNAs almost completely reversed the apoptotic effect of estradiol. Estradiol treatment also led to a loss of mitochondrial potential and a dramatic increase in the release of cytochrome *c* from the mitochondria, which resulted in activation of caspases and cleavage of PARP. Furthermore, overexpression of anti-apoptotic Bcl-x_L was able to protect MCF-7:5C cells from estradiol-induced apoptosis. This particular study was the first to show a link between estradiol-induced cell death and activation of the mitochondrial apoptotic pathway using a breast cancer cell model resistant to estrogen withdrawal (Lewis et al. 2005). Besides the action on the mitohodrial pathway, Bcl-2 overexpression increases cellular glutathione (GSH) level which is associated with increased resistance to chemotherapy-induced apoptosis (Voehringer 1999). GSH is a water-soluble tripeptide composed of glutamine, cysteine, and glycine. It is the most abundant intracellular small molecule thiol present in mammalian cells and it serves as a potent intracellular antioxidant protecting cells from toxins such as free radicals (Schroder et al. 1996; Anderson et al. 1999). Changes in GSH homeostasis have been implicated in the etiology and progression of some diseases and breast cancer (Townsend et al. 2003) and studies have shown that elevated levels of GSH prevent apoptotic cell death whereas depletion of GSH facilitates apoptosis (Anderson et al. 1999). Our laboratory has found evidence which suggests that GSH participates in retarding apoptosis in antihormone-resistant MCF-7:2A human breast cancer cells, which have ~60% elevated levels of GSH compared to wild-type MCF-7 cells and unable to undergo estrogen-induced apoptosis within 1 week unlike MCF-7:5C cells, and that depletion of GSH by 100 μM of L-buthionine sulfoximine (BSO), a potent inhibitor of glutathione biosynthesis, sensitizes these resistant cells to estradiol-induced apoptosis (Lewis-Wambi et al. 2008). However, the question arises as to the actual mechanism of the apoptotic trigger mediated by the ER complex.

5. Structure-function relationship studies for deciphering estrogen-induced apoptosis

The fact that SERMs do not affect the spontaneous growth of MCF-7:5C cells, but can completely block estradiol-induced apoptosis, was an important clue that the shape of the

ER can be modulated to prevent apoptosis. Extensive structure-function relationship studies were initially used to develop a molecular model of estrogen and antiestrogen action (Lieberman et al. 1983; Jordan et al. 1984; Jordan et al. 1986). The hypothetical model presumed the envelopment of a planar estrogen within the ligand-binding domain (LBD) of the ER complex. In contrast, the three-dimensional triphenylethylene binding in the LBD cavity prevents full ER's activation by keeping the LBD open. This structural perturbation of the ER complex is achieved by a correctly positioned bulky side chain on the SERM. This model was enhanced by the subsequent studies to solve the X-ray crystallography of the LBD ER's bound with an estrogen or an antiestrogen (Brzozowski et al. 1997; Shiau et al. 1998). The LBD of ERα is formed by H2-H11 helices and the hairpin β-sheet, while H12, in the agonist bound conformation closes over the LBD cavity filled with E2. E2 is aligned in the cavity by hydrogen bonds at both ends of the ligand, particularly the 3-OH group at the A-ring end of E2. This allows hydrophobic van der Waals contacts along the lipophilic rings of E2, in particular between Phe404 and E2's A-ring, to promote a low energy conformation (Brzozowski et al. 1997). This results in sealing of the ligand-binding cavity by H12, and exposes the AF-2 motif at the surface of the receptor for interaction with coactivators to promote transcriptional transactivation. In contrast, 4-hydroxytamoxifen binds to ER's LBD to block the closure of the cavity by relocating H12 away from the binding pocket, thus preventing coactivator molecules from binding to the appropriate site on the external surface of the complex, which produces an antiestrogenic effect (Shiau et al. 1998). Therefore, it is the external shape of the ERs that is being modulated by the ligand which dictates the binding of coactivator molecules. In other words, the shape of the ligand actually causes the receptor to change shape and programs the ER complex to be able to bind coregulator molecules. However, the simple model of a coregulator controlling the biology of an ER complex is not that simple. The modulation of the estrogen target gene is in fact, regulated by a dynamic process of assembly and destruction of transcription complex at the promoter site of a target gene. After ER is bound to an agonist ligand, its conformation changes allowing coregulator molecules to bind to the complex, for example, SRC-3. SRC-3 is a core coactivator that also attracts other coregulators that do not directly bind to ER, such as p300/CBP histone acetyltransferase, CARM1 methyltransferase, and ubiquitin ligases UbC and UbL. All of these coregulators perform specific subreactions within the protein complex of ER and DNA necessary for transcription of target genes, such as chromatin remodeling through methylation and acetylation modifications, and also direct their enzymatic activity towards adjacent factors, which promote dissociation of the coactivator complex and subsequent ubiquitinilation of select components for proteosomal degradation. As a result, this allows the next cycle of coactivator-receptor-DNA interactions to proceed and the binding and degradation of transcription complexes sustaining the gene transcription (Lonard et al. 2000). However, although AF-2 is deactivated by 4OHTAM, the 4OHTAM:ERα complex has estrogen-like activity (Levenson et al. 1998), whereas raloxifene does not (Levenson et al. 1997). This is believed to be because the side chain of raloxifene shields and neutralizes asp351 to block estrogen action (Levenson and Jordan 1998). In contrast the side chain of tamoxifen is too short. It appears that when helix 12 is not positioned correctly the exposed asp351 can interact with AF-1 to produce estrogen action. This estrogen-like activity can be inhibited by substituting asp351 for glycine an uncharged amino acid (MacGregor Schafer et al. 2000). However, knowledge of the structure of the

4OHTAM: ER LBD complex (Shiau et al. 1998) led to the idea that all estrogens may not be the same in their interactions with ER (Jordan et al. 2001). Previous studies suggest that non-planar TPEs with a bulky phenyl substituent prevents helix-12 from completely sealing the LBD pocket (Jordan et al. 2001). This physical event creates a putative 'anti-estrogen like' configuration within the complex. However, the complex is not anti-estrogenic because Asp351 is exposed to communicate with AF-1 thus causing estrogen-like action. Therefore, there are putative Class I (planar) and Class II (non-planar) estrogens (Jordan et al. 2001). A similar classification and conclusion has been proposed (Gust et al. 2001), but the biological consequences of this classification were unknown until recently.
To further address the hypothesis that the shape of the ER complex can be controlled by the shape of an estrogen, and thereby altering its functional properties, such as induction of apoptosis, a range of hydroxylated TPEs was synthesized (Figure 3) to establish new tools to investigate the relationship of shape with estrogenic activity through the exposure of asp351 (Maximov et al. 2010).

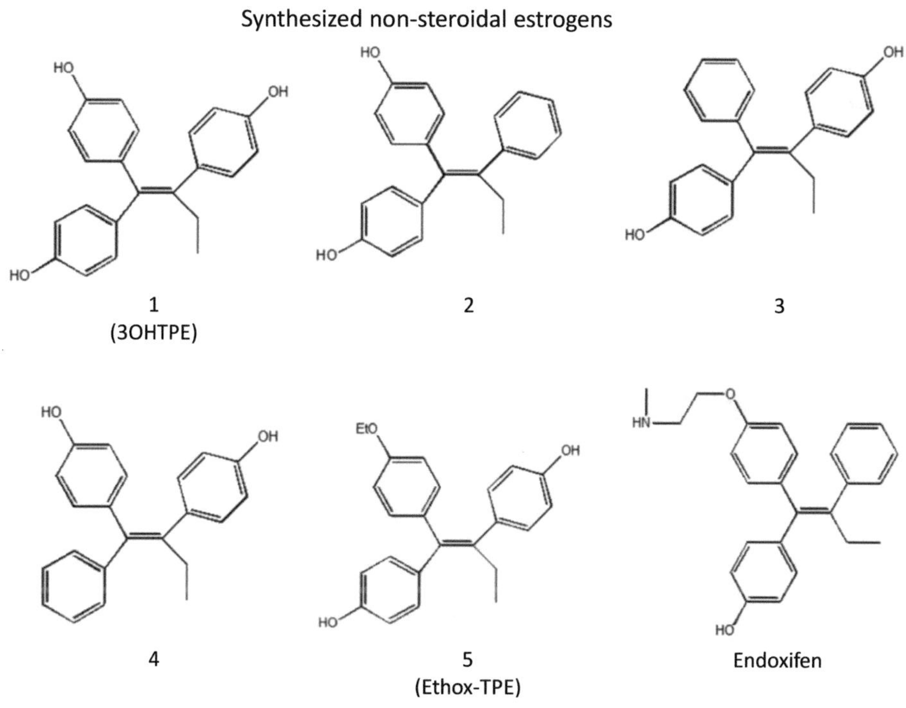

Fig. 3. Synthesized class II non-steroidal estrogens. All estrogens are hydroxylated derivatives of triphenylethylene; 1 – 3-hyrdoxytriphenylethylene (3OHTPE), 2- bisphenoltripenylethylene, 3 – E-dihydroxytriphenylethylene, 4- Z-dihydroxytriphenylethylene, 5- ethoxytripenylethylene, and Endoxifen (a metabolite of the antiestrogenic triphenylethylene tamoxifen with high affinity for the estrogen receprtor).

We compared and contrasted the estrogen-like properties of the hydroxylated TPEs to promote proliferation in the ERα-positive human breast cancer cell line MCF-7:WS8 cells (Figure 4A), which are hypersensitive to the proliferative actions of E2. Compounds were compared with the tamoxifen metabolites 4-OHT and endoxifen. Results show that our

MCF-7:WS8 human breast cancer cells were exquisitely sensitive to E2 which produced a concentration-dependent increase in growth, and all of the TPE's were potent agonists with the ability to stimulate MCF-7:WS8 breast cancer cell growth, however, their agonist potency was less compared to E2. The metabolites, 4-OHT and endoxifen, had no significant agonist effect in MCF-7:WS8 cells, however, these compounds at 1 μM were able to completely inhibit estradiol-stimulated MCF-7:WS8 breast cancer cell growth, thus confirming their role as antiestrogens (data not shown). To determine the ability of the test TPEs to activate the ER, MCF-7:WS8 cells were transiently transfected with an ERE-luciferase reporter gene encoding the firefly reporter gene with 5 consecutive Estrogen Responsive Elements (EREs) under the control of a TATA promoter. The binding of ligand-activated ER complex at the EREs in the promoter of the luciferase gene activates transcription. The measurement of the luciferase expression levels permits a determination of agonist activity of the TPE:ER complex. All the phenolic TPEs were estrogenic and induced the increase of ERE-luciferase activity, but were less potent compared to E2. To confirm and advance the hypothesis that the shape of the estrogen ER complex was different for planar and nonplanar (TPE –like) estrogens, series of tested phenolic TPEs were evaluated in the ER-negative breast cancer cell line T47D:C42 (Pink et al. 1996) which was transiently transfected with an ERE luciferase plasmid and either the wild-type ER or the D351G mutant ER plasmids. Previously it was found that the mutant D351G ER completely suppressed estrogen-like properties of 4-OHT at an endogenous TGFα target gene(MacGregor Schafer et al. 2000). We established that in the presence of the wild-type ER all of the tested TPE compounds were potent agonists with the ability to significantly enhance ERE luciferase activity (Figure 4C). In contrast, when the D351G mutant ER gene was transfected with the ERE luciferase reporter only the planar E_2 was estrogenic whereas the TPEs did not activate the ERE reporter gene (Figure 4D). These results confirm the importance of Asp351 in ER activation by TPE ligands to trigger estrogen action. To further confirm the hypothesis, the best "fits" of the tested TPEs and endoxifen, obtained from docking simulations ran against the antagonist conformation of the ER, were superimposed on the experimental agonist conformation of the ER. Overall the TPEs are unlikely to be accommodated in the agonist conformation of the ER due to the sterical clashes between "Leu crown", mostly Leu525 and Leu540, helix 12 and ligands, indicating, that these ligands most likely bind to ER's conformation more closely related with the antagonist form. X-ray crystallography of ER-4OHTAM and ER-Raloxifene complexes, demonstrating that the presence of the alkyaminoethoxy sidechain of 4OHTAM is crucial for the ER to gain an antagonistic conformation by displacing the H12 of the receptor by 4OHTAM's bulky sidechain, thus preventing the binding of the coactivators (Shiau et al. 1998). The absence of the alkyaminoethoxy sidechain on the tested TPEs does not allow these compounds to act as antiestrogens, like 4-OHT or endoxifen, which posseses the alkyaminoethoxy sidechain (Shiau et al. 1998). However, the fact that these TPEs were able to significantly induce growth and ERE activation in MCF-7:WS8 cells demonstrated that they are still full agonists, despite the changes in biological potencies of the tested TPEs, due to repositioning of the hydroxyl groups and addition of the ethoxy group. Thus cell growth is a very sensitive property of the ligand:ER complex and can occur minimally with an AF-1 function alone in the case of TPEs but also with the possibility for interacting with a perturbated LBD. 4OHT does not stimulate growth so possibly a corepressor binds in the case of a SERM:ER complex. An interesting aspect of the study (Maximov et al. 2010) is the importance of Asp351 in activation of the ER thereby acting as a molecular test for the presumed structure

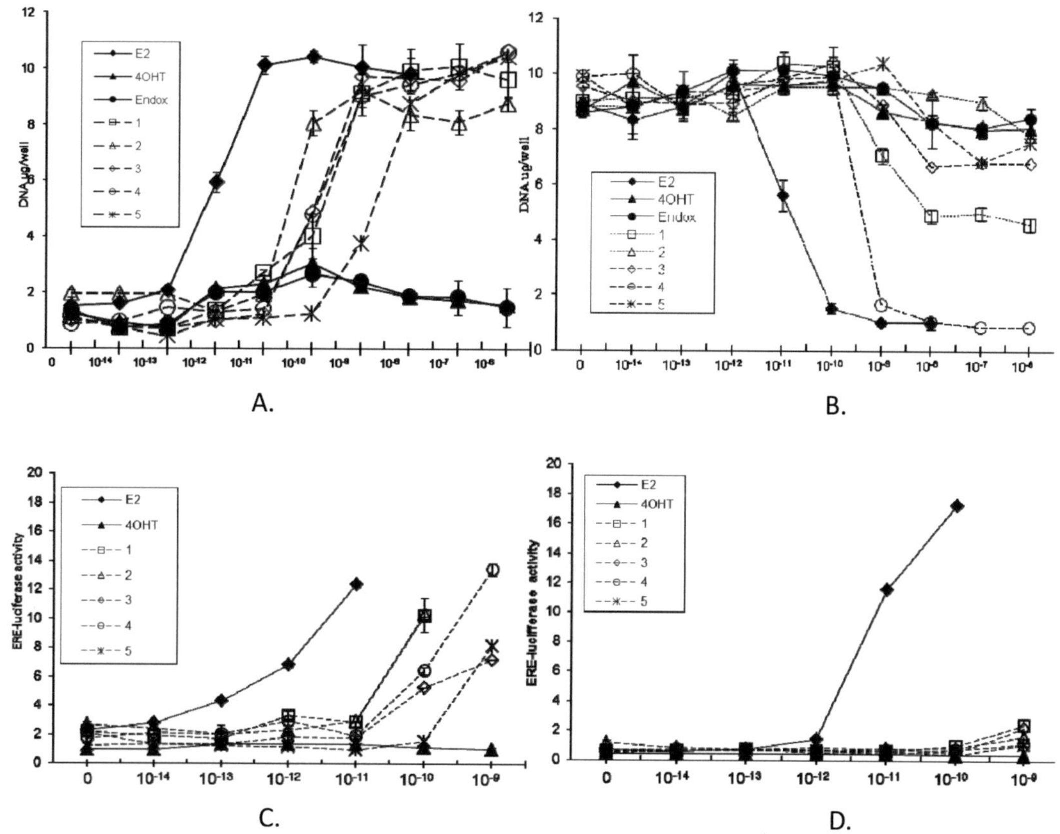

Fig. 4. A: Agonist activity in MCF-7:WS8 cells of synthesized TPEs and E2 and anti-estrogens 4-OHT and Endoxifen; B: E2 induces apoptosis in long-term estrogen deprived MCF-7:5C cells and synthesized TPEs are unable to act as full agonists resembling more anti-estrogens 4-OHT and Endoxifen; C: E2 and all TPEs are able to increase the activity of luciferase in T47D:C4:2 cells transiently transfected with wild-type ER DNA construct; D: E2 is the only agonist in D351G ER mutant T47D:C4:2 cells, as TPEs are unable to increase the luciferase activity in cells expressing the mutant form of ER, indicating the importance of Asp351 of the ER for activation with non-planar TPEs.

of the TPE:ER complex. Based on the X-ray crystallography of the ER in complex with 4OHTAM (Shiau et al. 1998) and raloxifene (Brzozowski et al. 1997), it was determined that the basic side chains of these antiestrogens are in proximity of Asp351 in the ER. It was hypothesized that this interaction with raloxifene actually neutralizes and shields Asp351 preventing it from interacting with ligand-independent activating function 1 (AF-1). In contrast, 4OHTAM possesses some estrogenic activity, because the side chain is too short (Shiau et al. 1998). Substitution of Asp351 with Glycine which is a non-charged aminoacid, leads to loss of estrogenic activity of the ER bound with 4OHTAM (MacGregor Schafer et al. 2000; Levenson et al. 2001). Results from ERE luciferase assays in T47:C4:2 cells transiently transfed with wild type and D351G mutant ER expression plasmids demonstrated that wild type ER was activated by all of the tested TPEs, however substitution of Asp351 by Gly prevented the increase of ERE luciferase activity by all TPEs and only planar E2, which does not interact with Asp351 at all, or exposes it on the surface of the complex, was able to activate ERE in D351G ER transfected cells. This confirms and expands the classification of estrogens, where planar estrogens such as E2 are classified as class I and all TPE-related estrogens are classified as class II estrogens based on the mechanism of activation of the ER (Jordan et al. 2001).

Further we tested the hypothesis that, the shape of the ER complex with either planar estrogens (Class I) or angular estrogens (Class II), can modulate the apoptotic actions of estrogen through the shape of the resulting complex. In this study MCF-7:5C cells were employed to investigate the actions of 4-OHT and our model TPEs on estradiol-induced apoptosis. As estrogen-induced apoptosis can be reversed in a concentration related manner by the nonsteroidal antiestrogen 4-OHT, paradoxically, all tested TPEs were able to reverse the apoptotic effect of estradiol in MCF-7:5C cells, at the same time the tested TPEs alone were not able to induce apoptosis in these cells significantly (Figure 4B). However, the tested TPEs have still retained their ability to induce ERE-luciferase activity in MCF-7:5C cells, indicating that these compounds are still agonists of the ER in these cells, but biologically acted as antagonists. Besides differences in biological effects of TPEs in MCF-7 cells and MCF-7:5C cells, biochemical effects of tested TPEs on ER complex similar to those with 4-OHT were studied. 4-OHT is known to retard the destruction of the 4-OHT ER complex (Pink and Jordan 1996; Wijayaratne and McDonnell 2001). Similarly, the TPEs do not facilitate the rapid destruction of the TPE:ER complex, as it was shown via Western blotting that the TPE:ER levels are analogous to 4-OHT:ER levels rather than estradiol ER-like, where ER is rapidly degraded. As it was noted previously, ER degradation plays a crucial role in estrogen-mediated gene expression. It was previously shown that ER protein degradation is proteosome mediated (Lonard et al. 2000; Reid et al. 2003), and ER coactivator SRC3/AIB1 links the transcriptional activity of the receptor and its proteosome degradation (Shao et al. 2004). Our results indicate that the transcriptional activity of ER, based on qRT-PCR results, is similar on the pS2 gene in both MCF-7:WS8 cells and MCF-7:5C cells with the tested TPE compounds, and based on our ChIP assay results for evaluating the ER's recruitment on the pS2 gene promoter, the E2:ER complex has robust binding in the promoter region and SRC-3 is detected presumably bound to the ER complex, however, 4-OHT:ER complexes only have modest binding of ERα and virtually no SRC-3 in the promoter region, at the same time, the TPEs permit some binding of the TPE:ER complexes in the promoter region but there are lower levels of SRC-3 and a reduced ability to stimulate PS2 mRNA synthesis (Figure 5).

We believe that the changed conformation of the TPE:ER complex, prevents the complete closure of H12 over the ligand-binding cavity and thus does not allow co-activators to bind to the incompletely open AF-2 motif on the ER's surface. Indeed, LeClercq's group (Bourgoin-Voillard et al. 2010) have recently confirmed and extended our molecular classifications of estrogens, with a larger series of compounds and have also shown that an angular TPE does not cause the destruction of the ER complex in a manner analogous to estradiol when MCF-7 cells are examined by immunohistochemistry for the ER, and that the putative Class II estrogens that do not permit the appropriate sealing of the LBD with helix 12 do not efficiently bind co-activators, therefore our respective studies are in agreement.

In summary, the proposed hypothesis that the TPE-ER complex significantly changes the shape of the ER to adopt a conformation that mimics that adopted by 4-OHT when it binds to the ER. A co-activator now has difficulty in binding to the TPE-ER complex appropriately, but whereas this does affect cell replication, it dramatically impairs the events that must be triggered to cause apoptosis. Future studies will confirm or refute our hypothesis based upon the known intrinsic activity of mutant ERs and their capacity to investigate estrogen-target genes.

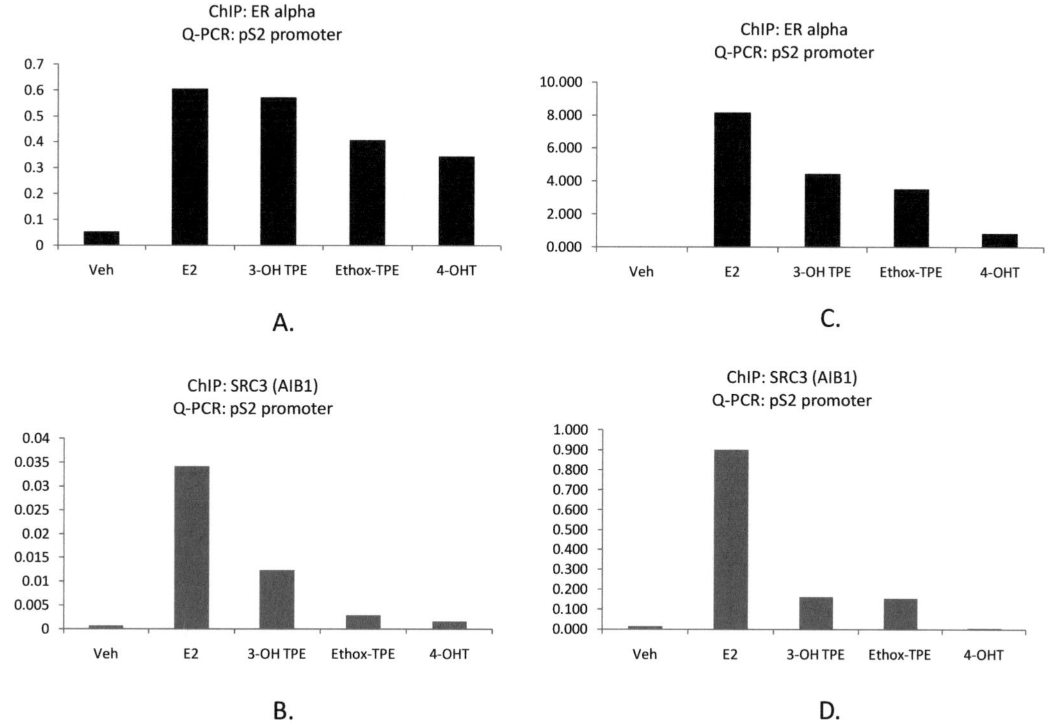

Fig. 5. A&B: ChIP analysis performed in MCF-7:WS8 cells with pS2 promoter region was pulled down via anti-ERα antibody (A) and anti-SRC3/AIB1 antibody (B); C&D: ChIP analysis performed in MCF-7:5C cells with pS2 promoter region pulled down via anti-ERα antibody (C) and anti-SRC3/AIB1 antibody (D). All results indicate that in both cell lines tested TPEs and E2 recruit ERα complex to the pS2 promoter region, but interestingly, class II estrogens are unable to co-recruit sufficient amount of SRC-3 co-activator, unlike E2.

6. Relevance to current clinical research

Laboratory studies show that low concentrations of estrogen can cause apoptotic death of breast tumor cells, following estrogen deprivation with antihormonal treatment. This has translated very well into the clinic, and recent clinical trials have demonstrated that low-dose estrogen treatment can effectively be utilized after the formation of resistance to antihormonal treatment. Ellis and colleagues (Ellis et al. 2009) have shown, that a daily dose of 6 mg of estradiol could stop the growth of tumors or even cause them to shrink in about 25% of women with metastatic breast cancer that had developed resistance to antihormonal therapy. At the same time, these results correlate with earlier results obtained by Loenning and coworkers (Lonning et al. 2001), who have studied the efficacy of high dose of DES on the responsiveness of metastatic breast cancer following exhaustive antihormonal treatment with tamoxifen, aromatase inhibitors and etc. 4 out of 32 patients had complete responses (Lonning et al. 2001) and 1 patient after 5 year treatment with DES had no recurrence for a following 6 years (Lonning 2009). The question at that moment remains whether estrogen at physiologic concentrations can be efficient as antitumor agent in estrogen-deprived breast tumors. As mentioned previously, Ellis and coworkers have demonstrated that an equivalent clinical benefit for high (30 mg daily) and low (6 mg daily) dose of estradiol in metastatic breast cancer patients who had failed aromatase inhibitor therapy, which is long-term estrogen deprivation. Overall, the results demonstrate that low dose estrogen therapy has fewer systemic sideffects, but the same efficacy as a treatment for long-term antihormone resistant breast cancer as high dode estrogen therapy. This can be seen as "replacement with" physiologic estrogen to premenopausal levels. The benefit-risk ratio is in favor of low-dose estrogen therapy. These results correlate well with results from WHI trial of estrogen-replacement therapy (ERT) in hysterectomized postmemopausal women (LaCroix et al. 2011). The WHI results show a sustained reduction in the incidence of breast cancer in postmenopausal women up to 5 years after the intervention with conjugated equine estrogens for 5 years prior. It was demonstrated that the group of patients receiving conjugated equine estrogens had incidence of breast cancer 0.27% in comparison to the control group of patients the incidence was 0.35%. The idea that woman's own estrogen can act as an antitumor agent after estrogen-deprivation to prevent metastization and tumor growth (Wolf and Jordan 1993) has lead to incorporation into the Study of Letrozole Extension (SOLE) trial. This trial is addressing the question whether regular drug holydays can decrease recurrence of breast cancer by physiologic estrogen after deprivation with aromatase inhibitor letrozole. Subsequent trials may have to use ERT for a few weeks to trigger apoptosis.

7. Conclusion

Taken together, the demonstrations of the apoptotic actions of estrogen as a potential anticancer agent in postmenopausal breast cancer patients, now provides a rationale to further explore and decipher mechanisms of estrogen-induced apoptosis. There is a possibility that future studies on the molecular mechanism of estrogen-induced apoptosis will help to indentify new more safer and specific agents for breast cancer therapy.

8. Acknowledgments

This work was supported by the Department of Defense Breast Program under Award number W81XWH-06-1-0590 Center of Excellence (principal investigator V. Craig Jordan); subcontract under the SU2C (AACR) Grant number SU2C-AACR-DT0409; the Susan G Komen For The Cure Foundation under Award number SAC100009 (international postdoctoral fellow Philipp Y. Maximov) and the Lombardi Comprehensive Cancer Center Support Grant (CCSG) Core Grant NIH P30 CA051008. The views and opinions of the author(s) do not reflect those of the US Army or the Department of Defense.

9. References

Allen, E., Doisy, E.A. (1923). An ovarian hormone: Preliminary reports on its localization extraction and partial purification and action in test animals. *JAMA* 81: 810-821.

Anderson, C. P., J. M. Tsai, et al. (1999). Depletion of glutathione by buthionine sulfoxine is cytotoxic for human neuroblastoma cell lines via apoptosis. *Exp Cell Res* 246(1): 183-192.

Balaburski, G. M., R. C. Dardes, et al. (2010). Raloxifene-stimulated experimental breast cancer with the paradoxical actions of estrogen to promote or prevent tumor growth: a unifying concept in anti-hormone resistance. *Int J Oncol* 37(2): 387-398.

Beatson, G. T. (1896). On the treatment of inoperable cases of carcinoma of the mamma: suggestions for a new method of treatment, with illustrative cases. *Lancet* 2: 162-165.

Bourgoin-Voillard, S., D. Gallo, et al. (2010). Capacity of type I and II ligands to confer to estrogen receptor alpha an appropriate conformation for the recruitment of coactivators containing a LxxLL motif-Relationship with the regulation of receptor level and ERE-dependent transcription in MCF-7 cells. *Biochem Pharmacol* 79(5): 746-757.

Boyd, S. (1900). On Oophorectomy in cancer of the breast. *British Medical Journal* 2: 134-141.

Brodie, A. H., D. Jelovac, et al. (2003). The intratumoral aromatase model: studies with aromatase inhibitors and antiestrogens. *J Steroid Biochem Mol Biol* 86(3-5): 283-288.

Brzozowski, A. M., A. C. Pike, et al. (1997). Molecular basis of agonism and antagonism in the oestrogen receptor. *Nature* 389(6652): 753-758.

Cummings, S. R., S. Eckert, et al. (1999). The effect of raloxifene on risk of breast cancer in postmenopausal women: results from the MORE randomized trial. Multiple Outcomes of Raloxifene Evaluation. *JAMA* 281(23): 2189-2197.

Dodds, E. C., Goldberg, L., Lawson, W., Robinson, R. (1938). Estrogenic activity of certain synthetic compounds. *Nature* 141: 247-248.

EBCTCG (2005). Effects of chemotherapy and hormonal therapy for early breast cancer on recurrence and 15-year survival: an overview of the randomised trials. *Lancet* 365(9472): 1687-1717.

Ellis, M. J., F. Gao, et al. (2009). Lower-dose vs high-dose oral estradiol therapy of hormone receptor-positive, aromatase inhibitor-resistant advanced breast cancer: a phase 2 randomized study. *JAMA* 302(7): 774-780.

Fisher, B., J. P. Costantino, et al. (1998). Tamoxifen for prevention of breast cancer: report of the National Surgical Adjuvant Breast and Bowel Project P-1 Study. *J Natl Cancer Inst* 90(18): 1371-1388.

Fisher, B., J. Dignam, et al. (1999). Tamoxifen in treatment of intraductal breast cancer: National Surgical Adjuvant Breast and Bowel Project B-24 randomised controlled trial. *Lancet* 353(9169): 1993-2000.

Folca, P. J., R. F. Glascock, et al. (1961). Studies with tritium-labelled hexoestrol in advanced breast cancer. Comparison of tissue accumulation of hexoestrol with response to bilateral adrenalectomy and oophorectomy. *Lancet* 2(7206): 796-798.

Gail, M. H., J. P. Costantino, et al. (1999). Weighing the risks and benefits of tamoxifen treatment for preventing breast cancer. *J Natl Cancer Inst* 91(21): 1829-1846.

Glascock, R. F. and W. G. Hoekstra (1959). Selective accumulation of tritium-labelled hexoestrol by the reproductive organs of immature female goats and sheep. *Biochem J* 72: 673-682.

Goss, P. E., J. N. Ingle, et al. (2005). Randomized trial of letrozole following tamoxifen as extended adjuvant therapy in receptor-positive breast cancer: updated findings from NCIC CTG MA.17. *J Natl Cancer Inst* 97(17): 1262-1271.

Gottardis, M. M. and V. C. Jordan (1987). Antitumor actions of keoxifene and tamoxifen in the N-nitrosomethylurea-induced rat mammary carcinoma model. *Cancer Res* 47(15): 4020-4024.

Gottardis, M. M. and V. C. Jordan (1988). Development of tamoxifen-stimulated growth of MCF-7 tumors in athymic mice after long-term antiestrogen administration. *Cancer Res* 48(18): 5183-5187.

Gottardis, M. M., M. E. Ricchio, et al. (1990). Effect of steroidal and nonsteroidal antiestrogens on the growth of a tamoxifen-stimulated human endometrial carcinoma (EnCa101) in athymic mice. *Cancer Res* 50(11): 3189-3192.

Gottardis, M. M., S. P. Robinson, et al. (1988). Contrasting actions of tamoxifen on endometrial and breast tumor growth in the athymic mouse. *Cancer Res* 48(4): 812-815.

Gust, R., R. Keilitz, et al. (2001). Investigations of new lead structures for the design of selective estrogen receptor modulators. *J Med Chem* 44(12): 1963-1970.

Haddow, A. (1950). The chemotherapy of cancer. *Br Med J* 2(4691): 1271-1272.

Haddow, A. (1970). David A. Karnofsky memorial lecture. Thoughts on chemical therapy. *Cancer* 26(4): 737-754.

Haddow, A., Watkinson, J.M., Paterson, E. (1944). Influence of synthetic oestrogens upon advanced malignant disease. *British Medical Journal*: 393-398.

Harper, M. J. and A. L. Walpole (1967). A new derivative of triphenylethylene: effect on implantation and mode of action in rats. *J Reprod Fertil* 13(1): 101-119.

Herman, M. E. and B. S. Katzenellenbogen (1996). Response-specific antiestrogen resistance in a newly characterized MCF-7 human breast cancer cell line resulting from long-term exposure to trans-hydroxytamoxifen. *J Steroid Biochem Mol Biol* 59(2): 121-134.

Howell, A., J. Cuzick, et al. (2005). Results of the ATAC (Arimidex, Tamoxifen, Alone or in Combination) trial after completion of 5 years' adjuvant treatment for breast cancer. *Lancet* 365(9453): 60-62.

Howell, A., D. J. Dodwell, et al. (1992). Response after withdrawal of tamoxifen and progestogens in advanced breast cancer. *Ann Oncol* 3(8): 611-617.

Ingle, J. N., D. L. Ahmann, et al. (1981). Randomized clinical trial of diethylstilbestrol versus tamoxifen in postmenopausal women with advanced breast cancer. *N Engl J Med* 304(1): 16-21.

Jensen, E. V., Jacobson, H.I. (1962). Basic guidelines to the mechanism of estrogen action. *Recent Progr. Hormone Res.* 18: 387-414.

Jensen, E. V. and V. C. Jordan (2003). The estrogen receptor: a model for molecular medicine. *Clin Cancer Res* 9(6): 1980-1989.

Jordan, V. C. (2001). Selective estrogen receptor modulation: a personal perspective. *Cancer Res* 61(15): 5683-5687.

Jordan, V. C. (2003). Tamoxifen: a most unlikely pioneering medicine. *Nat Rev Drug Discov* 2(3): 205-213.

Jordan, V. C. (2004). Selective estrogen receptor modulation: concept and consequences in cancer. *Cancer Cell* 5(3): 207-213.

Jordan, V. C. (2007). SERMs: meeting the promise of multifunctional medicines. *J Natl Cancer Inst* 99(5): 350-356.

Jordan, V. C. (2008). Tamoxifen: catalyst for the change to targeted therapy. *Eur J Cancer* 44(1): 30-38.

Jordan, V. C. and A. M. Brodie (2007). Development and evolution of therapies targeted to the estrogen receptor for the treatment and prevention of breast cancer. *Steroids* 72(1): 7-25.

Jordan, V. C. and L. G. Ford (2011). Paradoxical Clinical Effect of Estrogen on Breast Cancer Risk: A "New" Biology of Estrogen-induced Apoptosis. *Cancer Prev Res (Phila)* 4(5): 633-637.

Jordan, V. C., R. Koch, et al. (1986). Oestrogenic and antioestrogenic actions in a series of triphenylbut-1-enes: modulation of prolactin synthesis in vitro. *Br J Pharmacol* 87(1): 217-223.

Jordan, V. C., M. E. Lieberman, et al. (1984). Structural requirements for the pharmacological activity of nonsteroidal antiestrogens in vitro. *Mol Pharmacol* 26(2): 272-278.

Jordan, V. C., E. Phelps, et al. (1987). Effects of anti-estrogens on bone in castrated and intact female rats. *Breast Cancer Res Treat* 10(1): 31-35.

Jordan, V. C. and S. P. Robinson (1987). Species-specific pharmacology of antiestrogens: role of metabolism. *Fed Proc* 46(5): 1870-1874.

Jordan, V. C., J. M. Schafer, et al. (2001). Molecular classification of estrogens. *Cancer Res* 61(18): 6619-6623.

Kennedy, B. J. (1965). Hormone therapy for advanced breast cancer. *Cancer* 18(12): 1551-1557.

Kennedy, B. J. (1965). Systemic effects of androgenic and estrogenic hormones in advanced breast cancer. *J Am Geriatr Soc* 13: 230-235.

Kennedy, B. J. and I. T. Nathanson (1953). Effects of intensive sex steroid hormone therapy in advanced breast cancer. *J Am Med Assoc* 152(12): 1135-1141.

Lacassagne, A. (1936). Hormonal pathogenesis of adenocarcinoma of the breast. *Am J Cancer* 27: 217-225.

LaCroix, A. Z., R. T. Chlebowski, et al. (2011). Health outcomes after stopping conjugated equine estrogens among postmenopausal women with prior hysterectomy: a randomized controlled trial. *JAMA* 305(13): 1305-1314.

Lathrop, A. E. C., Loeb, L. (1916). Further Investigations on the Origin of Tumors in Mice. *J Cancer Res* 1(1): 1-19.

Lee, E. S., J. M. Schafer, et al. (2000). Cross-resistance of triphenylethylene-type antiestrogens but not ICI 182,780 in tamoxifen-stimulated breast tumors grown in athymic mice. *Clin Cancer Res* 6(12): 4893-4899.

Lerner, L. J., F. J. Holthaus, Jr., et al. (1958). A non-steroidal estrogen antiagonist 1-(p-2-diethylaminoethoxyphenyl)-1-phenyl-2-p-methoxyphenylethanol. *Endocrinology* 63(3): 295-318.

Lerner, L. J. and V. C. Jordan (1990). Development of antiestrogens and their use in breast cancer: eighth Cain memorial award lecture. *Cancer Res* 50(14): 4177-4189.

Levenson, A. S., W. H. Catherino, et al. (1997). Estrogenic activity is increased for an antiestrogen by a natural mutation of the estrogen receptor. *J Steroid Biochem Mol Biol* 60(5-6): 261-268.

Levenson, A. S. and V. C. Jordan (1998). The key to the antiestrogenic mechanism of raloxifene is amino acid 351 (aspartate) in the estrogen receptor. *Cancer Res* 58(9): 1872-1875.

Levenson, A. S., J. I. MacGregor Schafer, et al. (2001). Control of the estrogen-like actions of the tamoxifen-estrogen receptor complex by the surface amino acid at position 351. *J Steroid Biochem Mol Biol* 76(1-5): 61-70.

Levenson, A. S., D. A. Tonetti, et al. (1998). The oestrogen-like effect of 4-hydroxytamoxifen on induction of transforming growth factor alpha mRNA in MDA-MB-231 breast cancer cells stably expressing the oestrogen receptor. *Br J Cancer* 77(11): 1812-1819.

Lewis-Wambi, J. S., H. R. Kim, et al. (2008). Buthionine sulfoximine sensitizes antihormone-resistant human breast cancer cells to estrogen-induced apoptosis. *Breast Cancer Res* 10(6): R104.

Lewis, J. S., K. Meeke, et al. (2005). Intrinsic mechanism of estradiol-induced apoptosis in breast cancer cells resistant to estrogen deprivation. *J Natl Cancer Inst* 97(23): 1746-1759.

Lewis, J. S., C. Osipo, et al. (2005). Estrogen-induced apoptosis in a breast cancer model resistant to long-term estrogen withdrawal. *J Steroid Biochem Mol Biol* 94(1-3): 131-141.

Lieberman, M. E., J. Gorski, et al. (1983). An estrogen receptor model to describe the regulation of prolactin synthesis by antiestrogens in vitro. *J Biol Chem* 258(8): 4741-4745.

Liu, H., E. S. Lee, et al. (2003). Apoptotic action of 17beta-estradiol in raloxifene-resistant MCF-7 cells in vitro and in vivo. *J Natl Cancer Inst* 95(21): 1586-1597.

Lonard, D. M., Z. Nawaz, et al. (2000). The 26S proteasome is required for estrogen receptor-alpha and coactivator turnover and for efficient estrogen receptor-alpha transactivation. *Mol Cell* 5(6): 939-948.

Lonning, P. E. (2009). Additive endocrine therapy for advanced breast cancer - back to the future. *Acta Oncol* 48(8): 1092-1101.

Lonning, P. E., P. D. Taylor, et al. (2001). High-dose estrogen treatment in postmenopausal breast cancer patients heavily exposed to endocrine therapy. *Breast Cancer Res Treat* 67(2): 111-116.

MacGregor Schafer, J., H. Liu, et al. (2000). Allosteric silencing of activating function 1 in the 4-hydroxytamoxifen estrogen receptor complex is induced by substituting glycine for aspartate at amino acid 351. *Cancer Res* 60(18): 5097-5105.

Maximov, P. Y., C. B. Myers, et al. (2010). Structure-function relationships of estrogenic triphenylethylenes related to endoxifen and 4-hydroxytamoxifen. *J Med Chem* 53(8): 3273-3283.

O'Regan, R. M., C. Gajdos, et al. (2002). Effects of raloxifene after tamoxifen on breast and endometrial tumor growth in athymic mice. *J Natl Cancer Inst* 94(4): 274-283.

Osborne, C. K., V. Bardou, et al. (2003). Role of the estrogen receptor coactivator AIB1 (SRC-3) and HER-2/neu in tamoxifen resistance in breast cancer. *J Natl Cancer Inst* 95(5): 353-361.

Osborne, C. K., E. Coronado, et al. (1991). Acquired tamoxifen resistance: correlation with reduced breast tumor levels of tamoxifen and isomerization of trans-4-hydroxytamoxifen. *J Natl Cancer Inst* 83(20): 1477-1482.

Osipo, C., C. Gajdos, et al. (2003). Paradoxical action of fulvestrant in estradiol-induced regression of tamoxifen-stimulated breast cancer. *J Natl Cancer Inst* 95(21): 1597-1608.

Park, W. C., H. Liu, et al. (2005). Deregulation of estrogen induced telomerase activity in tamoxifen-resistant breast cancer cells. *Int J Oncol* 27(5): 1459-1466.

Pink, J. J., M. M. Bilimoria, et al. (1996). Irreversible loss of the oestrogen receptor in T47D breast cancer cells following prolonged oestrogen deprivation. *Br J Cancer* 74(8): 1227-1236.

Pink, J. J. and V. C. Jordan (1996). Models of estrogen receptor regulation by estrogens and antiestrogens in breast cancer cell lines. *Cancer Res* 56(10): 2321-2330.

Reid, G., M. R. Hubner, et al. (2003). Cyclic, proteasome-mediated turnover of unliganded and liganded ERalpha on responsive promoters is an integral feature of estrogen signaling. *Mol Cell* 11(3): 695-707.

Robinson, S. P. and V. C. Jordan (1989). Antiestrogenic action of toremifene on hormone-dependent, -independent, and heterogeneous breast tumor growth in the athymic mouse. *Cancer Res* 49(7): 1758-1762.

Robson, J. M., Schonberg, A. (1937). Estrous reactions, including mating, produced by triphenyl ethylene. *Nature* 140: 196.

Schroder, C. P., A. K. Godwin, et al. (1996). Glutathione and drug resistance. *Cancer Invest* 14(2): 158-168.

Shao, W., E. K. Keeton, et al. (2004). Coactivator AIB1 links estrogen receptor transcriptional activity and stability. *Proc Natl Acad Sci U S A* 101(32): 11599-11604.

Shiau, A. K., D. Barstad, et al. (1998). The structural basis of estrogen receptor/coactivator recognition and the antagonism of this interaction by tamoxifen. *Cell* 95(7): 927-937.

Song, R. X., G. Mor, et al. (2001). Effect of long-term estrogen deprivation on apoptotic responses of breast cancer cells to 17beta-estradiol. *J Natl Cancer Inst* 93(22): 1714-1723.

Toft, D. and J. Gorski (1966). A receptor molecule for estrogens: isolation from the rat uterus and preliminary characterization. *Proc Natl Acad Sci U S A* 55(6): 1574-1581.

Townsend, D. M., K. D. Tew, et al. (2003). The importance of glutathione in human disease. *Biomed Pharmacother* 57(3-4): 145-155.

Voehringer, D. W. (1999). BCL-2 and glutathione: alterations in cellular redox state that regulate apoptosis sensitivity. *Free Radic Biol Med* 27(9-10): 945-950.

Vogel, V. G., J. P. Costantino, et al. (2006). Effects of tamoxifen vs raloxifene on the risk of developing invasive breast cancer and other disease outcomes: the NSABP Study of Tamoxifen and Raloxifene (STAR) P-2 trial. *JAMA* 295(23): 2727-2741.

Vogel, V. G., J. P. Costantino, et al. (2010). Update of the National Surgical Adjuvant Breast and Bowel Project Study of Tamoxifen and Raloxifene (STAR) P-2 Trial: Preventing breast cancer. *Cancer Prev Res (Phila)* 3(6): 696-706.

Walpole, A. L., Patterson, E. (1948). Synthetic oestrogens in mammary cancer. *Lancet* 2(2583): 783-786.

Wijayaratne, A. L. and D. P. McDonnell (2001). The human estrogen receptor-alpha is a ubiquitinated protein whose stability is affected differentially by agonists, antagonists, and selective estrogen receptor modulators. *J Biol Chem* 276(38): 35684-35692.

Wolf, D. M. and V. C. Jordan (1993). A laboratory model to explain the survival advantage observed in patients taking adjuvant tamoxifen therapy. *Recent Results Cancer Res* 127: 23-33.

Yao, K., E. S. Lee, et al. (2000). Antitumor action of physiological estradiol on tamoxifen-stimulated breast tumors grown in athymic mice. *Clin Cancer Res* 6(5): 2028-2036.

2

Targeted Apoptosis in Breast Cancer Immunotherapy

Lin-Tao Jia[1] and An-Gang Yang[2]
[1]Department of Biochemistry and Molecular Biology,
[2]Department of Immunology, Fourth Military Medical University, Xi'an, China

1. Introduction

Apoptosis is programmed and precisely regulated cell death characterized by morphological and biochemical alterations distinct from necrosis (Edinger & Thompson, 2004). The development of breast cancers, like other processes of carcinogenesis, involves uncontrolled cell proliferation and insufficient apoptosis due to either the lack of pro-apoptotic stimuli in the in vivo environment or the disturbance of cellular apoptotic pathways (Brown & Attardi, 2005). Whereas both chemotherapy and radiation caused massive apoptotic cell death in the tumor tissues, we are far from conquering the breast malignancies until the establishment of targeted pro-apoptotic therapeutic protocols or the development of apoptosis-inducing drugs that target the tumor without causing severe impairment of the normal organism (Alvarez et al, 2010; Fulda & Debatin, 2006; Motyl et al, 2006; Muschel et al, 1998). However, thanks to the elucidation of mechanisms underlying physiological and pathological apoptosis, studies have been addressed in the development of pro-apoptotic strategies targeting the cancer cells, which has provided novel approaches to the successful immutherapy of breast cancers (Schlotter et al, 2008).

2. Unbalanced proliferation and apoptosis in breast cancers

Cells undergo consistent proliferation and apoptosis during ontogenesis and in maintenance of normal morphology and function of multiple organs. These vital behaviors of cells are regulated by requisite molecular mechanism so that they are balanced to avoid uncontrolled expanding or degeneration of certain tissues (Domingos & Steller, 2007). During carcinogenesis, however, these mechanisms were disturbed by or compromised to genetic alterations either occurring spontaneously or caused by environmental stress, resulting in over-proliferation and resistance to apoptosis (Brown & Attardi, 2005; de Bruin & Medema, 2008).

2.1 Apoptotic signaling pathways

As a process of cell death with hallmarks of morphological abnormalities, e.g. shrunken and bubbled cytoplasm, condensed nucleus, fragmented chromatin but intact membrane or organelle at the early stage, apoptosis is triggered by extracellular or intracellular stimuli, and results from intracellular signaling thereafter, which ultimately leads to the degradation of functional proteins, destroy of cytoskeletons and fragmentation of DNA (Hengartner, 2000; He et al, 2009). The major initiators, mediators and executioners involved in apoptotic signaling have been unraveled, which contribute to a better understanding of carcinogenesis in diverse tissues, e.g. the mammary gland (Johnstone et al, 2002).

Both extrinsic and intrinsic stimuli can initiate apoptotic signaling, which involves the activation of downstream mediators in diverse pathways, and converge on the processing of cysteine-dependent aspartate-directed proteases, caspases (Hengartner, 2000). Caspases exist as proenzymes in cells, and once activated they can cleave various cellular protein substrates at concensus amino acid sites, leading the cells to apoptosis (Hengartner, 2000). So far two types of caspases have been identified: initiator (apical) caspases, e.g. caspases-2, -8, -9 and -10, and effector caspases, e.g. caspases-3, -6 and -7 (Thornberry & Lazebnik, 1998). Initiator caspases processed and activated by upstream stimuli could cleave inactive pro-forms of effector caspases, and effector caspases in turn cleave other protein substrates including divergent proteins maintaining normal cell structure, metabolism and physiological function, e.g. poly ADP-ribose polymerase (PARP) involved in DNA repair, lamin A protein of the cytoskeleton, and the DNA-fragmentation factor DFF45 (Riedl & Shi, 2004; Timmer & Salvesen, 2007).

2.1.1 Extrinsic pathway: Death receptor-mediated signaling

Death receptors are a class of transmembrane receptors that, once engaged by their ligands, initiate intracellular signaling resulting in cell death. These receptors belong to a tumor-necrosis factor receptor (TNFR) superfamily binding to a homotrimeric TNF protein family, among which Fas ligand (FasL or CD95L)/Fas have been well-documented (Lavrik, 2005). As a type II transmembrane protein, FasL binds and induces the trimerization of Fas, which in turn recruits the adaptor molecule Fas-associated death domain (FADD) via interaction between their death domains (DD). FADD also contains a death effector domain (DED), which aggregates and activates another DED-containing protein, FADD-like interleukin-1β-converting enzyme (FLICE)/caspase-8. This is followed by a cascade of caspase activation and ultimately the cleavage of various protein substrates and apoptosis of the cell (Houston & O'Connell, 2004; Wajant, 2002).

In addition to FasL/Fas, other death receptors and ligands have also been found to play vital roles in mediating apoptotic signaling (Houston & O'Connell, 2004; Wajant, 2002). Of note are TNF/TNFR and TRAIL/TRAIL-R1, each of which triggers specific signaling pathways, thus resulting in apoptosis in a variety of cell types or physiological or pathological processes (Baud & Karin, 2001; Gonzalvez &Ashkenazi, 2010). Upon activated by TNF, TNFR1 interacts with various death domain-containing proteins, forming a complex comprising TRADD, TNF Receptor Associated Factor-2 (TRAF2), cellular inhibitor of apoptosis-1 (CIAP1), and the receptor-interacting protein-1 (RIP1). The complex then recruits I-kappaB-kinase (IKK) and releases and activates Nuclear Factor-KappaB (NF-κB), which actually promotes cell survival (Baud & Karin, 2001; Shen & Pervaiz, 2006). However, in a following step, the TRADD-based complex can also dissociate from the receptor and bind to FADD, which consequently causes the activation of Caspase-8 and end up with apoptosis (Baud & Karin, 2001; Shen & Pervaiz, 2006). The caspase-8 inhibitor FLIP, which is a target gene of NF-κB, dictates the outcome of TNF signaling, i.e. whether cells continue to survive or undergo apoptosis (Hyer et al, 2006).

Growth factors (GFs) represent pro-survival stimuli conteracting the apoptotic signaling. After associating with their receptors, GFs activate PI3K (Phosphatidylinositde-3 Kinase) and subsequently Akt. Akt suppresses apoptosis via disrupting Bad inhibition of Bcl-2/Bcl-X_L (Duronio, 2008). The protein kinase C (PKC) also inhibits Bad via activation of ribosomal S6 kinases (p90RSKs) (Thimmaiah et al, 2010).

2.1.2 Intrinsic pathway: Role of mitochondrion and endoplasmic reticulum-related signaling

The intrinsic pathway of apoptosis begins when an injury, such as oncogene activation and DNA damage, occurs within the cell, or alternatively, cells are in stress, e.g. hypoxia or survival factor deprivation (Fulda & Debatin, 2006). The mitochondrion plays a crucial role in sensoring and regulating intrinsic signaling pathway, in particular, by providing a platform for normal functioning of the Bcl-2 family proteins (Chipuk et al, 2010; Yip & Reed, 2008).

As a family of proteins containing one or more Bcl-2 homology (BH) domains, which share sequence homology and mediate heterodimeric interactions among different members, the Bcl-2 family proteins differentially affect mitochondrial outer membrane permeabilization, and thus can be divided as anti-apoptotic and pro-apoptotic protein subfamilies (Chipuk et al, 2010; Yip & Reed, 2008). The anti-apoptotic proteins, e.g., Bcl-2 and Bcl-X_L, are usually located on the surface of the mitochondrion and block cell death by preventing the activation and homo-oligomerization of the pro-apoptotic Bcl-2 family members. The pro-apoptotic family members, such as Bax, Bad, Bid and Bak, are often found in the cytosol and relocate to the surface of the mitochondria in response to cellular damage or stress (Chipuk et al, 2010; Yip & Reed, 2008). Consequently, an interaction between anti-apoptotic proteins and excessive pro-apoptotic proteins leads to the formation of pores in the mitochondria and the release of cytochrome C and other pro-apoptotic molecules from the intermembrane space. The released cytochrome C interacts with Apaf-1 to recruit pro-caspase 9 into a multi-protein complex called the apoptosome, where caspase-9 is activated. The activated caspase-9 thus induces the processing of effector caspases, the degradation of diverse substrates of caspases and ultimately the morphological and biochemical changes by which apoptosis is featured (Scorrano & Korsmeyer, 2003; Inoue et al, 2009).

Other proteins released from the mitochondria include the apoptosis-inducing factor (AIF), second mitochondria-derived activator of caspase (SMAC)/ Diablo, Arts and Omi/high temperature requirement protein-A2 (HTRA2). As a ubiquitous mitochondrial oxidoreductase, AIF could migrate into the nucleus, bind and cause the destruction of genomic DNA, and induce apoptosis in a caspase-independent manner (Modjtahedi, 2006), while SMAC/Diablo and HTRA2, once released from the damaged mitochondira, counteract the effect of inhibitor of Apoptosis Proteins (IAPs), which normally bind and prevent activation of Caspase-3 (Wang & Youle, 2009). The interaction between Bcl-2 family members, IAPs, SMAC and Omi/HTRA2 is central to the intrinsic apoptosis pathway (Wang & Youle, 2009).

The tumor suppressor p53 is also a sensor of cellular stress and is a critical activator of the intrinsic pathway. As a transcription factor, p53 is phosphorylated and stabilized by DNA checkpoint proteins in response to DNA damage, and transcriptionally activates pro-apoptotic proteins of Bcl-2 family, e.g. Bax and Bid, and other tumor suppressor such as PTEN, the outcome of which is cell cycle arrest to allow DNA repair, and apoptosis in cases of severe DNA damage (Manfredi, 2010; Robles & Harris, 2001). The mouse double minute-2

homolog (MDM2) protein negatively regulates p53 function by mediating the nuclear export and ubiquitination of p53 (Manfredi, 2010).
As an organelle mainly involved in correct protein folding and intracellular trafficking, the endoplasmic reticulum (ER) is highly sensitive to stresses that perturb cellular energy levels, the redox state or Ca2+ concentration. These ER stresses initiate unfolded protein responses (UPR), which promote cell survival and switch to pro-apoptotic signaling when the ER stress is prolonged (Rasheva & Domingos, 2009; Szegezdi et al, 2006). ER stress-induced apoptosis is a complicated process mediated by a series of specific proteins, in particular, the pancreatic ER kinase (PKR)-like ER kinase (PERK), activating transcription factor 6 (ATF6) and inositol-requiring enzyme 1 (IRE1) in the initiation phase, the transcription factor C/EBP homologous protein (CHOP), growth arrest and DNA damage-inducible gene 34 (GADD34), Tribbles-related protein 3 (TRB3) and Bcl-2 family members in the commitment phase, and ultimately caspases during the execution of apoptosis (Rasheva & Domingos, 2009; Szegezdi et al, 2006).

2.2 Alterations of apoptotic signaling in breast cancer cells

Breast cancer is a malignancy with a wide spectrum of genetic alterations, phenotypic heterogeneity, and a variety of contributing etiological factors like age, family history, parity, and age of menarche or menopause (McCready et al, 2010). While breast cancers share the characteristics, e.g. deregulated proliferation and apoptosis with carcinomas of other origins, the molecular mechanisms underlying these characteristics are quite different, or even unique for certain processes of breast cancer development or metastasis. To date, several molecular markers and related signaling pathways have been revealed to play key roles in breast carcinogenesis by causing persistent proliferation and blocked apoptosis of breast epithelial cells (McCready et al, 2010).

2.2.1 Attenuated or blocked signaling in classical apoptotic pathways

The neoplastic breast epithelial cells have evolved diverse mechanisms to resist apoptosis via the extrinsic or intrinsic pathway. The downregulation of Fas or Fas ligand is found in numerous breast cancers, and is implicated in prognosis evaluation of patients with breast malignancies (Mottolese et al, 2000). Meanwhile, the expression of FasL may also be upregulated in breast cancers, which contributes to excessive apoptosis of T cells and thus serves as a mechanism of immune escape (Muschen et al, 2000). Signaling by death receptors can also be negatively regulated by overexpression of their inhibitors, e.g. the FLICE-like inhibitory proteins (FLIP) which dampens caspase-8 activation after recruited to the death-inducing signaling complex (DISC) (Rogers et al, 2007). Another inhibitor of death receptors, phosphoprotein enriched in diabetes/phosphoprotein enriched in astrocytes-15 kDa (PED/PEA-15), has also been implicated in mediating AKT-dependent chemoresistance in human breast cancer cells (Eramo et al, 2005). As crucial regulators of mitochondrial apoptotic pathway, several Bcl-2 family members have been found aberrantly expressed or frequently mutated in breast cancers. For example, overexpression of Bcl-2 or Bcl-X_L is associated with the development or metastasis of breast carcinomas (Alireza et al, 2008; Martin et al, 2004). In contrast, the absence or inactivation of the pro-apoptotic Bcl-2 family members, such as Bax, Bid and Bim is involved in breast carcinogenesis (Sivaprasad et al, 2007; Sjöström-Mattson et al, 2009; Whelan et al, 2010). Among the caspase-recruiting adaptors, the downregulation of Apaf-1 was found to correlate with the progression of some clinical breast adenocarcinomas (Vinothini et al, 2011). Finally, the polymorphisms and loss of function mutations within caspase genes have also been detected in breast cancers (Ghavami et al, 2009).

2.2.2 Reinforced estrogen signaling in breast carcinogenesis

As a sex hormone, estrogens exert their actions by binding to the intracellular receptors-estrogen receptors (ER)-α or ER-β. While estrogen/ER regulates growth, differentiation and homeostasis of the normal mammary gland, sustained engagement of ER with endogenous or exogenous estrogen (E2) is well established to cause breast cancer (Hayashi et al, 2003). In fact, ER-positive breast cancers account for 70% of the nearly 200,000 new cases diagnosed annually in the USA. Activated ER promotes breast cancer development via three major mechanisms: stimulation of cellular proliferation through the receptor-mediated hormonal activity, direct genotoxic effects by increasing mutation rates through a cytochrome P450-mediated metabolic activation, and induction of aneuploidy (J. Russo & I.H. Russo, 2006). Estrogen-bound ERs become activated transcription factors via induced dimerization and translocation to the nucleus. This is followed by the recognition of the estrogen-responsive element (ERE) in the 5′ regulatory sequences of the target genes with the assistance of a "pioneer factor", FoxA1, and consequently the altered expression of the gene via recruitment of related transcriptional factors (Yamaguchi, 2007). A growing list of genes have proved to be the target of estrogen signaling, among which are cell cycle genes like E2F1 and cyclin D1, and those involved in cell survival and oriented differentiation. A systemic analysis suggested that estrogen/ER signaling is crucial for the regulation of genes involved in an evolutionarily conserved apoptosis pathway (Liu & Chen, 2010). It is also hypothesized that estrogen promotes the survival of ER-positive breast cancer cells mainly by suppressing the apoptotic machinery or upregulation of the anti-apoptotic molecules, e.g. Bcl-2 and Bcl-X_L (Gompel et al, 2000; Rana et al, 2010).

2.2.3 Elevated HER2 expression and signaling in breast carcinogenesis

Human epidermal growth factor receptor 2 (HER2) is a member of the avian erythroblastosis oncogene B (ErbB) protein family with alternative names ErbB2, neu, CD340 (cluster of differentiation 340) and p185. As a receptor tyrosine kinase encoded by the *ERBB2* proto-oncogene, HER2 over-expression has been found in a wide variety of cancers (Moasser, 2007). Approximately 30% of breast cancers exhibit an overexpression of HER2 due to aneuploidy or the amplification of the *ERBB2* gene. Transcriptional deregulation involving cis-acting element mutation or abnormal activation of transcription factors due to dysfunction of tumor suppressors like p53 also contribute to HER2 overexpression (Freudenberg et al, 2009; Moasser, 2007). HER2 gene amplification and over-expression are frequently detected in high-grade ductal carcinoma in situ (DCIS) and high-grade inflammatory breast cancer (IBC), but not in benign breast biopsies such as the terminal duct lobular units (TDLUs), suggesting that over-expression of HER2 usually occurs at the transition from hyperplasia to DCIS (Freudenberg et al, 2009; Moasser, 2007). HER2 overexpression in breast cancers correlates with high metastasis capacity, increased disease recurrence and worse prognosis, and are therefore routinely examined in breast cancer patients for a determination of therapeutic protocol and prediction of the treatment outcome (Eccles, 2001).

Despite its well-documented association with transformation of normal breast epithelial cells and metastasis and poor outcome of breast cancers, the detailed mechanisms underlying HER2-mediated signal events and cell behavior are far from being fully understood. Nevertheless, it is established that HER2 functions through homodimerization and more frequently forming heterodimers with other human epidermal growth factor receptors (HERs) (Moasser, 2007; Park et al, 2008). These HERs are commonly activated upon binding of a ligand in their extracellular domain, resulting in dimerization of HERs and triggering the intrinsic tyrosine kinase activity of the receptors responsible for a mutual or monodirectional phosphorylation between the dimerized HERs. The phosphorylated tyrosine-containing motif provides a docking station for intracellular signaling molecules (Moasser, 2007; Park et al, 2008). Given the existence of several tyrosine phosphorylation sites in the intracellular sites, the phosphorylation patterns are unique for a certain HER2 dimer, and thus trigger downstream signaling different from other dimers. Although none of the known HER ligands bind directly to HER2 with high affinity, heregulin, a cytokine secreted by the breast stromal cells, can activate HER2 by inducing or stabilizing heterodimers with other HER receptors. More importantly, HER2 is the preferred heterodimerization partner of other HER receptors like HER3, and strengthens their binding to a cognate ligand (Park et al, 2008).

The HER dimers containg HER2 modulate diverse signaling pathways involved in cell proliferation, apoptosis and migration. Adaptor proteins in Ras-MAPK pathway, e.g. Grb2 and Shc, and the p85 subunit of phosphatidylinositol 3-kinase (PI3K) can bind directly to the dimers, leading to prolonged signaling of both pathways (Moasser, 2007; Park et al, 2008). In addition to inducing cell over-proliferation via well-defined mechanisms like NF-kB activation downstream of PI3K, these signaling events also efficiently inhibit apoptosis via negatively regulating tumor suppressors p53 and PTEN, and cell cycle inhibitors p21 Cip1/WAF1 and p27Kip1 (Park et al, 2008). Whereas the molecular machinery utilized by HER2 to promote cell migration and invasion remains unclear, the upregulation of the chemokine CXCR4 and thus the stromal cell–derived factor-1 (SDF-1)/CXCR4 axis are believed to play a central role in mediating metastasis of HER2-positive cancers (Li et al, 2004).

2.2.4 Other genetic alterations

It is now widely accepted that all cancers are attributed to alterations of the genomic information or gene expression (Teixeira et al, 2002; Jovanovic et al, 2010). In this regard, both germline mutations that increase the risk of carcinogenesis and somatic chromatin alterations in specific gene locus have been implicated in the development of breast cancers (Teixeira et al, 2002; Jovanovic et al, 2010). Like malignancies in other tissues, breast cancer occurs as a result of the activation of oncogenes or dysfunction of a tumor suppressor gene. In addition to the well-documented cancer-related genes, e.g. c-Myc, Ras, ATM, p53 and PTEN, accumulated data have unraveled a class of genes whose functional abnormalities are specifically associated with the development of breast carcinoma (Geyer et al, 2009; Prokopcova et al, 2007; Teixeira et al, 2002). This is exemplified by the breast cancer-susceptibility genes BRCA1 and BRCA2, the mutation of which leads to a lifetime risk of as high as 80% of developing breast cancer and accounts for 15% of total breast cancer cases. Germline mutations in the BRCA1 and BRCA2 genes result in chromosome instability and deficient repair of DNA double-strand breaks by homologous recombination. BRCA-mediated homologous recombination and DNA repair require their interaction with ataxia telangiectasia mutated gene (ATM), RAD51C, BRIP1, Checkpoint kinase 2 (CHEK2) and the partner and localizer of BRCA2 (PALB2), the mutations of which have also been found in breast cancer development (Byrnes, 2008; Fulda & Debatin, 2006; Venkitaraman, 2009). PIK3CA, an oncogene encoding the PI3K catalytic subunit, exhibits a high frequency of gain-of-function mutations in breast cancers, leading to constitutive PI3K/AKT pathway activation in breast cancer. PIK3CA mutations have been observed in more than 30% of ERα-positive breast cancers (Cizkova et al, 2010).

3. Strategies of targeted apoptosis in breast cancer cells

Given that resistance to apoptosis is a major causative factor of breast carcinogenesis, correction of the deregulated apoptotic process or enforced induction of apoptosis will be beneficial in the treatment of breast cancers. However, an ideal apoptosis-based therapeutic protocol must be cancer cell-specific in order to avoid impairment of adjacent normal tissues or a systemic cytotoxicity of the therapeutics. This could be achieved either by targeted delivery of pro-apoptotic molecules in the cancer cells, or by strategies that confer the candidate therapeutics apoptosis-inducing activity specifically in the cancer cells (Alvarez et al, 2010).

3.1 Therapeutics that trigger apoptosis in breast cancers

3.1.1 Apoptosis-inducing chemicals

Despite a relatively late elucidation of molecular mechanisms of apoptosis, chemical drugs or radiation traditionally used for cancer therapy have proved efficient in apoptosis induction. DNA-damaging agents like doxorubicin, etoposide, cisplatin or bleomycin may induce apoptosis via both extrinsic and intrinsic apoptotic pathways (Fulda & Debatin, 2006). Treatment of patients with some of these anticancer drugs causes an increase in the expression of CD95L/FasL, which stimulates the receptor pathway in an autocrine or paracrine manner; conventional chemotherapeutic agents also trigger intrinsic apoptotic pathway by eliciting mitochondrial permeabilization (Fulda & Debatin, 2006). In addition, detailed mechanism underlying the apoptosis-inducing effect of chemicals may include the perturbations of intermediate metabolism, increased expression or activity of p53 or an apoptotic mediator, or changes in the ratios of the anti-apoptotic and pro-apoptotic Bcl-2 family members. For example, paclitaxel treatment causes the accumulation of BH3-only Bcl-2 family protein Bim and induces Bim-dependent apoptosis in epithelial tumors (Tan et al., 2005); paclitaxel also causes hyperphosphorylation and inactivation of Bcl-2, and facilitates the opening of the permeability transition (PT) pore (Ruvolo et al., 2001).

3.1.2 Apoptosis initiators, mediators and executioners

The past two decades has witnessed an increasingly clear depiction of the molecular machinery of apoptosis, which facilitated the development of strategies aiming at apoptosis induction of breast cancer cells (Brown & Attardi, 2005). Theoretically, introduction of any active molecule in the irreversible apoptotic pathway is sufficient to trigger apoptosis of cancer cells (Waxman & Schwartz, 2003). These active molecules involve extracellular cytokines or ligands representing death stimuli, e.g. FasL, tumor necrosis factor-α (TNF-α) or the TNF-related apoptosis-inducing ligand (TRAIL), and cellular mediators in the apoptotic pathway such as the pro-apoptotic members of Bcl-2 family and adaptors that link death signal sensors and caspases. Finally, introduction of apoptotic executioners, in

particular, effector caspases in cancer cells, will directly trigger apoptosis independently of upstream apoptotic signaling machinery (Ashkenazi, 2008; Fulda & Debatin, 2006).
While a simple overexpression or accumulation of the apoptotic proteins could commit killing of cancer cells, it is also common that a structural modification is needed before delivery or ectopic expression in cancer cells due to the following reasons. First, a tumoricidal dose of the pro-apoptotic protein, e.g. TNF-α, may also be very closer to a dose that causes systemic toxicity. In this case, screening from the mutated or modulated counterparts to obtain a lowerly toxic mutant is necessary (Meany et al, 2008). Second, the mediators or executioners of apoptosis, such as the Bcl-2 family memebers and caspases, exist as inactive zymogen or precursors in the cells, and will not trigger apoptosis unless activated (Yip & Reed, 2008). Constitutively active caspases-3 and -6 have been generated by removal of the prodomain and rearrangement of the large and small subunits (Srinivasula et al, 1998a). Active forms of Bax or Bid can be acquired by deletion of an amino-terminal domain, whereas an amino-terminal moiety of AIF is sufficient to trigger the caspase-independent apoptosis (Yu et al, 2006). Finally, strategies to generate cancer-targeted molecules are beneficial to improving the tumoricidal efficacy while alleviating the side effect, and therefore add weight to the applicability of the antitumor studies from bench to bedside (Alvarez et al, 2010).

3.1.3 Therapeutics targeting apoptosis inhibitors and growth signals

During carcinogenesis or acquiring resistance to chemotherapy, many breast epithelial cells have developed apoptosis-escaping mechanisms by upregulating a class of apoptosis inhibitors (Hyer et al, 2006; Liston et al, 2003). These involve the anti-apoptotic members of Bcl-2 family, e.g. Bcl-2 and Bcl-X_L, as well as endogenous inhibitors of caspases, e.g. the IAP family and c-FLIP proteins (Hyer et al, 2006; Liston et al, 2003). Among the IAPs, both survivin and X-linked inhibitor of apoptosis (XIAP) have been targeted in breast cancer treatment (Liston et al, 2003). Therefore, antisense oligonucleotides or small interfering RNAs (siRNAs) targeted to these inhibitors holds out great promise to counteract these inhibitors and possibly restore the apoptotic signaling in these cells (Crnkovic-Mertens, 2003; Li et al, 2006). The targeting of growth signals that counteract the cellular apoptotic machinery was also widely exploited. Of note are the monoclonal antibodies or chemical agents which target HER2, vascular endothelial growth factor (VEGF) and the epidermal growth factor receptor (EGFR) (Alvarez et al, 2010; Ludwig et al, 2003). Also targeted are the heat shock proteins (HSPs), the molecular chaperones required for the stability and function of the growth factor signaling and anti-apoptotic proteins (Sánchez-Muñoz et al, 2009).

3.2 Targeted introduction of apoptosis-inducing proteins

It has been an inherent challenge to selectively introduce the therapeutics or cytotoxic mechanism into the malignant cells in cancer therapy (Alvarez et al, 2010). Theoretically, targeted apoptosis induction in breast cancer cells could be achieved via two basic approaches. First, pro-apoptotic molecules could be delivered specifically into breast cancer cells. Thanks to the characteristic expression of a class of cell surface markers by breast cancer cells, antibodies that recognize these markers have been utilized to construct apoptosis-eliciting recombinant proteins, or alternatively, to generate targeted delivery system for pro-apoptotic genes (Alvarez et al, 2010). Second, the regulatory element, e.g. promoter of a gene specifically expressed in breast cancer cells could be used to control the expression of an apoptosis-inducing gene, which results in the tumor-specific expression of the gene (Lee, 2009). Despite an overall limited clinical application of these targeted strategies, both approaches have proved effective in vitro or in xenograft breast cancer models (Alvarez et al, 2010; Lee, 2009).

In our study, a series of cancer-targeted pro-apoptotic fusion proteins were generated based on the active apoptosis mediators or executioners and a single chain antibody, e23sFv, which binds HER2 with high affinity (Jia et al, 2003; Xu et al, 2004; Zhao et al, 2004). These fusion proteins, designated "immunoapoptotins" after the well documented immunotoxins, consist of e23sFv in the amino terminal, a translocation domain and a constitutively active apoptotic protein (Pastan et al, 2006). The constitutively active apoptotic proteins were obtained by reversing the large and small subunits of caspases-3 or -6, or through generating a truncated form of granzyme B, AIF or the pro-apoptotic Bcl-2 family member, Bid (Figure 1; Jia et al, 2003; Qiu et al, 2008; Xu et al, 2004; Zhao et al, 2004). A translocation domain originating from a protein toxin, Pseudomonas Exotoxin A (PEA), was embedded in the fusion protein to mediate a translocation of the apoptotic proteins from an intracellular vesicle to the cytosol, which is required for apoptosis execution by a majority of apoptotic proteins (Jia et al, 2003; Qiu et al, 2008; Wang et al, 2010; Wang et al, 2007; Xu et al, 2004; Zhao et al, 2004). In principle, the single chain antibody mediates the recognition of HER2-overexpressing breast cancer cells and internalization of the fusion protein via endocytosis. In the endosome, the fusion protein undergoes proteolytic processing by a proprotein convertase, furin, which is enriched in the intracellular vesicles like lysosome, endosome or Golgi apparatus (Wang et al, 2010; Wang et al, 2007). This results in the generation of a carboxyl-terminal fragment encompassing the active apoptotic protein, which is released into the cytosol and triggers the apoptosis of the cells (Figure 1). Unless processed inside the cells, these recombinant proteins are nontoxic due to a steric hindrance of pro-apoptotic moiety by the N-terminal antibody and translocation domain (Wang et al, 2010; Wang et al, 2007). Unlike previously reported tumor killer proteins, such as immunotoxins, the cytotoxic activities of the immunoapoptotins are based on human endogenous proteins that kill tumor cells in an intrinsic physiologic manner, resulting in relatively weak immunogenicity and minor systemic toxicity over repeated treatments (Chen et al, 1997; Jia et al, 2003; Pastan et al, 2006).

These immunoapoptotins could be prepared by engineered bacteria or mammalian cells. Alternatively, the construct expressing the immunoapoptotins could be delivered into in vivo cells via a retroviral vector or non-viral systems (Jia et al, 2003; Wang, 2010; Xu et al, 2004). In addition, we also generated lymphocytes that could secrete immunoapoptotins after genetic modifications (Jia et al, 2003; Zhao et al, 2004). The apoptosis-inducing capacities of the immunoapoptotins were examined in vitro by incubation of the fusion proteins with the target cancer cells, coculture of the immunoapoptotin-secreting lymphoma Jurkat cells with target cells, or direct transfection of target cells with the construct of an amino-terminal signal sequence-containing immunoapototins, which is anticipated to exert their tumoricidal effect via an autocrine pattern (Jia et al, 2003; Qiu et al, 2008; Wang et al, 2010). As a result, the immunoapoptotins selectively induce apoptosis of HER2-positive breast cancer SKBr-3 and ovary cancer SKOv-3 cell lines, but not of those that barely express HER2. Xenograft tumor models were next generated via subcutaneous injection of the nude mice with HER2-positive or -negative breast cancer cells (Jia et al, 2003; Qiu et al, 2008; Wang et al, 2010). Intratumoral injection of the immunoapoptotin-producing adenovirus resulted in dramatic suppression of tumor growth and significantly prolonged mice survival. In addition, intravenous administration of either the immunoapoptotin-producing adenovirus or the lymphocytes that secrete these recombinant proteins also accounted for marked tumor suppression in vivo (Jia et al, 2003; Qiu et al, 2008; Wang et al, 2010; Xu et al, 2004; Zhao et al, 2004). A distribution of immunoapoptotin in the tumor tissue but not other major organs was observed, consistent with the detection of redundant apoptosis specifically in the xenograft tumors (Jia et al, 2003; Wang et al, 2010; Xu et al, 2004; Zhao et al, 2004). These results indicate that the immunoapoptotins, which combines the properties of a tumor-specific antibody with the potent tumoricidal activity of apoptotic mediators or executioners, may provide novel approaches to immunotherapy or gene therapy of HER2-positive breast cancers. The genetically modified somatic cells, especially lymphocytes, are expected to suppress primary tumors and micrometastases, owing to continuous secretion of the fusion proteins and their diffusion through blood and lymph fluid. These modified cells remain viable because they are HER2-negative and the immunoapoptotins are directed to the lumen of the endoplasmic reticulum and secreted co-translationally (Jia et al, 2003; Xu et al, 2004; Zhao et al, 2004).

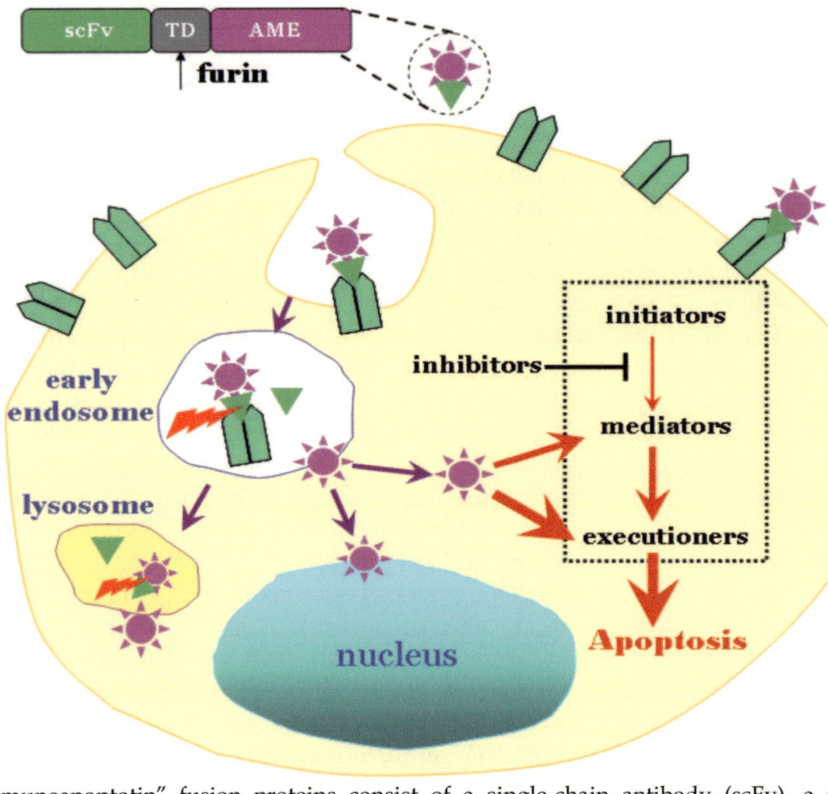

The "immunoapoptotin" fusion proteins consist of a single-chain antibody (scFv), a translocation domain (TD) and a constitutively active apoptosis mediator/executioner (AME). The antibody recognizes a distinguished surface marker (e.g. HER2) of breast cancer cells, and internalizes via endocytosis; the translocation domain mediates the processing of the fusion protein in the endosome or lysosome by furin to release into the cyotsol a C-terminal moiety; the released moiety containing the AME triggers apoptosis of the cell independently of the endogenous upstream apoptotic machinery.

Fig. 1. Immunoapoptotins specifically induce apoptosis of breast cancer cells.

Another constituent in the immunoapoptotins that need to be addressed is the translocation domain, which is exogenous to human and thus has potentials to elicit immunological responses, resulting in either systemic toxicity or neutralization of the killer protein (Wang et al, 2010; Wang et al, 2007). To ameliorate the primary structure of the killer protein, we generated truncated variants of PEA or diphtheria toxin (DT) translocation domains to identify the minimal sequence required for furin processing and translocation (Wang et al, 2010; Wang et al, 2007). Consequently, we found that peptides encompassing the 273rd to 282nd amino acids of PEA (TRHRQPRGWE), or 187th to 196th amino acids of DT (AGNRVRRSVG) are furin-sensitive sequences, and immunoapoptotins based on these translocation sequences exhibited relatively low systemic toxicity while maintaining potent pro-apoptotic activities when applied to HER2-positive cancers (Wang et al, 2010; Wang et al, 2007). Considering that cancer specific antigens other than HER2 can also be targeted by an antibody, our immunoapoptotin strategy would have a versatile applicability in the treatment of breast cancers with distinguished cell surface biomarkers.

Estrogen receptor overexpression and estrogen-dependence are found in a majority of breast cancer cases (Ghazoui et al, 2011). A class of selective estrogen receptor modulators (SERMs), as represented by tamoxifen (TAM), have been used for targeted therapy of these breast cancers with encouraging outcomes at least partially via reversing the anti-apoptotic effect of estrogen receptor signaling (Jordan & O'Malley, 2007). Unfortunately, use of SERMs is associated with de novo and acquired resistance and some undesirable side effects (Jordan & O'Malley, 2007). In contrast, a targeted introduction or activation of a cellular apoptosis executioner will elicit irreversible cell death without inducing drug resistance (Waxman & Schwartz, 2003). According to the well-documented "induced proximity model", the activation of the initiators occurs only when they are recruited by upstream oligomerization inducers, which bring the procaspases into close proximity and thus allow intramolecular processing (Shi, 2004). This model has been applied in developing pro-apoptotic strategies in cancer treatment based on the oligomerization capacity of either mouse IgG Fc portion or the tandem FK506-binding domain (FKBP) plus its dimeric ligand FK1012 (Muzio et al, 1998; Shi, 2004; Srinivasula et al, 1998b). In a study focusing on ER-positive breast cancer treatment, we generated a fusion gene encoding the chimeric protein of caspase-8 and the ligand-binding domain (LBD) of ERα and introduced the gene into breast cancer cell lines (Zhao et al, 2011). Upon administration of estrogen, the fusion protein will be induced to form a dimer, which triggers the activation of caspase-8 and apoptosis (Tamrazi et al, 2002; Shi, 2004). Indeed, incubation of estradiol with the chimeric gene-modified breast cancer cells induced a rapid dimerization of the chimeric protein, which in turn caused the activation of caspase-8 within the chimeric protein and leads to apoptosis of the modified cells (Zhao et al, 2011). Estradiol also significantly impaired the development of the xenograft breast cancers derived from the chimeric gene-modified SKBr-3 cells, and inhibited the growth of in vivo tumors originating from MCF-7 cells when administered in combination with the chimeric gene recombinant adenovirus (Zhao et al, 2011).

Unlike previously reported artificial caspase recruitment models, our study employed the receptor of endogenous estrogenic hormones, which otherwise promote the growth of breast cancer cells, to trigger the apoptotic signaling in breast cancers, thus switching the estrogenic hormones from potential mitogens to apoptosis inducers in breast cancers (Shi, 2004; Zhao et al, 2011). Therefore, the caspase-8 and estrogen receptor-based chimeric protein has implications in developing novel therapeutics of estrogen-dependent and -independent breast cancers. Despite the effectiveness of the chimeric protein, optimization of this suicidal system using an accurate dimerization-related domain of ERα is necessary for preventing inappropriate autoactivation of chimeric caspase-8; given that the estrogen antagonist, tamoxifen, is also found to induce the formation of ER dimers in a much lower efficiency, it remains elusive whether tamoxifen in place of estradiol could trigger dimerization and activation of caspase-8 conjugated to the ER ligand-binding domain (Tamrazi et al, 2002; Zhao et al, 2011).

In addition to the generation of fusion/chimeric proteins, the pro-apoptotic gene regulatory elements, as well as the gene construct carriers, either non-viral or viral particles, have also been modified to target breast cancers. The antibody-drug conjugate, Trastuzumab-DM1 is currently in a late clinical trial for treatment of HER2-positive breast cancers (Alley et al, 2010; Senter, 2009). Breast cancer-targeted delivery systems are also constructed by modifying the envelop of viral particles, liposomes or other nanomaterials with tumor cell-binding phage peptides, or with ligands or antibodies that recognize HER2, E-selectin, transferrin or erythropoietin-producing hepatocellular receptor tyrosine kinase receptor class A2 (EphA2) (Alvarez et al, 2010; Mann et al, 2010; Normanno et al, 2009; Sarkar et al, 2005; Tandon et al, 2011). Tumor-specific regulatory elements, such as promoters of human telomerase reverse transcriptase (hTERT), survivin, Muc1 and the homologous recombination-related protein Rad51, as well as the hypoxia-responsive elements (HRE) have been employed in the regulation of pro-apoptotic genes like Bax and truncated Bid in the development of breast cancer-targeted therapeutic strategies (Lee, 2009; Kazhdan et al, 2006; Hine et al, 2008).

3.3 Selective blockade of anti-apoptotic signaling

It is widely accepted that intracellular apoptosis-inhibitory mechanisms account for a rapid progression and chemotherapy resistance of a variety of breast cancers. Therefore, targeted restoration of the apoptotic signaling by suppression of the anti-apoptotic factors helps reverse the malignant phenotype of breast cancers (Fulda & Debatin, 2006; Waxman & Schwartz, 2003). This could be achieved in the post-transcriptional level by targeted siRNA or in the post-translational level via targeted degradation of the anti-apoptotic proteins (Fulda & Debatin, 2006; Waxman & Schwartz, 2003). Considering that the short hairpin RNA (shRNA) expression is commonly driven by an RNA polymerase III promoter, which somehow excludes a modification of the promoter using a tumor-specific elements, specific delivery of siRNAs instead of selective expression of the shRNAs in neoplastic cells would be appropriate to targeting breast cancer cells (Couto and High, 2010; Wen et al, 2008). Again, the antibodies or ligands that recognize breast cancer cells are utilized in these targeted delivery systems (Couto and High, 2010; Wen et al, 2008). In one of our studies, a subset of siRNA delivery systems were generated by fusing a tumor-targeting antibody with the nucleic acid-binding peptide derived from the arginine-rich protein, protamine. The targeted delivery of the synthesized siRNA or shRNA-expressing cassette in cells expressing the corresponding antigen was corroborated in in vivo models (Wen et al, 2008).

The protein ubiquitination process governs the degradation of unfavored endogenous proteins in the cells. In an attempt to trigger targeted degradation of the breast cancer-related proteins, Li et al generated a series of chimeric molecules in which the Src homology 2 (SH2) domain of the ubiquitin ligase Cbl was replaced with that from growth factor receptor binding protein 2 (Grb2), Grb7, p85 or Src (Li et al, 2007). These chimeric proteins could interact with HER2 and accelerate the degradation of this oncoprotein, suggesting a novel approach to the targeted therapy of HER2-overexpressing cancers (Li et al, 2007).

4. Targeted apoptosis in clinical treatment of breast cancers

The development of targeted pro-apoptotic strategies in laboratory studies on breast cancer treatment is in parallel with the emerging of novel targeted agents for clinical breast cancer therapy (Fulda & Debatin, 2006; Waxman & Schwartz, 2003). As aforementioned, monoclonal antibodies or small molecule inhibitors targeting HER2 (Herceptin/trastuzumab), EGFR (Gefitinib/Iressa) and VEGF (Avastin/Bevacizumab) have found their clinical applications in the war against breast cancers (Schlotter et al, 2008). In particular, as a well-documented adjuvant drug for metastatic breast cancer therapy, Herceptin has provided startling benefits to patients by reducing suffering and mortality of breast cancers, although frequent resistance development and cardiovascular toxicity have limited its repeated administration (Paik et al, 2008). In clinical trials of breast cancers, the death receptor ligands recombinant TNF-α and TRAIL have exhibited notable apoptosis-inducing potentials (Gonzalvez &Ashkenazi, 2010; Li et al, 2010). Intriguingly, TRAIL has displayed minimal adverse effects on normal tissues and the most striking therapeutic benefits in patients with HER2, ER and progesterone receptor (PR) triple-negative breast cancers (Oakman et al, 2010; 19: 312). Targeted expression of TRAIL under the control of a radiation-inducible RecA promoter delivered by Salmonella typhimurium significantly improved the survival of mice bearing breast cancers (Ganai et al, 2009).

Small RNAs or chemicals targeting the anti-apoptotic genes are also on their way towards the prescription for breast cancer patients. However, as a pioneering anticancer nucleic acid drug, G3139- the antisense oligonucleotide targeting Bcl-2 showed limited therapeutic efficacy when combined with doxorubicin and docetaxel in phage I/II studies on breast cancers (Moulder et al, 2008). Inhibitors to poly(ADP-ribose) polymerase-1 (PARP-1), a well-defined substrate of caspase-3, have showed single agent activity in treatment of breast cancers in a phase I trial, and conferred therapeutic benefits in combination with chemotherapy in triple-negative breast cancers without an increase in normal tissue toxicity in a phase II clinical trial. (Drew & Plummer, 2010).

5. Conclusion and perspective

Accumulating evidence on breast malignancies has supported that insufficient apoptosis contributes crucially to the occurrence and progression of breast cancers, and apoptosis resistance accounts for failure of traditional anticancer therapy on a majority of clinical breast cancers (Brown & Attardi, 2005; Evan & Vousden, 2001). In recent years, an extensive understanding of the canonical apoptosis signaling mechanisms has allowed the development of novel approaches to reversing or compensating for the apoptosis deficiency of cancer cells, either by introduction of a pro-apoptotic molecule or via blockade of the anti-apoptotic signals in breast cancers (Fulda & Debatin, 2006; Waxman & Schwartz, 2003). Given the distinguished expression of the definitive tumor-specific antigens (TSA) in breast carcinomas, strategies targeting these cells could be developed based on specific recognition mediated by antigen/antibody or ligand/receptor binding or on a selective expression of the therapeutic genes under the control of the TSA regulatory elements (Rakha et al, 2010; Schlotter et al, 2009). Despite a successful clinical application of the targeted drugs, e.g. antibodies or chemical reagents to trigger apoptosis in numerous breast cancer cases, modifications to these drugs are probably necessary for two purposes (Alley et al, 2010; Fulda & Debatin, 2006). First, combination of the therapeutic antibodies or chemicals with other potent cytotoxic mechanisms will improve their apoptosis-inducing efficacy in breast cancers. Second, additional approaches to achieving a "genuine" breast cancer targeting in drug delivery or gene expression facilitate reducing a systemic cytotoxicity or other adverse effects on patients (Alley et al, 2010; Lee, 2009). Nevertheless, the ongoing studies aiming at targeted apoptosis induction in breast cancers have opened new avenues to successful breast cancer immunotherapy.

6. References

Alireza, A., Raheleh, S., Abbass, R., Mojgan, M., Mohamadreza, M., Gholamreza, M. & Shadi, B. (2008) An immunohistochemistry study of tissue bcl-2 expression and its serum levels in breast cancer patients. *Ann N Y Acad Sci*, Vol. 1138, (Sep 2008), pp. (114-120), ISSN 0077-8923

Alley, S.C., Okeley, N.M. & Senter, P.D. (2010) Antibody-drug conjugates: targeted drug delivery for cancer. *Curr Opin Chem Biol*, Vol. 14, No. 4, (Aug 2010), pp. (529-537), ISSN 1367-5931

Alvarez, R.H., Valero, V. & Hortobagyi, G.N. (2010) Emerging targeted therapies for breast cancer. *J Clin Oncol*, Vol. 28, No. 20, (Jul 2010), pp. (3366-3379), ISSN 0732-183X

Ashkenazi, A. (2008) Targeting the extrinsic apoptosis pathway in cancer. *Cytokine Growth Factor Rev*, Vol. 19, No. 3-4, (Jun-Aug 2008), pp. (325-331), ISSN 1359-6101

Baud, V. & Karin, M. (2001) Signal transduction by tumor necrosis factor and its relatives. *Trends Cell Biol*, Vol. 11, No. 9, (Sep 2001), pp. (372-377), ISSN 0962-8924

Brown, J.M. & Attardi, L.D. (2005) The role of apoptosis in cancer development and treatment response. *Nat Rev Cancer*, Vol. 5, No. 3, (Mar 2005), pp. (231-237), ISSN 1474-175X

Byrnes, G.B., Southey, M.C. & Hopper, J.L. (2008) Are the so-called low penetrance breast cancer genes, ATM, BRIP1, PALB2 and CHEK2, high risk for women with strong family histories? *Breast Cancer Res*, Vol. 10, No. 3, (Jun 2008), pp. (208-214), ISSN 1465-5411

Chen, S.Y., Yang, A.G., Chen, J.D., Kute, T., King, C.R., Collier, J., Cong, Y., Yao, C. & Huang, X.F. (1997) Potent antitumour activity of a new class of tumour-specific killer cells. *Nature*, Vol. 385, No. 6611, (Jan 1997), pp. (78-80), ISSN 0028-0836

Chipuk, J.E., Moldoveanu, T., Llambi, F., Parsons, M.J. & Green, DR. (2010) The BCL-2 family reunion. *Mol Cell*, Vol. 37, No. 3, (Feb 2010), pp. (299-310). ISSN 1097-2765

Cizkova, M., Cizeron-Clairac, G., Vacher, S., Susini, A., Andrieu, C., Lidereau, R. & Bièche, I. (2010) Gene expression profiling reveals new aspects of PIK3CA mutation in ERalpha-positive breast cancer: major implication of the Wnt signaling pathway. *PLoS One*, Vol. 5, No. 12, (Dec 2010), pp. (e15647), ISSN 1932-6203

Cory, S., Huang, D.C. & Adams, J.M. (2003) The Bcl-2 family: roles in cell survival and oncogenesis. *Oncogene*, Vol. 22, No. 53, (Nov 2003), pp. (8590-8607), ISSN 0950-9232

Cosimo, S.D. & Baselga, J. (2008) Targeted therapies in breast cancer: Where are we now? *Eur J Cancer*, Vol. 44, No. 18, (Nov 2008), pp. (2781-2790), ISSN 0959-8049

Couto, L.B. & High, K.A. (2010) Viral vector-mediated RNA interference. *Curr Opin Pharmacol*, Vol. 10, No. 5, (Oct 2010), pp. (534-542, ISSN 1471-4892

Crnkovic-Mertens, I., Hoppe-Seyler, F. & Butz, K. (2003) Induction of apoptosis in tumor cells by siRNA-mediated silencing of the livin/ML-IAP/KIAP gene. *Oncogene,* Vol. 22, No. 51, (Nov 2003), pp. (8330-8336), ISSN 0950-9232

de Bruin, E.C. & Medema, J.P. (2008) Apoptosis and non-apoptotic deaths in cancer development and treatment response. *Cancer Treat Rev,* Vol. 34, No. 8, (Dec 2008), pp. (737-749), ISSN 0305-7372

Domingos, P.M. & Steller, H. (2007) Pathways regulating apoptosis during patterning and development. *Curr Opin Genet Dev,* Vol. 17, No. 4, (Aug 2007), pp. (294-299), ISSN 0959-437X

Drew, Y. & Plummer, R. (2010) The emerging potential of poly(ADP-ribose) polymerase inhibitors in the treatment of breast cancer. *Curr Opin Obstet Gynecol,* Vol. 22, No. 1, (Feb 2010), pp. (67-71), ISSN 1040-872X

Duronio, V. (2008) The life of a cell: apoptosis regulation by the PI3K/PKB pathway. *Biochem J,* Vol. 415, No. 3, (Nov 2008), pp. (333-344), ISSN 0264-6021

Eccles, S.A. (2001) The role of c-erbB-2/HER2/neu in breast cancer progression and metastasis. *J Mammary Gland Biol Neoplasia,* Vol. 6, No. 4, (Oct 2001), pp. (393-406), ISSN 1083-3021

Edinger, A.L. & Thompson, C.B. (2004) Death by design: apoptosis, necrosis and autophagy. *Curr Opin Cell Biol,* Vol. 16, No. 6, (Dec 2004), pp. (663-669), ISSN 0955-0674

Eramo, A., Pallini, R., Lotti, F., Sette, G., Patti, M., Bartucci, M., Ricci-Vitiani, L., Signore, M., Stassi, G., Larocca, L.M., Crinò, L., Peschle, C. & De Maria, R. (2005) Inhibition of DNA methylation sensitizes glioblastoma for tumor necrosis factor-related apoptosis-inducing ligand-mediated destruction. *Cancer Res,* Vol. 65, No. 24, (Dec 2005), pp. (11469-11477), ISSN 0008-5472

Evan, G.I. & Vousden, K.H. (2001) Proliferation, cell cycle and apoptosis in cancer. *Nature,* Vol. 411, No. 6835, (May 2001), pp. (342-348), ISSN 0028-0836

Freudenberg, J.A., Wang, Q., Katsumata, M., Drebin, J., Nagatomo, I. & Greene, M.I. (2009) The role of HER2 in early breast cancer metastasis and the origins of resistance to HER2-targeted therapies. *Exp Mol Pathol,* Vol. 87, No. 1, (Aug 2009), pp. (1-11), ISSN 0014-4800

Fulda, S. & Debatin, K.M. (2006) Extrinsic versus intrinsic apoptosis pathways in anticancer chemotherapy. *Oncogene,* Vol. 25, No. 34, (Aug 2006), pp. (4798-4811), ISSN 0950-9232

Ganai, S., Arenas, R.B. & Forbes, N.S. (2009) Tumour-targeted delivery of TRAIL using Salmonella typhimurium enhances breast cancer survival in mice. *Br J Cancer,* Vol. 101, No. 10, (Nov 2009), pp. (1683-1691), ISSN 0007-0920

Geyer, F.C., Lopez-Garcia, M.A., Lambros, M.B. & Reis-Filho, J.S. (2009) Genetic characterization of breast cancer and implications for clinical management. *J Cell Mol Med,* Vol. 13, No. 10, (Oct 2009), pp. (4090-4103), ISSN 1582-1838

Ghavami, S., Hashemi, M., Ande, S.R., Yeganeh, B., Xiao, W., Eshraghi, M., Bus, C.J., Kadkhoda, K., Wiechec, E., Halayko, A.J. & Los, M. (2009) Apoptosis and cancer: mutations within caspase genes. *J Med Genet,* Vol. 46, No. 8, (Aug 2009), pp. (497-510), ISSN 0022-2593

Ghazoui, Z., Buffa, F.M., Dunbier, A.K., Anderson, H., Dexter, T., Detre, S., Salter, J., Smith, I.E., Harris, A.L. & Dowsett, M. (2011) Close and stable relationship between proliferation and a hypoxia metagene in aromatase inhibitor treated ER-positive breast cancer. *Clin Cancer Res,* 2011 Feb 15. [Epub ahead of print], ISSN 1078-0432

Gompel, A., Somaï, S., Chaouat, M., Kazem, A., Kloosterboer, H.J., Beusman, I., Forgez, P., Mimoun, M. & Rostène, W. (2000) Hormonal regulation of apoptosis in breast cells and tissues. *Steroids,* Vol. 65, No. 10-11, (Oct-Nov, 2000), pp. (593-598), ISSN 0039-128X

Gonzalvez, F. & Ashkenazi, A. (2010) New insights into apoptosis signaling by Apo2L/TRAIL. *Oncogene,* Vol. 29, No. 34, (Aug 2010), pp. (4752-4765), ISSN 0950-9232

Hayashi, S.I., Eguchi, H., Tanimoto, K., Yoshida, T., Omoto, Y., Inoue, A., Yoshida, N. & Yamaguchi, Y. (2003) The expression and function of estrogen receptor alpha and beta in human breast cancer and its clinical application. *Endocr Relat Cancer,* Vol. 10, No. 2, (Jun 2003), pp. (193-202), ISSN 1351-0088

He, B., Lu, N. & Zhou, Z. (2009) Cellular and nuclear degradation during apoptosis. *Curr Opin Cell Biol,* Vol. 21, No. 6, (Dec, 2009), pp. (900-912), ISSN 0955-0674

Hengartner, M.O. (2000) The biochemistry of apoptosis. *Nature,* Vol. 407, No. 6805, (Oct 2000), pp. (770-776), ISSN 0028-0836

Hine, C.M., Seluanov, A. & Gorbunova, V. (2008) Use of the Rad51 promoter for targeted anti-cancer therapy. *Proc Natl Acad Sci U S A,* Vol. 105, No. 52, (Dec 2008), pp. (20810-20815), ISSN 0027-8424

Houston, A. & O'Connell, J. (2004) The Fas signalling pathway and its role in the pathogenesis of cancer. *Curr Opin Pharmacol,* Vol. 4, No. 4, (Aug 2004), pp. (321-326), ISSN 1471-4892

Hyer, M.L., Samuel, T. & Reed, J.C. (2006) The FLIP-side of Fas signaling. *Clin Cancer Res,* Vol. 12, No. 20 Pt 1, (Oct 2006), pp. (5929-5931), ISSN 1078-0432

Inoue, S., Browne, G., Melino, G. & Cohen, G.M. （2009） Ordering of caspases in cells undergoing apoptosis by the intrinsic pathway. *Cell Death Differ,* Vol. 16, No. 7, (Jul 2009), pp. (1053-1061), ISSN 1350-9047

Jia, L.T., Zhang, L.H., Yu, C.J., Zhao, J., Xu, Y.M., Gui, J.H., Jin, M., Ji, Z.L., Wen, W.H., Wang, C.J., Chen, S.Y. & Yang, A.G. (2003) Specific tumoricidal activity of a secreted pro-apoptotic protein consisting of HER2 antibody and constitutively active caspase-3. *Cancer Res,* Vol. 63, No.12, (Jun 2003), pp. (3257-3262), ISSN 0008-5472

Johnstone, R.W., Ruefli, A.A. & Lowe, S.W. (2002) Apoptosis: a link between cancer genetics and chemotherapy. *Cell,* Vol. 108, No. 2, (Jan 2002), pp. (153-164), ISSN 0092-8674

Jordan, V.C. & O'Malley, B.W. (2007) Selective estrogen-receptor modulators and antihormonal resistance in breast cancer. *J Clin Oncol,* Vol. 25, No. 36, (Dec 2007), pp. (5815-5824), ISSN 0732-183X

Jovanovic, J., Rønneberg, J.A., Tost, J. & Kristensen, V. (2010) The epigenetics of breast cancer. *Mol Oncol,* Vol. 4, No. 3, (Jun 2010), pp. (242-254), ISSN 1574-7891

Kazhdan, I., Long, L., Montellano, R., Cavazos, D.A. & Marciniak, R.A. (2006) Targeted gene therapy for breast cancer with truncated Bid. *Cancer Gene Ther,* Vol. 13, No. 2, (Feb 2006), pp. (141-149), ISSN 0929-1903

Lavrik, I., Golks, A. & Krammer, P.H. (2005) Death receptor signaling. *J Cell Sci,* Vol. 118, No. Pt 2, (Jan 2005), pp. (265-267), ISSN 0021-9533

Lee M. (2009) Hypoxia targeting gene expression for breast cancer gene therapy. *Adv Drug Deliv Rev,* Vol. 61, No. 10, (Aug 2009), pp. (842-849), ISSN 0169-409X

Lessene, G., Czabotar, P.E. & Colman, P.M. (2008) BCL-2 family antagonists for cancer therapy. *Nat Rev Drug Discov,* Vol. 7, No. 12, (Dec 2008), pp. (989-1000), ISSN 1474-1776

Li, M., Qin, X., Xue, X., Zhang, C., Yan, Z., Han, W., Komarck, C., Wang, T.D. & Zhang, Y. (2010) Safety evaluation and pharmacokinetics of a novel human tumor necrosis factor-alpha exhibited a higher antitumor activity and a lower systemic toxicity. *Anticancer Drugs,* Vol. 21, No. 3, (Mar 2010), pp. (243-251), ISSN 0959-4973

Li, Q.X., Zhao, J., Liu, J.Y., Jia, L.T., Huang, H.Y., Xu, Y.M., Zhang, Y., Zhang, R., Wang, C.J., Yao, L.B., Chen, S.Y. & Yang, A.G. (2006) Survivin stable knockdown by siRNA inhibits tumor cell growth and angiogenesis in breast and cervical cancers. *Cancer Biol Ther,* Vol. 5, No. 7, (Jul 2006), pp. (860-866), ISSN 1538-4047

Li, X., Shen, L., Zhang, J., Su, J., Shen, L., Liu, X., Han, H., Han, W. & Yao, L. (2007) Degradation of HER2 by Cbl-based chimeric ubiquitin ligases. *Cancer Res,* Vol. 67, No. 18, (Sep 2007), pp. (8716-8724), ISSN 0008-5472

Li, Y.M., Pan, Y., Wei, Y., Cheng, X., Zhou, B.P., Tan, M., Zhou, X., Xia, W., Hortobagyi, G.N., Yu, D. & Hung, M.C. (2004) Upregulation of CXCR4 is essential for HER2-mediated tumor metastasis. *Cancer Cell,* Vol. 6, No. 5, (Nov 2004), pp. (459-469), ISSN 1535-6108

Liston, P., Fong, W.G. & Korneluk, R.G. (2003) The inhibitors of apoptosis: there is more to life than Bcl2. *Oncogene,* Vol. 22, No. 53, (Nov 2003), pp. (8568-8580), ISSN 0950-9232

Liu, Z. & Chen, S. (2010) ER regulates an evolutionarily conserved apoptosis pathway. *Biochem Biophys Res Commun,* Vol. 400, No. 1, (Sep 2010), pp. (34-38), ISSN 0006-291X

Ludwig, D.L., Pereira, D.S., Zhu, Z., Hicklin, D.J. & Bohlen, P. (2003) Monoclonal antibody therapeutics and apoptosis. *Oncogene,* Vol. 22, No. 56, (Dec 2003), pp. (9097-106), ISSN 0950-9232

Manfredi, J.J. (2010) The Mdm2-p53 relationship evolves: Mdm2 swings both ways as an oncogene and a tumor suppressor. *Genes Dev,* Vol. 24, No. 15, (Aug 2010), pp. (1580-1589), ISSN 0890-9369

Mann, A.P., Somasunderam, A., Nieves-Alicea, R., Li, X., Hu, A., Sood, A.K., Ferrari, M., Gorenstein, D.G. & Tanaka, T. (2010) Identification of thioaptamer ligand against E-selectin: potential application for inflamed vasculature targeting. *PLoS One,* Vol. 5, No. 9, (Sep 2010), pp. (e13050). ISSN 1932-6203

Martin, S.S., Ridgeway, A.G., Pinkas, J., Lu, Y., Reginato, M.J., Koh, E.Y., Michelman, M., Daley, G.Q., Brugge, J.S. & Leder, P. (2004) A cytoskeleton-based functional genetic screen identifies Bcl-xL as an enhancer of metastasis, but not primary tumor growth. *Oncogene,* Vol. 23, No. 26, (Jun 2004), pp. (4641-4645), ISSN 0950-9232

McCready, J., Arendt, L.M., Rudnick, J.A. & Kuperwasser, C. (2010) The contribution of dynamic stromal remodeling during mammary development to breast carcinogenesis. *Breast Cancer Res,* Vol. 12, No. 3, (Jun 2010), pp. (205-213), ISSN 1465-5411

Meany, H.J., Seibel, N.L., Sun, J., Finklestein, J.Z., Sato, J., Kelleher, J., Sondel, P. & Reaman, G. (2008) Phase 2 trial of recombinant tumor necrosis factor-alpha in combination with dactinomycin in children with recurrent Wilms tumor. *J Immunother,* Vol. 31, No. 7, (Sep 2008), pp. (679-683), ISSN 1524-9557

Moasser, M.M. (2007) The oncogene HER2: its signaling and transforming functions and its role in human cancer pathogenesis. *Oncogene,* Vol. 26, No. 45, (Oct 2007), pp. (6469-6487), ISSN 0950-9232

Modjtahedi, N., Giordanetto, F., Madeo, F. & Kroemer, G. (2006) Apoptosis-inducing factor: vital and lethal. *Trends Cell Biol,* Vol. 16, No. 5, (May 2006), pp. (264-272), ISSN 0962-8924

Mottolese, M., Buglioni, S., Bracalenti, C., Cardarelli, M.A., Ciabocco, L., Giannarelli, D., Botti, C., Natali, P.G., Concetti, A. & Venanzi, F.M. (2000) Prognostic relevance of altered Fas (CD95)-system in human breast cancer. *Int J Cancer,* Vol. 89, No. 2, (Mar, 2000), pp. (127-132), ISSN 0020-7136

Motyl, T., Gajkowska, B., Zarzyńska, J., Gajewska, M. & Lamparska-Przybysz, M. (2006) Apoptosis and autophagy in mammary gland remodeling and breast cancer chemotherapy. *J Physiol Pharmacol,* Vol. 57, No. Suppl 7, (Nov 2006), pp. (17-32), ISSN 0867-5910

Moulder, S.L., Symmans, W.F., Booser, D.J., Madden, T.L., Lipsanen, C., Yuan, L., Brewster, A.M., Cristofanilli, M., Hunt, K.K., Buchholz, T.A., Zwiebel, J., Valero, V., Hortobagyi, G.N. & Esteva, F.J. (2008) Phase I/II study of G3139 (Bcl-2 antisense oligonucleotide) in combination with doxorubicin and docetaxel in breast cancer. *Clin Cancer Res,* Vol. 14, No. 23, (Dec 2008), pp. (7909-7916), ISSN 1078-0432

Muschel, R.J., Soto, D.E., McKenna, W.G. & Bernhard, E.J. (1998) Radiosensitization and apoptosis. *Oncogene,* Vol. 17, No. 25, (Dec, 1998), pp. (3359-3363), ISSN 0950-9232

Müschen, M., Moers, C., Warskulat, U., Even, J., Niederacher, D. & Beckmann, M.W. (2000) CD95 ligand expression as a mechanism of immune escape in breast cancer. *Immunology,* Vol. 99, No. 1, (Jan 2000), pp.(69-77), ISSN 0019-2805

Muzio, M., Stockwell, B.R., Stennicke, H.R., Salvesen, G.S. & Dixit, V.M. (1998) An induced proximity model for caspase-8 activation. *J Biol Chem,* Vol. 273, No. 5, (Jan 1998), pp. (2926-2930), ISSN 0021-9258

Normanno, N., Morabito, A., De Luca, A., Piccirillo, M.C., Gallo, M., Maiello, M.R. & Perrone, F. (2009) Target-based therapies in breast cancer: current status and future perspectives. *Endocr Relat Cancer,* Vol. 16, No. 3, (Sep. 2009), pp. (675-702), ISSN 1351-0088

Oakman, C., Viale, G. & Di Leo, A. (2010) Management of triple negative breast cancer. *Breast,* Vol. 19, No. 5, (Oct 2010), pp. (312-321), ISSN 0960-9776

Paik, S., Kim, C. & Wolmark, N. (2008) HER2 status and benefit from adjuvant trastuzumab in breast cancer. *N Engl J Med,* Vol. 358, No. 13, (Mar 2008), pp. (1409-1411), ISSN 0028-4793

Park, J.W., Neve, R.M., Szollosi, J. & Benz C.C. (2008) Unraveling the Biologic and Clinical Complexities of HER2. *Clin Breast Cancer,* Vol. 8, No. 5, (Oct 2008), pp. (392-401), ISSN 1526-8209

Pastan, I., Hassan, R., Fitzgerald, D.J. & Kreitman, R.J. (2006) Immunotoxin therapy of cancer. *Nat Rev Cancer,* Vol. 6, No. 7, (Jul 2006), pp. (559-565), ISSN 1474-175X

Prokopcova, J., Kleibl, Z., Banwell, C.M. & Pohlreich, P. (2007) The role of ATM in breast cancer development. *Breast Cancer Res Treat,* Vol. 104, No. 2, (Aug 2007), pp. (121-128), ISSN 0167-6806

Qiu, X.C., Xu, Y.M., Wang, F., Fan, Q.Y., Wang, L.F., Ma, B.A., Jia, L.T., Zhao, J., Meng, Y.L., Yao, L.B., Chen, S.Y. & Yang, A.G. (2008) Single-chain antibody/activated BID chimeric protein effectively suppresses HER2-positive tumor growth. *Mol Cancer Ther,* Vol. 7. No. 7, (Jul 2008), pp. (1890-1899), ISSN 1535-7163

Rakha, E.A., Reis-Filho, J.S. & Ellis, I.O. (2010) Combinatorial biomarker expression in breast cancer. *Breast Cancer Res Treat,* Vol. 120, No. 2, (Apr 2010), pp. (293-308), ISSN 0167-6806

Rana, A., Rangasamy, V. & Mishra, R. (2010) How estrogen fuels breast cancer. *Future Oncol,* Vol. 6, No. 9, (Sep 2010), pp. (1369-1371), ISSN 1479-6694

Rasheva, V.I. & Domingos, P.M. (2009) Cellular responses to endoplasmic reticulum stress and apoptosis. *Apoptosis,* Vol. 14, No. 8, (Aug 2009), pp. (996-1007), ISSN 1360-8185

Riedl, S.J. & Shi, Y. (2004) Molecular mechanisms of caspase regulation during apoptosis. *Nat Rev Mol Cell Biol,* Vol. 5, No. 11, (Nov 2004), pp. (897-907), ISSN 1471-0072

Robles, A.I. & Harris, C.C. (2001) p53-mediated apoptosis and genomic instability diseases. *Acta Oncol,* Vol. 40, No. 6, pp. (696-701), ISSN 0284-186X

Rogers, K.M., Thomas, M., Galligan, L., Wilson, T.R., Allen, W.L., Sakai, H., Johnston, P.G. & Longley, D.B. (2007) Cellular FLICE-inhibitory protein regulates chemotherapy-induced apoptosis in breast cancer cells. *Mol Cancer Ther,* Vol. 6, No. 5, (May 2007), pp. (1544-1551), ISSN 1535-7163

Russo, J. & Russo, I.H. (2006) The role of estrogen in the initiation of breast cancer. *J Steroid Biochem Mol Biol,* Vol. 102. No. 1-5, (Dec 2006), pp. (89-96), ISSN 0960-0760

Ruvolo, P.P., Deng, X. & May, W.S. (2001) Phosphorylation of Bcl2 and regulation of apoptosis. *Leukemia,* Vol. 15, No. 4, (Apr 2001), pp. (515-522), ISSN 0887-6924

Sánchez-Muñoz, A., Pérez-Ruiz, E., Jiménez, B., Ribelles, N., Márquez, A., García-Ríos, I. & Alba Conejo, E. (2009) Targeted therapy of metastatic breast cancer. *Clin Transl Oncol,* Vol. 11, No. 10, (Oct 2009), pp. (643-650), ISSN 1699-048X

Sarkar, D., Su, Z.Z., Vozhilla, N., Park, E.S., Gupta, P. & Fisher, P.B. (2005) Dual cancer-specific targeting strategy cures primary and distant breast carcinomas in nude mice. *Proc Natl Acad Sci U S A,* Vol. 102, No. 39, (Sep 2005), pp. (14034-14039), ISSN 0027-8424

Schlotter, C.M., Vogt, U., Allgayer, H. & Brandt, B. (2008) Molecular targeted therapies for breast cancer treatment. *Breast Cancer Res,* Vol. 10, No. 4, (Jul 2008), pp. (211-222), ISSN 1465-5411

Scorrano, L. & Korsmeyer, S.J. (2003) Mechanisms of cytochrome c release by pro-apoptotic BCL-2 family members. *Biochem Biophys Res Commun,* Vol. 304, No. 3, (May 2003), pp. (437-444), ISSN 0006-291X

Senter, P.D. (2009) Potent antibody drug conjugates for cancer therapy. *Curr Opin Chem Biol,* Vol. 13, No. 3, (Jun 2009), pp. (235-244). ISSN 1367-5931

Shen, H.M. & Pervaiz, S. (2006) TNF receptor superfamily-induced cell death: redox-dependent execution. *FASEB J*, Vol. 20, No. 10, (Aug 2006), pp. (1589-1598), ISSN 0892-6638

Shi Y. (2004) Caspase activation: revisiting the induced proximity model. *Cell*, Vol. 117, No. 7, (Jun 2004), pp. (855-858), ISSN 0092-8674

Sivaprasad, U., Shankar, E. & Basu, A. (2007) Downregulation of Bid is associated with PKCepsilon-mediated TRAIL resistance. *Cell Death Differ*, Vol. 14, No. 4, (Apr 2007), pp. (851-860), ISSN 1350-9047

Sjöström-Mattson, J., Von Boguslawski, K., Bengtsson, N.O., Mjaaland, I., Salmenkivi, K. & Blomqvist, C. (2009) The expression of p53, bcl-2, bax, fas and fasL in the primary tumour and lymph node metastases of breast cancer. *Acta Oncol*, Vol. 48, No. 8, pp. (1137-1143), ISSN 0284-186X

Srinivasula, S.M., Ahmad, M., MacFarlane, M., Luo, Z., Huang, Z., Fernandes-Alnemri, T. & Alnemri, E.S. (1998a) Generation of constitutively active recombinant caspases-3 and -6 by rearrangement of their subunits. *J Biol Chem*, Vol. 273, No. 17, (Apr 1998), pp. (10107-10111), ISSN 0021-9258

Srinivasula, S.M., Ahmad, M., Fernandes-Alnemri, T. & Alnemri, E.S. (1998b) Autoactivation of procaspase-9 by Apaf-1-mediated oligomerization. *Mol Cell*, Vol. 1, No. 7, (Jun 1998), pp. (949-957), ISSN 1097-2765

Szegezdi, E., Logue, S.E., Gorman, A.M. & Samali, A. (2006) Mediators of endoplasmic reticulum stress-induced apoptosis. *EMBO Rep*, Vol. 7, No. 9, (Sep 2006), pp. (880-885), ISSN 1469-221X

Tamrazi, A., Carlson, K.E., Daniels, J.R., Hurth, K.M. & Katzenellenbogen, J.A. (2002) Estrogen receptor dimerization: ligand binding regulates dimer affinity and dimer dissociation rate. *Mol Endocrinol*, Vol. 16, No. 12, (Dec 2002), pp. (2706–2719), ISSN 0888-8809

Tan, T.T., Degenhardt, K., Nelson, D.A., Beaudoin, B., Nieves-Neira, W., Bouillet, P., Villunger, A., Adams, J.M. & White, E. (2005) Key roles of BIM-driven apoptosis in epithelial tumors and rational chemotherapy. *Cancer Cell*, Vol. 7, No. 3, (Mar 2005), pp. (227-238), ISSN 1535-6108

Tandon, M., Vemula, S.V. & Mittal, S.K. (2011) Emerging strategies for EphA2 receptor targeting for cancer therapeutics. *Expert Opin Ther Targets*, Vol. 15, No. 1. (Jan 2011), pp. (31-51), ISSN 1472-8222

Teixeira, M.R., Pandis, N. & Heim, S. (2002) Cytogenetic clues to breast carcinogenesis. *Genes Chromosomes Cancer*, Vol. 33, No.1, (Jan 2002), pp. (1-16), ISSN 1045-2257

Thimmaiah, K.N., Easton, J.B. & Houghton, P.J. (2010) Protection from rapamycin-induced apoptosis by insulin-like growth factor-I is partially dependent on protein kinase C signaling. *Cancer Res*, Vol. 70, No. 5, (Mar 2010), pp. (2000-2009), ISSN 0008-5472

Thornberry, N.A. & Lazebnik, Y. (1998) Caspases: enemies within. *Science*, Vol. 281, No.5381, (Aug 1998), pp. (1312-1316), ISSN 0036-8075

Timmer, J.C. & Salvesen, G.S. (2007) Caspase substrates. *Cell Death Differ*, Vol. 14, No. 1, (Jan 2007), pp. (66-72), ISSN 1350-9047

Venkitaraman, A.R. (2009) Linking the Cellular Functions of BRCA Genes to Cancer Pathogenesis and Treatment. *Annu Rev Pathol Mech Dis,* Vol. 4, (Oct 2008), pp. (461-487), ISSN 1553-4006

Vinothini, G., Murugan, R.S. & Nagini, S. (2011) Mitochondria-mediated apoptosis in patients with adenocarcinoma of the breast: Correlation with histological grade and menopausal status. *Breast,* Vol. 20, No. 1, (Feb 2011), pp. (86-92), ISSN 0960-9776

Wajant, H. (2002) The Fas signaling pathway: more than a paradigm. *Science,* Vol. 296, No. 5573, (May 2002), pp. (1635-1636), ISSN 0036-8075

Wang, C. & Youle, R.J. (2009) The role of mitochondria in apoptosis. *Annu Rev Genet,* Vol. 43, pp. (95-118), ISSN 0066-4197

Wang, F., Ren, J., Qiu, X.C., Wang, L.F., Zhu, Q., Zhang, Y.Q., Huan, Y., Meng, Y.L., Yao, L.B., Chen, S.Y., Xu, Y.M. & Yang, A.G. (2010) Selective cytotoxicity to HER2-positive tumor cells by a recombinant e23sFv-TD-tBID protein containing a furin cleavage sequence. *Clin Cancer Res,* Vol. 16, No. 8, (Apr 2010), pp. (2284-2294), ISSN 1078-0432

Wang, T., Zhao, J., Ren, J.L., Zhang, L., Wen, W.H., Zhang, R., Qin, W.W., Jia, L.T., Yao, L.B., Zhang, Y.Q., Chen, S.Y. & Yang, A.G. (2007) Recombinant immunopro-apoptotic proteins with furin site can translocate and kill HER2-positive cancer cells. *Cancer Res,* Vol. 67, No. 24, (Dec 2007), pp. (11830-11839), ISSN 0008-5472

Waxman, D.J. & Schwartz, P.S. (2003) Harnessing apoptosis for improved anticancer gene therapy. *Cancer Res,* Vol. 63, No. 24, (Dec 2003), pp. (8563-8572), ISSN 0008-5472

Wen, W.H., Liu, J.Y., Qin, W.J., Zhao, J., Wang, T., Jia, L.T., Meng, Y.L., Gao, H., Xue, C.F., Jin, B.Q., Yao, L.B., Chen, S.Y. & Yang A.G. (2007) Targeted inhibition of HBV gene expression by single-chain antibody mediated small interfering RNA delivery. *Hepatology,* Vol. 46, No.1, (Jul 2007), pp. (84-94), ISSN 0270-9139

Whelan, K.A., Caldwell, S.A., Shahriari, K.S., Jackson, S.R., Franchetti, L.D., Johannes, G.J. & Reginato, M.J. (2010) Hypoxia suppression of Bim and Bmf blocks anoikis and luminal clearing during mammary morphogenesis. *Mol Biol Cell,* Vol. 21, No. 22, (Nov 2010), pp. (3829-3837), ISSN 1059-1524

Xu, Y.M., Wang, L.F., Jia, L.T., Qiu, X.C., Zhao, J., Yu, C.J., Zhang, R., Zhu, F., Wang, C.J., Jin, B.Q., Chen, S.Y. & Yang, A.G. (2004) A caspase-6 and anti-human epidermal growth factor receptor-2 (HER2) antibody chimeric molecule suppresses the growth of HER2-overexpressing tumors. *J Immunol,* Vol. 173, No.1, (Jul 2004), pp. (61-67), ISSN 0022-1767

Yamaguchi, Y. (2007) Microenvironmental regulation of estrogen signals in breast cancer. *Breast Cancer,* Vol. 14, No. 2, pp. (175-181), ISSN 1074-6900

Yip, K.W. & Reed, J.C. (2008) Bcl-2 family proteins and cancer. *Oncogene,* Vol. 27, No. 50, (Oct 2008), pp. (6398-6406), ISSN 0950-9232

Yu, C.J., Jia, L.T., Meng, Y.L., Zhao, J., Zhang, Y., Qiu, X.C., Xu, Y.M., Wen, W.H., Yao, L.B., Fan, D.M., Jin, B.Q., Chen, S.Y. & Yang, A.G. (2006) Selective pro-apoptotic activity of a secreted recombinant antibody/AIF fusion protein in carcinomas overexpressing HER2. *Gene Ther,* Vol. 13, No. 4, (Feb 2006), pp. (313-320), ISSN 0969-7128

Zhao, J., Zhang, L.H., Jia, L.T., Zhang, L., Xu, Y.M., Wang, Z., Yu, C.J., Peng, W.D., Wen, W.H., Wang, C.J., Chen, S.Y. & Yang, A.G. (2004) Secreted antibody/granzyme B fusion protein stimulates selective killing of HER2-overexpressing tumor cells. *J Biol Chem,* Vol. 279, No. 20, (May 2004), pp. (21343-21348), ISSN 0021-9258

Zhao, Z.N., Zhou, Q., Bai, J.X., Yan, B., Qin, W.W., Wang, T., Li, Y., Yang, A.G. & Jia, L.T. (2011) Estrogen-induced dimerization and activation of ERα-fused caspase-8: Artificial reversal of the estrogenic hormone effect in carcinogenesis. *Cancer Biol Ther,* Vol. 11, No. 9, (May 2011), pp. (816-825), ISSN 1538-4047

3

Induction of Apoptosis in Human Cancer Cells by Human Eb- or Rainbow Trout Ea4-Peptide of Pro-Insulin-Like Growth Factor-I (Pro-IGF-I)

Maria J. Chen, Chun-Mean Lin and Thomas T. Chen
Department of Molecular and Cell Biology, University of Connecticut, Storrs, CT, USA

1. Introduction

Insulin-like growth factors (IGFs)-I and -II are members of the insulin family that play essential roles in regulating growth, development and metabolism in all vertebrates (de Pablo et al., 1990, 1993; Stewart and Rotwein, 1996). Like many peptide hormones, IGFs are initially produced as pre-pro-hormones containing an amino-terminal signal peptide, followed by the mature peptide of B, C, A, and D domains, and a carboxyl terminal E-domain. Via post-translational processing, the signal peptide and the E-peptide are proteolytically cleaved off from the pre-pro-peptide, and both the mature IGFs and E-peptides are secreted into the circulation (Rotwein et al., 1986; Duguay 1999). From molecular characterization of IGF-I gene and its transcription products, multiple isoforms of IGF-I mRNA were identified from fish to mammals. In human, three different species of IGF-I mRNAs which encode three isoforms of pro-IGF-I (i.e., pro-IGF-Ia, -Ib and Ic) were identified (Rotwein et al., 1986; Duguay 19995). These three isoforms of pro-IGF-I contain an identical mature IGF-I with 70 amino acid residues (aa) and different E-peptides with 30 aa (Ea), 77 aa (Eb) and 40 aa (Ec), respectively. The a-type E-domains are highly conserved among vertebrates but the b-type E-peptides are conserved in the first 15 amino acids and different thereafter among human, rats and mice (variable region).

In fish, multiple isoforms of IGF-I transcripts have also been identified. These different isoforms of IGF-I transcripts encode an identical mature IGF-I but different E-peptides. Shamblott and Chen (1992, 1993) reported the presence of four different IGF-I transcripts encoding four different isoforms of pro-IGF-I for rainbow trout (*Oncorhynchus mykiss*). Similar to the isoforms of human pro-IGF-I, the four different isoforms of the rainbow trout pro-IGF-I contain an identical mature IGF-I (70 aa) and four different lengths of E-peptides (i.e., rtEa1, 35 aa; rtEa2, 47 aa; rtEa3, 62 aa; rtEa4, 74 aa). The first 15 amino acid residues of these four E-peptides are identical among themselves and the a-type E-peptides of mammals, and the 20 amino acid residues at the C-termini share 70% identity with their human counterparts. The rtEa1-peptide is composed of the first 15 and the last 20 amino acid residues. Insertion of either 12 or 27 amino acid residues between the first and the last segments of rtEa1-peptide results in rtEa2- or rtEa3-peptide, whereas insertion of both segments into rtEa1-peptide gives rise to rtEa4-peptide. Similar to rainbow trout, four different forms of Ea-peptides of pro-IGF-I have also been identified in Chinook salmon,

Coho salmon (Duguay et al., 1992: Willis and Devlin, 1993), and red drum (Faulk et al., 2010). However, not all teloests possess four different E-peptides. While gilthead seabream possesses three different E-peptides (namely Ea1, Ea2 and Ea4), zebrafish and grouper each has only one Ea-peptide: Ea2-peptide in zebrafish and Ea4-peptide in grouper (Chen et al., 2001; Shi et al., 2002; Tiago et al., 2008).

Although the biological activity of the mature IGF-I has been extensively studied, the biological activity of E-peptides has been over-looked until recently. It was generally assumed that E-peptides of pro-IGF-I may be biologically inert; however the following lines of evidence suggest that E-peptides may possess biological activity. First, many peptide hormones are initially synthesized as complex pro-hormone molecules and following post-translational processing to generate multiple peptides with distinct or similar biological activities. Examples are pro-opiomelanocortin (Civelli et al., 1986), pro-glucaogon (Bell et al., 1983) and pro-insulin (Ido et al., 1997), just to name a few. In a similar manner, generation of E-peptides from pro-IGF-I may suggest a pluripotential role for these peptides. Second, the E-domains of pro-IGF-I are evolutionally conserved. Third, different isoforms of pro-IGF-I transcripts are expressed in a tissue-specific and developmental stage-specific manner, and exhibiting differential responses to growth hormone (Shamblott and Chen 1993; Duguay 1994; Yang and Goldspink 2002). Siegfried et al. (1992) reported the first evidence that hEb-peptide contained biological activity. In their studies, Siegfried and colleagues showed that a synthetic peptide amide with 23 amino acid residues (Y-23-R-NH_2) of the hEb-peptide (a.a. 103-124) at 2-20 nM exerted mitogenic activity in normal and malignant human bronchial epithelial cells. They further demonstrated that Y-23-R-NH_2 bound to specific high affinity receptors ($K_d = 2.8 \pm 1.4 \times 10^{-11}$M) present at 1-2 x 10^4 binding sites per cell and the ligand binding was not inhibited by recombinant insulin or IGF-I. Several investigators have reported recently that the Eb-peptide of rodent pro-IGF-I peptide (same sequence as hEc-peptide) possessed activity in promoting proliferation of rodent myoblasts, whereas Ea-peptide stimulated differentiation of mature myoblasts (Yang and Goldspink 2002; Matheny et al., 2010). Besides exerting mitogenic activity in rodent myoblasts by rodent Eb-peptide, murine Ea-peptide of pro-IGF-I also modulates the entry of mature IGF-I protein into C2C12, a murine skeletal muscle cell line (Pfeffer et al., 2009).

Evidence documenting the biological activity of E-peptides of rainbow trout pro-IGF-I came from studies conducted by Tian et al. (1999). Tian et al. reported that recombinant rtEa2-, rtEa3- and rtEa4-peptides but not Ea1-peptide exhibited a dose dependent mitogenic activity in NIH 3T3 cells and carprine mammary gland epithelial cells (CMEC). Recently, Mark Chen in Taiwan also demonstrated that Ea2-peptide of zebrafish exerted a stimulatory effect on incorporation of ^{35}S-sulfate into zebrafish gill bronchial cartilage in a sulfation assay (personal communication). These results are consistent with those reported in mammals (Siegfried et al., 1992; Matheny et al., 2010; Yang and Goldspink 2002). Further studies conducted in our laboratory showed that both recombinant rtEa4- or synthetic hEb-peptide exerted unexpected anti-cancer cell activities in established human cancer cell lines such as MDA-MB-231, HT-29, HepG2, SK-N-F1, SKOV-3A, PC-3 and OVCAR-3B (Chen et al., 2002, 2007; Kuo and Chen 2002). These activities include: (i) induction of morphological differentiation and inhibition of anchorage-independent growth, (ii) inhibition of invasion and metastasis, and (iii) inhibition of cancer-induced angiogenesis.

Programmed cell death, i.e., apoptosis, is a crucial process of eliminating unwanted cells in animal life, and it is vital for embryonic development, homeostasis and immune defense (Elmore 2007, for review). Apoptosis is characterized by typical morphological and biochemical hallmarks, such as cell shrinkage, nuclear DNA fragmentation and plasma membrane blebbing (Hengartner, 2000). Results of extensive studies revealed that two pathways, extrinsic pathway (death receptor triggered pathway) and intrinsic pathway (mitochondrial pathway) can lead to apoptosis (Hengartner, 2000; Fulda and Debatin, 2006). Furthermore, there is ample evidence indicating that these two pathways are linked, and molecules from one pathway can influence the other pathway. One striking feature of cancer cells is that they do not readily undergo apoptosis due to reduction of expression or mutation of pro-apoptotic genes such as caspase genes (Ghavani et al., 2009) while increasing expression of anti-apoptotic genes such as Bcl-2 family genes (Youle and Strasser, 2008). Certain anti-cancer drugs and agents which have been identified as potential effective cancer treatment can restore normal apoptotic pathways (Fulda and Debatin, 2006; Yang et al., 2008). Since rtEa4- and hEb-peptides have been shown to possess anti-cancer activities in vitro in a variety of human cancer cells (Kuo and Chen, 2002; Chen et al., 2007), it would be of great interest to determine if these peptides can also induce apoptosis in human cancer cells. In this paper, we report that rtEa4- and hEb-peptide of pro-IGF-I induces apoptosis in various human cancer cell lines via both extrinsic and intrinsic pathways.

2. Materials and methods

2.1 Cell culture

Single-cell subclones were isolated from the aggressive breast cancer cells (MDA-MB-231), ovarian cancer cells (OVCAR and SKOV), neuroblastoma cells (SK-N-SH and SK-N-F1) and non-cancerous foreskin cells (CCD-1112SK) [all purchased from ATCC, Mannassas, VA] were routinely maintained in F12/DMEM (Gibco-BRL, Rockville, MD) supplemented with 10% fetal bovine serum (FBS, Gibco-BRL) at 37°C under a humidified atmosphere of 5% CO_2. Each cell line was sub-cultured every 3 days.

2.2 Preparation of rtEa4- and hEb-peptides

Recombinant rtEa4-peptide, hEb-peptide and control protein were prepared following the method described by our laboratory (Tian et al., 1999; Kuo and Chen, 2002; Chen et al., 2007). Briefly, E. coli cells, transformed with an expressing vector pET-15b (Novagen, EMD Chemicals, Gibbstown, NJ) containing the coding sequence of rtEa4-peptide or hEb-peptide, were cultured in 5 ml of LB broth for 4 h, diluted to 500 ml LB broth and allow the culture to grow at 37 °C. The culture was induced with 1 mM isopropyl β-D-thiolactopyranoside (IPTG) at an OD_{600} of 0.6-0.8 for 2 h. Induced cells were harvested by low speed centrifugation and resuspended in 10 ml of a binding buffer (50 mM imidazole, 0.5 M NaCl, 20 mM Tris-HCl, pH 7.9). Following ultrasonication, the cell lysate was obtained by centrifugation at 39,000g for 20 min. The recombinant protein, containing His-tags, was isolated by affinity chromatography on His-bind resin (Novagen) and followed by extensive dialysis in 1X PBS buffer to remove immidazole. The purity of the recovered recombinant protein was accessed to be about 80% by electrophoresis on SDS-polyaccrylamide gels. The control protein was prepared from E. coli cells harboring the backbone of the expression vector without E-peptide insert following the same method as described above.

2.3 Microscopic observation of apoptotic cells induced by recombinant rtEa4-peptide

Cancer cells (MDA-MB-231C and SKOV-3A) in serum free medium were treated with various concentrations (1.4 μM or 2.8 μM) of recombinant rtEa4-peptide or control protein for 2 h, and were observed under an inverted phase contrast microscope (Olympus IX50) to determine apoptotic cells. SKOV-3A cells, after treated with 1.5 μM or control protein for 3 days, were stained with H33258 and observed under an inverted phase contrast microscope (Olympus IX50).

MDA-MB-231C cells in serum free medium were treated with rtEa4-peptide (3.0 μM) or same concentration of control protein for 48 h. One sample was treated with H_2O_2 for 16 h to induce apoptosis to serve as a positive control. TUNEL assay was carried out following the protocol supplied by the manufacturer (Roche Diagnostics Corp., Indianapolis, IN). MDA-MB-231C cells treated with rtEa4-peptide or control protein were stained with Rodamine Red labeled mono-specific polyclonal rabbit anti-activated capase 3 immunoglobulin (Biocompare, South San Francisco, CA) following conditions provided by the manufacturer. All images were observed under an inverted microscope (Olympus IX50) equipped with epifluorescence attachment.

2.4 Quantitative relative real-time RT-PCR analysis

Cancer cells (MDA-MB-231C, SKOV-3A, OVCAR-3B, SK-N-SH, and SK-N-F1) and non-immortalized foreskin cells (CCD-1112SK) were treated with recombinant rtEa4-peptide (2.0 μM), hEb-peptide (0.5 μM) or control protein for 6 h and RNA samples were prepared from these cells using Trizol reagent following the manufacturer's protocol (Invitrogen, Carlsbad, CA). Each RNA sample was treated with RNase-free DNase to remove any DNA contamination during isolation. To confirm that the RNA samples were free of DNA contamination, RNA samples were used as templates for direct amplification of β-actin sequence without prior reverse transcription. One micrograsm of total RNA was reverse transcribed in a 20 μl reaction volume, containing 100 ng of oligo$(dT)_{18}$, 10 nM dNTP, 200mM DTT, 1 x reverse transcription buffer, and 1 μl SuperScrip^R III reverse transcriptase (Invitrogen) for 90 min at 42 ^oC, and the reverse transcription product was diluted to 100 μl with buffer. The PCR reaction was carried out in a 96-well plate with a final volume of 20 μl per well. The reaction mixture consists 1 X Sso fast EvaGreen Supermix (BioRad) containing Sso7d-fusion polymerase (BioRad), 500 nM of each forward and reverse primers (Table 1), and 4 μl of cDNA products. The amplification profile is as the following: 1 cycle of 95 ^oC for 2 min, 40 cycles of 95 ^oC for 2 sec and 60 ^oC for 10 sec annealing and synthesis (conditions provided by BioRad). The cycle threshold, CT, was determined from the fluorescence value which was 10 times the mean standard deviation of fluorescence of the base line cycles, and the efficiency of amplification in all of the genes determined is 95-98%. The relative expression was determined using the arithmetic formula:

$2^{-[(S\Delta CT - C\Delta CT)]}$, where SΔCT is the difference in CT values between the gene of interest in cells treated with rtEa4- or hEb-peptide and the house keeping gene (hGAPDH) in the sample, and CΔCT is the difference in CT values between the gene of interest in cells treated with control protein and the housekeeping gene (hGAPDH) of the control sample. Each experiment was repeated three times (n=3).

3. Results and discussion

Earlier studies conducted in our laboratory showed that recombinant rtEa4- or synthetic hEb-peptide of pro-IGF-I inhibited anchorage-independent growth and invasion of established human breast cancer cells (MDA-MB-231C), colon cancer cells (HT-29), ovarian cancer cells

(OVCAR-3A and SKOV-3B), neuroblastoma cells (SK-N-F1), human hepatoma cells (HepG-2) and rainbow trout hepatoma cells (RTH) in vitro (Chen et al., 2002; Kuo and Chen 2002). Chen et al. (2007) also showed that seeding of aggressive human breast cancer cells (MDA-MB-231C) onto the chorioallantoic membrane (CAM) of five-day old chicken embryos resulted in rapid growth of MDA-MB-231C cells into cancer nodules, invasion of the cancer cells and induction of the blood vessel formation in and around the cancer mass. The growth, invasion and angiogenesis by MDA-MB-231C cells on the chicken CAM was inhibited by treatment with a single or multiple doses rtEa4 or hEb-peptide. By microarray and quantitative relative real-time RT-PCR analyses, Chen et al. (2007) have further shown that a group of genes related to cancer cell activities were up- or down-regulated in MDA-MB-231C cells transfected with a cDNA encoding rtEa4-peptide. Together, these results suggest that rtEa4-or hEb-peptide may be developed as therapeutics for treating human cancers.

Gene	Sequence	Amplification Size (bp)
hGAPDH	(Fd): 5'GAAGGTGAAGGTCGGAGT-3' (Re): 5'-GAAGATGGTGATGGGATTTC-3'	207
hBcl-XL	(Fd): 5'-GCCACTTACCTGAATGACCACC-3' (Re): 5'-GGGAGGGTAGAGTGGATGGTCAG-3'	222
hCaspase-8	(Fd): 5'-GGTCTCACTCTGTTGCCCA-3' (Re): 5'-CAGGCGGATCACTTGAGGTC-3'	223
hCaspase-9	(Fd): 5'-GGGACAGATGAATGCCGTGGA-3' (Re): 5'-GGCACCACTCAGGAAGACGC-3'	229
hFADD	(Fd): 5'-CAGAGCGTGTGCGGGAGTC-3' (Re): 5'-GCTTCGGAGGTAGATGCGTC-3'	208
hMCL-1	(Fd): 5'-AGGAGGAGGGAGTGGTGGG-3' (Re): 5'-GTCCTAACCCTTCCTGGCACA-3'	279
hTRAIL-R1	(Fd): 5'-GCTGTTGGTGGCTGTGCTGA-3' (Re): 5'-CAGAGACGAAAGTGGACAGCGA-3'	179
hCytochromeC	(Fd): 5'-GGCAGGCAGATCACTTGAGG-3' (Re): 5-TCACTCGTCACCCAGGCTTG-3'	220
hBcl-2A	(Fd): 5'-TCCGACCACTAATTGCCAAGC-3' (Re): 5'-TCTCCCCAGCCTCCAGCAGC-3'	176
hCaspase-3	(Fd): 5'-GCAATAAATGAATGGGCTGAG-3' (Re): 5'-GCGTATGGAGAAATGGGCTG-3'	139
P53	(Fd): 5'-CCCAGCCAAAGAAGAAACCA-3' (Re): 5'-CTCGGAACATCTCGAAGCG-3'	81
hPTEN	(Fd): 5'-CAAGATGATGTTTGAAACTATTCCAATG-3' (Re): 5-CCTTTAGCTGGCAGACCACAA-3'	77

Table 1. Gene specific primers used in comparative real-time RT-PCR analysis

Cancer cells do not undergo apoptosis because they bypass apoptosis through a series of complex mechanisms involving dynamic interplays between cancer causing genes, oncogens, and/or mutated suppressor genes (Fulda and Debatin, 2004; Lowe and Lin, 2000). Apoptosis dysregulation in many cancers is one of the major hindrances towards the destruction of cancers in cancer therapy. Therefore, drugs and agents which can restore the normal apoptosis signaling pathways are considered as effective therapeutic agents for treating cancers (Evan and Vousden, 2001; Finkel 1999; Max 2002). Since rtEa4- or hEb-peptide suppresses anchorage-independent growth, invasion and angiogenesis of many different cancer cells in vitro (Chen et al., 2002, 2007; Chen and Kuo, 2002), it would be of great interest to know whether the protein can induce apoptosis in cancer cells. Treatment of ovarian cancer cells (SKOV-3A) or breast cancer cells (MDA-MB-231C) cells with recombinant rtEa4-peptide (1.4 and 2.8 μM) for 2 h, many cells exhibited distinct morphology of membrane blebbing, cell shrinkage, and chromatin condensation and disintegration (Fig 1). These morphological characteristics are consistent with those reported for apoptosis (Hacker 2000, for review). While these morphological changes in the rtEa4-peptide treated cells were further enhanced with time, no such morphological changes were observed in untreated cells or cells treated with control protein even after 48 h of culture. To confirm that rtEa4-peptide treated cancer cells exhibited apoptosis, MDA-MB-231C cells were treated with 3.0 μM of recombinant rtEa4-peptide for 48 h, and the treated cells were subjected to TUNEL assay or immuno-cytochemical staining with a mono-specific antibody against activated caspase 3. As shown in Figure 2, after incubation for 48 h in a serum free medium containing 3.0 μM of recombinant rtEa4-peptide, most of the cells showed positive in TUNEL assay (Fig 2A) as well as in immuno-cytochemical staining for activated caspase 3 (Fig 2B). Furthermore, apoptosis was also observed in ovarian cancer cells, SKOV 3A, treated with 1.5 μM of recombinant rtEa4-peptide (Fig 3). These results confirmed that rtEa4-peptide induced apoptosis in human breast cancer cells and ovarian cancer cells.

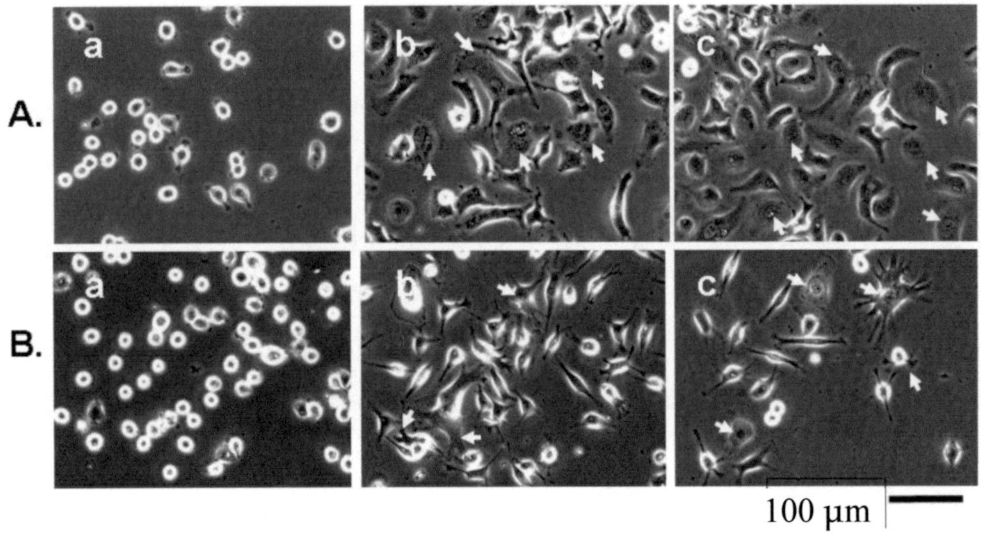

Fig. 1. Induction of apoptosis in ovarian cancer cells (A, SKOV-3A) and breast cancer cells (B, MDA-MB-231C) by recombinant rtEa4-peptide. Cancer cells in serum free medium were treated with or without rtEa4-peptide for 2 h, and observed under an inverted phase contrast microscope (Olympus IX50). a, control protein; b, 1.4 μM rtEa4-peptide ; c, 2.8 μM rtEa4-peptide. Arrows indicate apoptotic cells.

Generally speaking, apoptosis can be stimulated via extrinsic and intrinsic pathways. Does rtEa4-peptide or hEb-peptide induce apoptosis in cancer cells via both extrinsic and intrinsic pathways? It has been reported by many investigators that if apoptosis is induced via extrinsic pathway, up-regulation of expression of *TRAIL-RI, FADD* and *pro-Casp-8* genes will be observed. On the other hand, if apoptosis is induced via intrinsic pathway, down-regulation of expression of *Bcl-2, Bcl-XL and Mcl-1* genes and up-regulation of expression of

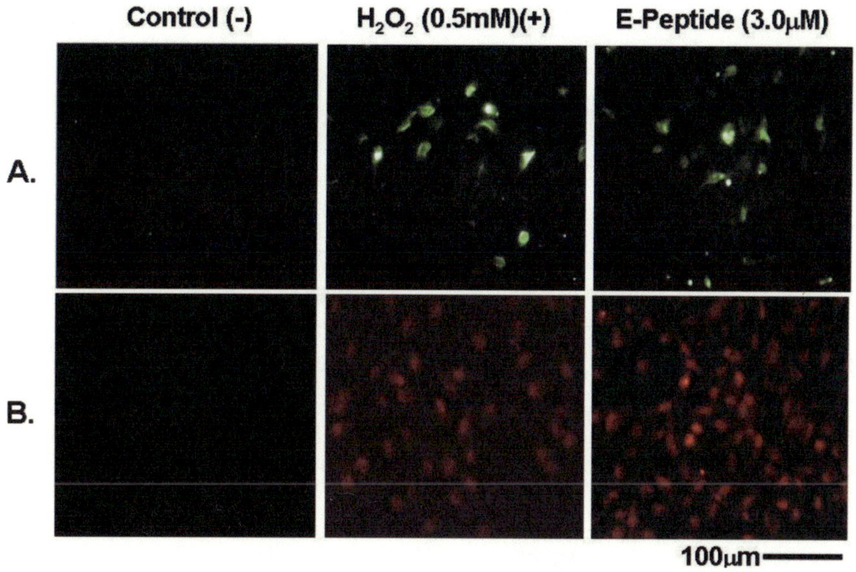

Fig. 2. Apoptotic cells identified by TUNEL assay (A) and immunostaining with monospecific antibody to activated capase-3 (B). MDA-MB-231C cells in serum free medium were treated with (3.0μM) rtEa4-peptide or control protein for 48 h. One sample was treated with H_2O_2 for 16 h to induce apoptosis as a positive control. TUNEL assay was carried out following the protocol supplied by the manufacturer. Monospecific polyclonal rabbit anti-activated caspase 3 immunoglobulin was labeled with Rodamine Red and used to stain recombinant rtEa4 peptide treated or positive control cells. The immuno-stained cells were observed under an inverted microscope (Olympus IX50) with epifluorescence attachment.

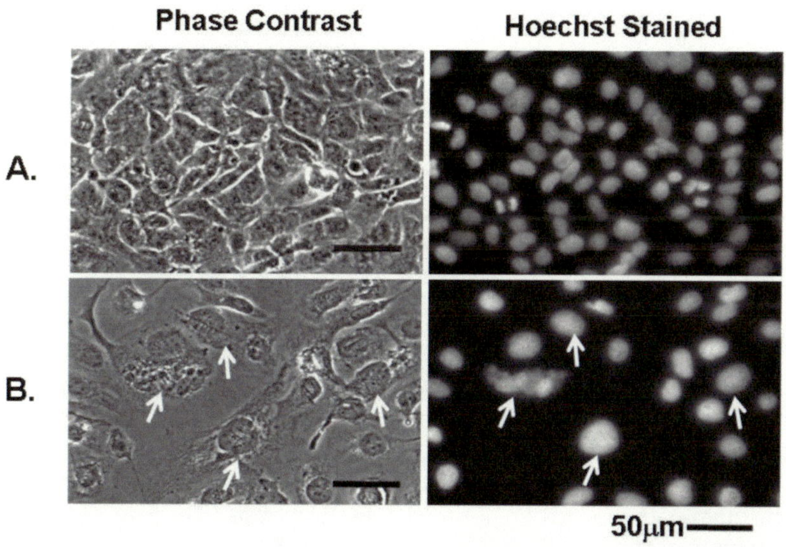

Fig. 3. Induction of apoptosis in ovarian cancer cells (SKOV-3A) by rtEa4-peptide. SKOV-3A cells in serum free medium were treated with control protein (A) or 1.5 μM of rtEa4-peptide (B) for 3 d, and cells were stained with H33258. Arrows indicate apoptotic cells.

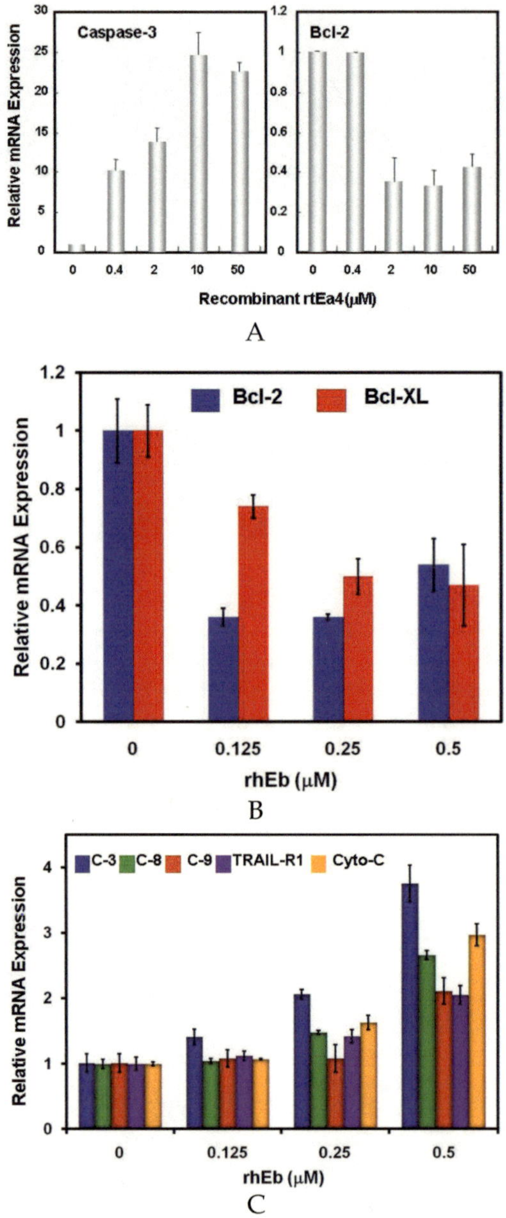

Fig. 4. Effect of recombinant rtEa4- (A) or hEb-peptide (B and C) on levels of Casp-3, Casp-8, Casp-9, TRAIL-R1 and Cyt-C mRNAs in MDA-MB-231C cells. MBA-MD-231C cells in serum free medium were treated with various concentrations of recombinant rtEa4- or hEb-peptide for 6 h, and total RNA samples were isolated from the treated cells. The levels of mRNA were determined by quantitative relative real-time RT-PCR analysis. The level of GAPDH mRNA was used as an internal control. Relative Expression Level = $2^{-(S\Delta CT - C\Delta CT)}$, where S$\Delta$CT is the difference between the CT number of the sample (cancer cells treated with E-peptide) and GAPDH, and the CΔCT is the difference between the CT of cancer cells without E-peptide treatment and the CT of GAPDH. Error bars indicate standard deviation (n=3).

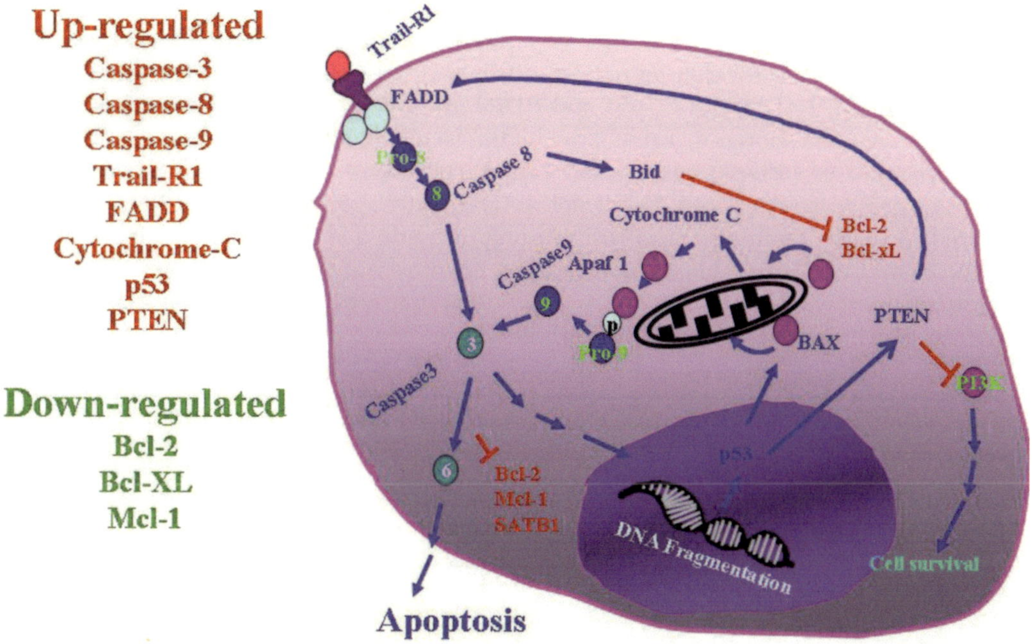

Fig. 5. A schematic presentation of extrinsic and intrinsic pathways of apoptosis. Apoptosis can be initiated via stimulation at the plasma membrane by death receptor (extrinsic pathway) or at mitochondria (intrinsic pathway). Stimulation of death receptors will result in aggregation and recruitment of the adaptor molecule Fas-associated protein with death domain (FADD) and pro-caspase 8. Upon recruitment, pro-caspase 8 is activated to caspase 8 and initiates apoptosis by direct activating downstream caspases (caspases 3 and 9). Intrinsic pathway is initiated by a variety of stress stimuli in which the mitochondrial membrane permeability is regulated by balance of opposing action of pro-apoptotic and antiapoptotic Bcl family members (Bax, Bak, Bcl2, Bcl-XL and Mcl-1). Following mitochondril permeabilization, mitochondrial proapoptotic proteins such as cytochrome C, Samc/Diablo, Omi/HrtA2, AIF and Endo G are released via transmembrane channels across the mitochondriasl outer membrane. This figure was redrawn from information provided by Fulda and Debatin (2006).

Cyt-C gene will be observed (Figure 5) (Fulda and Debatin, 2006; O'Brien and Kirby, 2008 for review). Therefore, to address the question whether rtEa4-peptide and hEb-peptide can induce apoptosis in cancer cells through both extrinsic and intrinsic pathways, levels of Bcl-2, Bcl-XL, Casp-3, Casp-8, Casp-9, TRAIL-R1 and Cyt-C mRNAs were measured by quantitative relative real-time RT-PCR analysis in MBA-MD-231C cells following treatment with recombinant rtEa4- or hEb-peptide. As shown in Figures 4A, 4B and 4C, upon treatment of MDA-MB-231C cells with various doses of recombinant rtEa4- or hEb-peptide, a dose-dependent up-regulation on levels of Casp-3, Casp-8, Casp-9, TRAIL-R1 and Cyt-C mRNAs and a dose-dependent down-regulation on levels of Bcl-2 and Bcl-XL mRNAs were observed. These results suggest that E-peptide may induce apoptosis in breast cancer cells via both extrinsic and intrinsic pathways. To further confirm that rtEa4- or hEb-peptide can also induce apoptosis in other cancer cells, human ovarian cancer cells (OVCAR-3A, SKOV-

3B), neuroblastoma cells (SK-N-SH and SK-N-F1) and non-cancerous foreskin cells (CCD-1112SK) were treated with 2.0 μM of rtEa4-peptide or 0.5 μM hEb-peptide for 6 h and RNA samples were extracted for determination of levels of Bcl-2, Bcl-XL, Mcl-1, Casp-3, Casp-8, Casp-9, TRAIL-R1, FADD, Cyt-C, p53 and PTEN mRNAs by quantitative relative real-time RT-PCR analysis. As shown in Table 2, while the levels of Bcl-2, Bcl-XL and Mcl-1 mRNAs in rtEa4-peptide or hEb-peptide treated cancer cells were down-regulated significantly, those of Casp-3, Casp-8, Casp-9, TRAIL-R1, FADD, Cyt-C, p53 and PTEN mRNAs were up-regulated. Results presented in Table 2 not only provide a strong evidence to support the hypothesis that rtEa4- or hEb-peptide induces apoptosis in cancer cells via both extrinsic and intrinsic pathways, but also confirm the notion that E-peptide can induce apoptosis in many cancer cells other than MBA-MD-231C cells.

Genes	Cell Lines (Relative Expression Levels)						
	rtEa4 (2μM)						hEb (0.5μM)
	CCD-1112SK*	MDA-MB-231C	OVCAR-3B	SKOV-3A	SKNSH	SKNF1	MDA-MB-231C
Bcl-2	1.08 ± 0.55	0.19 ± 0.03	0.66 ± 0.10	0.20 ± 0.05	0.79 ± 0.34	0.08 ± 0.02	0.54 ± 0.09
Bcl-XL	0.96 ± 0.04	0.33 ± 0.00	0.49 ± 0.01	0.21 ± 0.01	0.50 ± 0.04	0.18 ± 0.00	0.47 ± 0.14
Mcl-1	0.92 ± 0.04	0.60 ± 0.00	0.29 ± 0.01	0.15 ± 0.02	0.38 ± 0.08	0.07 ± 0.01	-
Casp-3	0.96 ± 0.12	3.48 ± 0.27	26.07 ± 2.50	12.18 ± 2.61	3.32 ± 0.10	13.91 ± 1.81	3.75± 0.28
Casp-8	0.91 ± 0.03	3.74 ± 0.28	2.44 ± 0.04	2.67± 0.06	5.49 ± 0.56	7.96 ± 0.01	2.66± 0.07
Casp-9	1.08 ± 0.01	2.18 ± 0.10	3.13 ± 0.021	1.98 ± 0.02	6.16 ± 0.18	8.70 ± 1.12	2.11 ± 0.2
TRAIL-R1	1.01 ± 0.11	2.04 ± 0.16	2.24 ± 0.01	1.37 ± 0.06	6.50 ± 0.16	7.47 ± 0.78	2.05± 0.14
FADD	1.04 ± 0.11	3.61 ± 0.09	1.42 ± 0.03	2.67 ± 0.03	3.31 ± 0.05	8.33 ± 1.14	1.49± 0.22
Cyt-C	1.02 ± 0.05	2.54 ± 0.18	1.40 ± 0.00	1.72 ± 0.01	4.31 ± 1.02	10.59 ± 8.20	2.97 ± 0.17
p53	1.08 ± 0.06	2.37 ± 0.05	3.09 ± 0.29	1.03 ± 0.51	3.99 ± 0.47	6.93 ± 1.75	1.57 ± 0.03
PTEN	--	8.30 ± 0.73	--	4.61 ± 0.11	4.09 ± 0.20	30.80 ± 0.15	--

Relative Expression Level $2^{-[(S\Delta CT-C\Delta CT)]}$ and standard deviation (n=3) vhere SΔCT is the difference between the CT number of the sample (cancer cells treated with E-peptide) and the house keeping gene (GAPDH), and the CΔCT is the difference between the CT of cancer cells without E-peptide treatment and the CT of GAPDH $2^{-[(S\Delta CT-C\Delta CT)]}>1$, up-regulation; $2^{-[(S\Delta CT-C\Delta CT)]}<1$, down-regulation *CCD-1112SK, non-immortalized human fibroblast cells.

Table 2. Relative Expression Levels of Apoptosis Genes by E-peptide of Pro-IGF I

It is very interesting to note that treatment of non-cancerous foreskin cells (CCD-1112SK) with the same concentration of recombinant rtEa4-peptide or hEb-peptide (result not shown) did not result in significant changes in the levels of Bcl-2, Bcl-XL, Mcl-1, Casp-3, Casp-8, Casp-9, TRAIL-R1, FADD, Cyt-C, p53 and PTEN mRNAs when compare to non-treatment control (Table 2). This observation suggests that rtEa4- or hEb-peptide only induces apoptosis in cancer cells. The resistance of cancer cells to apoptosis is one of the major concerns in cancer therapy. So in searching for effective chemotherapeutic drugs, the effectiveness of the drugs to induce apoptosis in a wide variety of cancer types will be the top choice. Although there are numerous chemotherapeutic drugs available on the market that have been shown to induce apoptosis in cancer cells, unfortunately these drugs also induce apoptosis in non-cancerous cells. In this study we have shown that rtEa4- or hEb-peptide can induce apoptosis in a variety of human cancer cells but not in non-cancerous cells. Therefore, we believe that rtEa4- or hEb-peptide could be developed as an ideal therapeutic agent for treating human cancers.

4. Acknowledgement

This work was supported by funds from US Department of Agriculture (CONS-9803641) to T.T.C.

5. References

Bell GI, Sanchez-Pescador R, Laybourn PJ, Najarian RC. 1983. Exon duplication and divergence in the human preproglucagon gene. Nature 304:716-718.

Chen MHC, Lin GH, Gong HY, Weng CF, Chang CY, Wu JH. 2001. The characterization of prepro-insulin-like growth factor-I Ea-2 expression and insulin-like growth factor-I genes(devoid 81 bp) in the zebrafish (*Danio reio*). Gene 268:67-75.

Chen MJ, Kuo Ya Huei, Tian XC, Chen TT. 2002. Anti-tumor activities of pro-IGF-I E-peptides: studies on morphological changes, anchroage-dependent cell division, and invasiveness in tumor cells. Gen. Comp. Endocrinol. 126:342-351.

Chen MJ, Chiou PP, Lin P, Lin C-M, Siri S, Peck K, Chen TT. 2007. Suppression of growth and cancer-induced angiogenesis of aggressive human breast cancer cells (MDA-MB-231) on the chorioallantoic membrane of developing chicken embryos by E-peptide of pro-IGF-I. J Cell Biochem 101:1316-1327.

Civelli O, Douglass J, Rosen H, Martens G, Herbert E. 1986. Biosynthesis of opioid peptides. In "Opioid Peptides: Molecular Pharmacology, Biosynthesis, and Analysis (ed by Rapaka RS and Hawaks RL) NDA Research Monograph 70:21-34.

de Pablo F, Scott LA, Roth J. 1990. Insulin and insulin-like growth factor I in early development: peptides, receptors and biological events. Endocr Rev 11:558-577.

de Pablo F, Perez-Villami B, Serna J, Gonzalez-Guerrero PR, Lopez-Carranza A, de la Rosa EJ, Alemany J, Caldes T. 1993. IGF-I and the IGF-I receptor in development of nonmammalian vertebrates. Mol Repro Deve 35:427-432; discussion 432-433.

Duguay SJ, Park LK, Samadpour M, Dickhoff WW. 1992. Nucleotide sequences and tissue distribution of three different insulin-like growth factor I prohormone in salmon. Mol Endocr 6: 1202-1210.

Duguay SJ. 1999. Post-translational processing of insulin-like growth factors. Horm Metab Res 31:43-49.

Elmore S. 2007. Apoptosis: A review of programmed cell death. Toxicol Pathol 35:495-516.

Evan GI, Vousden KH. 2001. Proliferation, cell cycle and apoptosis in cancer. Nature 411:342-348.

Finkel E. 1999. Does cancer therapy trigger cell suicide? Science 286:2256-2258.

Fulda S, Debatin KM. 2004. Apoptosis signaling in tumor therapy. Ann N Y Acad Sci 2004 1028: 150-156.

Fulda S, Debatin K-M 2006. Extrinsic verse intrinsic apoptosis pathways in anticancer chemotherapy. Oncogene 25: 4798-4811.

Faulk CK, Perez-Dominguez R, Webb Jr KA, Holt GJ. 2010. The novel finding of four distinct prepro-IGF-I E domains in a perciform fish, *Sciaenops ocellatus*, during ontogeny. Gen Comp Endocr 169:75-81.

Hacker G. 2000. The morphology of apoptosis. Cell Tissue Res 301:5-17.

Hengartner MO. 2000. The biochemistry of apoptosis. Nature 407:770-776.

Ghavami S, Hashemi M, Ande SR, Yeganeh B, Xiao W, Eshraghi M, Bus CJ, Kadkhoda K, Wiechec E, Halayke AJ, Los M. 2009. Apoptosis and cancer: mutation with caspase genes. J Med Genet 46: 497-510.

Ido Y, Vindigni A, Chang K, Stramm L, Chance R, Heath WF, DiMarchi RD, Di Cera E, Williamson JR. 1997. Precvention of vascular and neuraldysfunction in diabetic rats by C-peptide. Science 277:563-566.

Kuo YH, Chen TT.2002. Novel activities of pro-IGF-I E-peptides: regulation of morphological differentiation and anchorage-independent growth in human neuroblastoma cells. Exp Cell Res 280:75-89.

Lowe SW, Lin AW. 2000. Apoptosis in cancer. Carcinogenesis 21:485-495.

Matheny RW Jr, Nindl BC, Adamo ML. 2010. Minireview: mechano factor: a putative product of IGF-I gene expression involved in tissue repair and regeneration. Endocrinology 151: 865-875.

Marx J. 2002. Cancer research obstacle for promising cancer therapy. Science 295:1444.

O'Brien, MA, Kirby R. 2008. Apoptosis: a review of pro-apoptotic and anti-apoptotic pathways and dysregulation in disease. J Vet. Emergency and Crit Care 18: 572-586.

Pfeffer LA, Brisson, BK, Lei H, Barton ER. 2009. The insulin-like growth factor (IGF)-I E-peptides modulate cell entry of the mature IGF-I protein. Mol Biol Cell 20:3810-3817.

Rotein P, Pollock KM, Didier DK, Krivi GG. 1986. Organization and sequence of the human insulin-like growth factor I gene: Alternative RNA processing produces two insulin-like growth factor I precursor peptides. J Biol Chem 261:4828-4832.Shamblott MJ, Chen TT. 1992. Identification of a second insulin-like growth factor in a fish species. Proc Natl Acad Sci USA 89:8913-8971.

Shamblott MJ, Chen TT. 1993. Age-related and tissue-specific levels of five forms of insulin-like mRNA in a teleost. Mol Mar Biol Biotechnol 2:351-361.

Shi FT, Li WS, Bai CH, Lin HR. 2002. IGF-I of orange spotted grouper *Epinephelus coioides*: cDNA cloning, sequencing and expression in *Escherichia coli*. Fish Physiol Biochem 27:147-156.

Siegfried JM, Kasprzyk PG, Treston AM, Mulshine JL, Quinn KA, Cuttitta F. 1992. A mitogenic peptide amide encoded within the E-peptide domain of the insulin-like growth factor IB prohormone. Proc Natl Acad Sci USA 89:8107-8111.

Stewart CE, Rotwein P. 1996. Growth, differentiation, and survival: multiple physiological functions for insulin-like growth factors. Physiol Rev 76:1005-1026.

Tiago DM, Laize V, Cancela ML. 2008. Alternatively spliced transcripts of *Sparus aurata* insulin-like growth factor 1 are differentially expressed in adult tissu4s and during early development. Gem Comp Endocrinol 157:107-115.

Wallis AE and Devlin RH. 1993. Duplicate insulin-like growth factor-I genes in salmon display alternative splicing pathways. Mol Endocr 7:409-422.

Yang SY, Goldspink G. 2002. Different roles of the IGF-I Ec peptide (MGF) and mature IGF-I in myoblast proliferation and differentiation. FEBS Letters 522:156-160.

Yang SY, Sales KM, Fuller BJ, Seifalian AM, Winslet MC. 2008. Inducing apoptosis of human colon cancer by an IGF-I D domain analogue peptide. Molecular Cancer 7: 17-28.

Youle RJ, Strasser A. 2008. The BCL-2 protein family: opposing activities that mediate cell death. Nature Reviews / Molecular Cell Biology 9: 47-59.

4

Induction of Autophagic Cell Death by Targeting Bcl-2 as a Novel Therapeutic Strategy in Breast Cancer

Bulent Ozpolat, Neslihan Alpay and Gabriel Lopez-Berestein
Department of Experimental Therapeutics, The University of Texas-MD Anderson Cancer Center, Houston TX, USA

1. Introduction

Breast cancer is the second leading cause of tumor related death in women in Western countries. It has been estimated in recent reports that this year about 207.000 women will be diagnosed with breast cancer and about 40.000 will die of it in the US. (Jemal et al., 2010). While 5 year survival in early stages is about 90 %, it is as low as 15 % in metastatic stage. Despite the fact that there are many agents to treat the breast cancer, most of the tumors ultimately become unresponsive to these systemic therapeutics (Alvarez et al., 2010). Therefore new therapeutic strategies either alone or in combination with conventional therapies are required to improve the survival rates of breast cancer patients.

2. Autophagy

Autophagy (Greek, meaning self eating) is an evolutionary conserved process whereby damaged or excess organelles, long-lived or unfolded proteins, protein aggregates and invasive microbes are subjected to lysosomal degradation. There are three autophagy types, macroautophagy (autophagy from now on in this chapter) takes cytoplasmic components to the lysosome in a double-membrane vesicle (autophagosome); micro-autophagy, lysosome itself takes the cytoplasmic material inside by invagination of lysosome membrane, and in chaperone mediated autophagy the proteins are targeted to the lysosome by a chaperone protein such as Hsp-70 which is recognized by lysosome membrane proteins (Glick et al., 2010). Autophagy includes some other selective autophagy types such as mitophagy, autophagy for mitochondria, reticulophagy for endoplasmic reticulum), pexophagy for peroxisome, ribophagy for ribosome, aggrephagy for protein aggregates (Beau et al., 2008). Autophagy starts from endoplasmic reticulum as phagophore and expands towards the cytoplasmic content and forms autophagosome, then autophagosome fuses with lysosome and forms autophagolysosome (Klionsky & Emr, 2000). Autophagy takes place in most cells at a basal level to eliminate protein aggregates and damaged organelles, therefore, to maintain the cellular homeostasis (Scarlatti et al., 2009).

2.1 Autophagy as a survival pathway

Autophagy is induced by nutrient or growth factor deprivation, hypoxia, oxidative stress, radiation, hormonal and chemotherapeutic agents (He & Klionsky, 2009). During nutrient deprivation, autophagy produces energy from the recycling of the organelles or the proteins and prevents the cells to undergo apoptosis by sequestering mitochondria and preventing cytochrome c release - this protective role of autophagy is not limited to apoptosis but also extends to necrosis (Scarlatti et al., 2009).In the tumor hypoxic and acidic microenvironment, autophagy helps the cells to survive. Numerous anticancer agents such as doxorubicin, temozolomide, etoposide, arsenic trioxide, histone deacetylase inhibitors as well as TNF alpha, IFN gamma, imatinib, rapamycin, anti-estrogen tamoxifen and radiation therapy have also been shown to induce autophagy in various human cancer cells as a protective mechanism (Dalby et al.). But, if the stress leads to continuous or excessively induced autophagy, autophagic cell death may occur. Autophagic cell death (programmed cell death type II) is independent of caspase activation and DNA laddering presenting in apoptotic cell death. (Shen & Codogno). But it occurs depending on the nature of stimuli, cell type, presence or activation other autophagy related factors (Shen & Codogno). It has been shown that bax/bak double knockout mice embryonic fibroblasts which are resistant to apoptosis, could undergo autophagic cell death after starvation, etoposide and radiotherapy (Moretti et al., 2007). These studies suggests that autophagic cell death has been induced by growth-factor deprivation and cytosine arabinoside in sympathetic neurons (Xue et al., 1999), etoposide and staurosporine in mouse embryonic fibroblasts (Shimizu et al., 2004), rottlerin in pancreatic cancer cells (Akar et al., 2007), zoledronic acid in prostate cancer cell lines (Lin et al.). Although there is no marker for autophagic cell death, it can be shown, indirectly, by reduced cell death after inhibition of autophagy in two different ways such as pharmacological inhibition (for example 3-methyladenine) or siRNA based silencing of the autophagy genes such as Beclin-1, ATG5, ATG8.

2.2 Autophagy as tumor suppressor mechanism

Recently, autophagy has been shown to function as a tumor suppressor mechanism. Liang et al. reported that one of the autophagy promoting genes, Beclin-1, could inhibit tumorigenesis and is expressed at lower levels in human breast cancers and they suggested that low expression of autophagy proteins may play a role in the development or progression of breast and other malignancies (Liang et al., 1999). Yue et al. reported that Beclin-1 haploinsufficient mice had higher incidence and different spectrum of tumor formation including B cell lymphomas, hepatocellular carcinomas, lung adenocarcinoma (Yue et al., 2003). They showed that tumors were also larger in Beclin-1$^{+/-}$ mice than wild type ones, suggesting that the tumors developed at an earlier age. It has also been shown that heterozygous disruption of beclin-1 resulted in cell proliferation in vivo suggesting beclin-1 as a tumor suppressor (Qu et al., 2003). It has been suggested that autophagy cleans up unwanted proteins to keep genomic stability (Mathew et al., 2007) and prevent the cells to transform into malignant cells. Therefore, the induction of autophagy may help to reverse the malignant phenotype.

2.3 Autophagy as a pro-death and type II programmed cell death mechanism

Apoptosis (programmed cell death-type I, PCD-type I) and necrosis are well known mechanism of cell death induced by anticancer therapies (Dalby et al, 2010). Until recently, apoptosis was a synonym for programmed cell death and thought to be the major mechanism of cell death in response to chemo- and radiotherapy. However, emerging studies have demonstrated the existence of a non-apoptotic form of programmed death called autophagic cell death, which is now considered as a PCD-type II. In contrast to apoptosis, autophagic cell death, in general, is caspase-independent and does not involve classic DNA laddering and believed to be a result of an extensive autophagic degradation of intracellular content (Lockshin RA, Zakeri Z, 2007). Studies showed that cytotoxic signals can induce autophagy in cells that are resistant to apoptosis (apoptosis defective), such as those expressing high Bcl-2 or Bcl-XL, those lacking Bax and Bak or those being exposed to pan-caspase inhibitors, such as zVAD-fmk (Shimizu et al, 2004). Proapoptotic Bcl-2 family member proteins, *Bak* and *Bax*, regulate intrinsic apoptotic pathway by causing mitochondrial outer membrane permeabilization and cyctochrome c release. Bax and Bak (-/-) knockout fibroblast cells have been shown to be resistant to apoptosis and undergo an autophagic cell death after the induction of death, following starvation, growth factor withdrawal, chemotherapy (etoposide) or radiation (Moretti et al, 2007). The evidence suggests that autophagy leads to cell death in response to several compounds, including rottlerin (Akar et al, 2007) cytosine arabinoside (Xue et al, 1999), etoposide and staurosporine as well as growth factor deprivation (Xue et al, 1999). A link between autophagy and related autophagic cell death has been demonstrated using pharmacological (e.g. 3-MA) and genetic (silencing of *ATG5, ATG7 and Beclin-1*) approaches for suppression of autophagy. For example, the knockdown of ATG5 or Beclin-1 in cancer cells containing defects in apoptosis lead to a marked reduction in autophagic cell death (and autophagic response) in response to cell death stimuli with no sign of apoptosis (Akar et al, 2007). Studies also suggest that apoptosis and autophagy are linked by effector proteins (e.g., Bcl-2, Bcl-XL, Mcl-1, ATG5, p53) and common pathways (e.g., PI3K/Akt/mTOR, NF-kB, ERK) (Akar et al,2007; Yousefi et al, 2006, Shimizu S et al,2004; Akar U et al 2008)). Overall, there is evidence that autophagy may function as a type II PCD in cancer cells in which apoptosis is defective or hard to induce. Therefore it is reasonable to propose the notion that the induction of autophagic cell death may be used as a therapeutic strategy to treat cancer (Dalby et al, 2010, Ozpolat et al 2007).

2.4 Targeting autophagy as a novel cancer therapy

Autophagy can be used as a new therapeutic strategy either by inducing the autophagic cell death or inhibiting protective autophagy depending on the context (Dalby et al, 2010). Apoptosis defects such as a lack of caspase 3 or apoptosis resistance such as having overexpression of ant apoptotic proteins lead to resistance to chemotherapy, radiotherapy or some other anticancer agents. Up regulation of the expression of several antiapoptotic Bcl-2 family protein members, including Bcl-2, Bcl-XL, prevents cell to undergo apoptosis induced by death ligands or chemotherapeutic drugs (Bardeesy & DePinho, 2002; Simoes-Wust et al., 2002) Either the induction or the inhibition of autophagy can provide therapeutic benefits to patients and that the design and synthesis of modulators of autophagy may provide novel therapeutic tools and may ultimately lead to new therapeutic strategies in cancer. Defects in apoptosis leads to increased resistance to chemotherapy, radiotherapy, some anticancer agents and targeted therapies. Therefore, induction of autophagic cell death may be an ideal approach in those cancers that are resistant to apoptosis by anticancer therapies (e.g., chemotherapy, radiation). As explained in the previous section cancer cells can undergo autophagic cell death when their apoptosis is inhibited, or they are resistant to therapy-induced apoptosis (e.g. in response to DNA-damaging agents such as etoposide), suggesting that autophagic cell death can be induced as an alternative cell death mechanism when cells fail to undergo apoptosis. Therefore, induction of autophagic cell death may serve as a novel therapeutic tool to eliminate cancer cells with defective apoptosis, which is the case in many advanced, drug resistant and metastatic cancers (Dalby et al, 2010). We have recently demonstrated that the inhibition of some protein kinases (e.g., PKCδ in pancreatic cancer) or the targeting of key proteins that are involved in the suppression of autophagy (e.g. Bcl-2, TG2) can trigger autophagic cell death without any other treatment (Akar et al., 2008; Akar et al., 2007; Ozpolat et al., 2007). On the other hand, because a number of cancer therapies, such as radiation therapy, chemotherapy and targeted therapies (e.g. imatinib) induce autophagy as a protective resistance mechanism against anticancer therapies for cancer cell survival, the inhibition of autophagy can be used to enhance the efficacy of anticancer therapies.

3. Bcl-2

The Bcl-2 gene encodes a 26-kDa Bcl-2 proto-oncogene is overexpressed in 40-80 % of breast cancer patients and more than half of all human cancers (Hellemans et al., 1995; Oh et al.2011). Bcl-2 is a gene family consisting of several anti-apoptotic (such as Bcl-2, Bcl-XL, Mcl-1) and pro-apoptotic members (such as Bax, Bak, puma). The balance between pro- and anti-apoptotic proteins determines the cell's fate, to survive or die. Although some studies suggest that enhanced Bcl-2 expression is associated with improved survival in human colon cancer (Buglioni et al., 1999; Meterissian et al., 2001) and breast cancer studies (Cheng et al., 2004). The role of Bcl-2 in cancer cells was shown to be related to its ability to promote the tumorigenesis through interfering with apoptosis and autophagy (Reed et al, 1995, Oh et al.2011). It has been demonstrated that Bcl-2 overexpression leads to an aggressive tumor phenotype in patients with a variety of cancers as well as to the resistance of cancer cells against chemotherapy, radiation, and hormone therapy (Bishop, 1991; Reed, 1995). Recently, Buchholz et al, found 61% of the breast cancer patients treated at MD Anderson Cancer Center were Bcl-2 positive and they had a poor response to chemotherapy compared to those had less Bcl-2 expression (Buchholz et al., 2005). Figure below summarizes the novel functions of Bcl-2 in cancer cells, including metastasis, survival and tumor progresion, these functions will be explained in the following sections. Overall, Bcl-2 over expression confers drug resistance, an aggressive clinical course, and poor survival in patients (Patel et al., 2009; Pusztai et al., 2004).

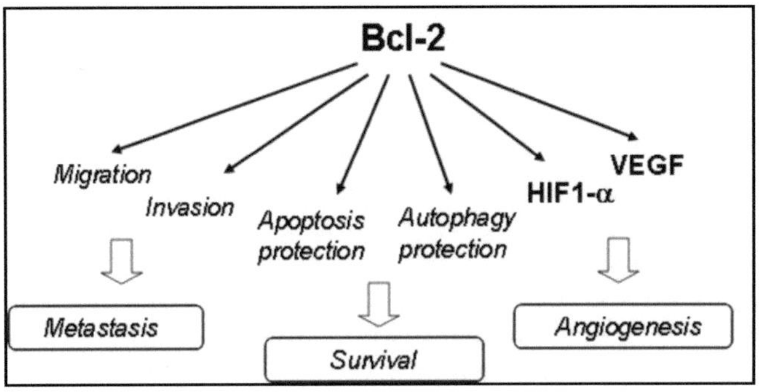

3.1 Bcl-2 as an inhibitor of apoptosis and autophagy

Bcl-2 family proteins work in pairs with their proapoptotic counterparts for example Bcl-2 heterodimerize with BAX, Bcl-XL with BAK. Proapoptotic members of this family mostly localized to cytosol. Following a death signal the proapoptotic members undergo a conformational change that enables them to target and integrate into membranes, particularly mitochondrial outer membrane (Gross et al., 1999). But anti-apoptotic Bcl-2 is predominantly a mitochondrial protein, and it can prevent mitochondrial changes which take place with apoptosis, including loss of mitochondria membrane potential, release of mitochondria proteins cytochrome c and apoptosis-inducing factor (AIF), and opening of the mitochondria permeability transition pore which is a large conductance pore that evolves in mitochondria after necrotic and apoptotic signals then cytochrome c is released and caspase 9 and 3 are activated (Gross et al., 1999). Therefore, downregulation of Bcl-2 leads to induction of apoptosis, reduction of the apoptotic threshold. Tormo et al. have shown the induction of apoptosis by lipid incorporated Bcl-2 antisense in transformed follicular lymphoma cells (Tormo et al., 1998). An siRNA based inhibition of Bcl-2 is also increased apoptosis in MCF7 breast cancer cells (Lima et al., 2004).

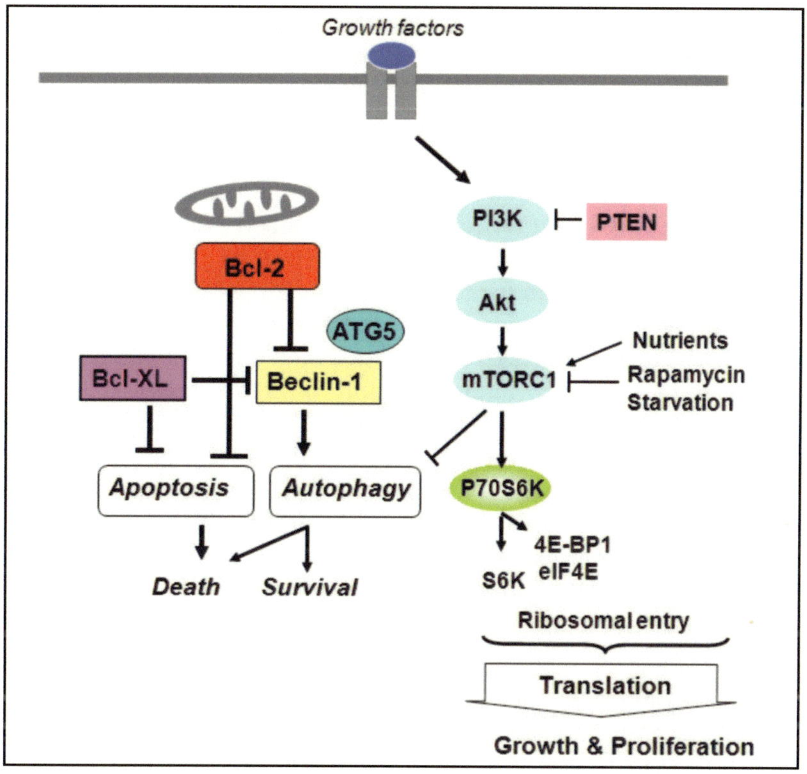

Regulation of autophagy and apoptosis through the crosstalk between Bcl-2 and Bcl-XL may determine the predominant response to anticancer therapies.

Recently, Pattingre et al., have reported that stable transfection of Bcl-2 in HT29 colon carcinoma cells inhibited starvation induced autophagy, decreased the association of beclin-1 and Vps34 and magnitude of beclin-1 associated class III phosphoinositol-3- kinase activity (Pattingre & Levine, 2006). The proposed mechanism is that Beclin-1 has a BH3 domain that is required to bind to Bcl-2 and bcl-XL for Bcl-2 mediated inhibition of autophagy (Boya & Kroemer, 2009) (Please see the Figure)(Dalby et al, 2010). It has been shown that the pharmacological BH3 mimetic ABT737 competitively inhibited the interaction between Beclin-1 and Bcl-2/Bcl-XL, antagonized autophagy inhibition by Bcl-2/Bcl-XL and hence stimulated autophagy (Maiuri et al., 2007). A recent study demonstrated that anti-autophagic property of Bcl-2 is a key feature of Bcl-2-mediated tumorigenesis (Oh et al, 2011). MCF7 cells expressing Bcl-2 mutant defective in apoptosis inhibition but competent for autophagy suppression grew *in vitro and in vivo* as efficiently as wild-type Bcl-2. The growth-promoting activity of this Bcl-2 mutant is strongly correlated with its suppression of autophagy in xenograft tumors, suggesting that oncogenic effect of Bcl-2 arises from its ability to inhibit autophagy but not apoptosis.

Recent studies also suggested that silencing of Bcl-2 by siRNA induced autophagic cell death (up to 55%) in estrogen receptor (+) MCF7 breast cancer cell line, but not apoptotic cell death (Akar et al., 2008). An increase in autophagy with increased number of punctates in GFP-LC3 transfected cells, increased LC3-II formation and acridine orange accumulation in autophagosomes as well as induction of autophagy genes (e.g., *ATG5* and *BECN1*) were observed in response to Bcl-2 silencing. We further blocked autophagy with ATG5 siRNA - autophagy related gene 5- and inhibition of ATG5 significantly blocked Bcl-2-siRNA-induced cell killing, suggesting the autophagic cell death(Akar et al., 2008). Bcl-2 mediated-autophagic cell death pathway induction is most likely related to MCF-7 cells caspase 3-deficiency thus, presenting a higher threshold for the induction of apoptosis, additionally; we reported that doxorubicin induces autophagy and apoptosis. These findings led to the hypothesis that apoptosis resistant cancer cells can be killed by autophagic cell death as an alternative death mechanism and this strategy may be uses as a therapeutic intervention for targeted silencing of genes for induction of autophagic cell death. It is important to recognize the conditions and genetic make up of the cells in order for the induction of autophagic cell death. Furthermore, doxorubicin at a high dose (IC95) induced apoptosis but at a low dose (IC50) induced only autophagy and Beclin-1 expression. In addition, when combined with chemotherapy (doxorubicin), therapeutic targeting of Bcl-2 by siRNA induced significant growth inhibition (83%) and autophagy in about 80% of the MCF-7 breast cancer cells(Akar et al., 2008). We also found that in vivo targeted silencing of Bcl-2 by systemically administrated nanoliposomal Bcl-2 siRNA induced autophagy and tumor growth inhibition in mice bearing MDA-MB231 tumors (Tekedereli et al, in press). These results provided the first evidence that targeted silencing of Bcl-2 induces autophagic cell death in breast cancer cells and that Bcl-2 siRNA may be used as a therapeutic strategy alone or in combination with chemotherapy in breast cancer cells that overexpress Bcl-2.

3.2 Bcl-2 induces cell proliferation and cell cycle progression

We have shown that silencing Bcl-2 decreased the clonogenicity and induced cell proliferation inhibition either alone or in combination with doxorubicin, which is a widely used anti-cancer agent, in estrogen receptor (+) MCF7 breast cancer cell line (Akar et al., 2008). We did not observe growth inhibition in Bcl-2-negative MDA-MB-453 cells after treatment with the siRNA, suggesting that Bcl-2 siRNA specifically inhibits growth of Bcl-2-overexpressing breast cancer cells (Akar et al., 2008). We also showed that Bcl-2 knockdown inhibited clonogenicity and cell proliferation in estrogen receptor (-) MDA-MB-231 cells (unpublished data). Emi et al. reported 50-70 % proliferation inhibition by Bcl-2 antisense oligonucleotides (ASO) in BT-474 and ZR-75-1 breast cancer cells. They also showed that pretreatment with bcl-2 antisense led to 2.5 to 10 fold increase in sensitivity to chemotherapy with either doxorubicin, mitomycin C, docetaxel or paclitaxel in MDA-MB-231, BT-474 and ZR-75-1 breast cancer cell lines in vitro (Emi et al., 2005). Inhibition of bcl-2 expression by

ASO has been shown to inhibit colony formation in AML progenitor cells (Konopleva et al., 2000). Inhibition of bcl-2 by ASO led the cells to arrest in G1 phase of cell cycle in PC3 prostate cancer cell line (Anai et al., 2007). Some other recent studies in breast cancer experimental models have also demonstrated that in vitro and in vivo downregulation of Bcl-2 by ASO enhanced the sensitivity to chemotherapeutic drugs, such as doxorubicin, paclitaxel, mitomycin C and cyclophosphamide suggesting the downregulation of Bcl-2 may be a useful strategy to prevent drug resistance and enhance-chemosensitivity (Emi et al., 2005; Tanabe et al., 2003). In melanoma, lymphoma and breast cancer xenografts pretreatment with Bcl-2 antisense enhanced antitumor activity of various chemotherapeutic agents such as cyclophosphamide, dacarbazine and docetaxel (Nahta & Esteva, 2003). George et. al., reported that bcl-2 siRNA combine with taxol (100 nM) increased the apoptotic cells in Tunel assay up to 70 % when compared to 30 % in taxol alone (100 nM) group in human glioma cells (George et al., 2009).

There are several conflicting studies on the effect of Bcl-2 on cell proliferation. Huang et al. (Huang et al., 1997) have shown that mutated Bcl-2 on BH4 domain which didn't interfere the ability of Bcl-2 to inhibit apoptosis led starved quiescent cells to enter the cell cycle much faster than wild type protein expressing cells on stimulation with cytokine or serum. It has also been suggested that whereas Bcl-2 deficiency caused the accelerated cell cycle progression, increased levels of Bcl-2 led to retarded G0 to S transition in T cells (Linette et al., 1996). It has also been reported that Bcl-2 delayed cell cycle progression by regulating S phase in ovarian carcinoma cells (Belanger et al., 2005). On the other hand, it has been reported that downregulation of Bcl-2 expression by anti-sense oligonucleotide did not change prostate cancer cells proliferation (Anai et al., 2007). Lima et al. have reported that inhibition of Bcl-2 by siRNA led to a decrease in viable cells when compared to control group. However, they further analyzed the cells with BrdU proliferation assay and there was no significant difference between the groups, concluding that decreased cell number was due to the spontaneous induction of apoptosis in MCF7 breast cancer cell line (Lima et al., 2004). Holle et al., used A T7 promoter driven siRNA expression vector system that targets Bcl-2 mRNA in MCF-7 human cancer cells, and inhibition of Bcl-2 expression inhibited cell proliferation and induced apoptosis (Holle et al., 2004).

3.3 Bcl-2 induces angiogenesis and metastasis

Recent studies suggested that Bcl-2 plays roles in metastasis, angiogenesis and autophagy. It is now established that angiogenesis plays an important role in the growth of solid and hematological tumors. Bcl-2 has been shown to induce VEGF expression, which plays a main role of in angiogenesis by regulating differentiation, migration and proliferation of endothelial cells by interacting with its receptors. Moreover, VEGF has also been recently shown to be a survival factor for both endothelial and tumor cells, preventing apoptosis through the induction of Bcl-2 expression (Biroccio et al., 2000; Fernandez et al., 2001; Iervolino et al., 2002; Nor et al., 2001). Anai et al (Anai et al., 2007) recently showed for the first time that knock-down of Bcl-2 by ASO leads to inhibition of angiogenesis in human prostate tumor xenografts. Bcl-2 ASO decreases rates of angiogenesis and proliferation by inducing G_1 cell cycle arrest and apoptosis. This was the first study which shows that therapy directed at Bcl-2 affects tumor vasculature. An increase in angiogenic potential of tumor cells after Bcl-2 transfection was also observed using different in vivo assays. In addition, Bcl-2 overexpression increases VEGF promoter activity through the HIF-1α transcription factor and transcription factors (Iervolino et al., 2002). Indeed, Bcl-2 increases

nuclear factor κB (NF-κB) transcriptional activity in the MCF7 ADR line (Ricca et al., 2000). Since NF-κB signaling blockade has been demonstrated to inhibit in vitro and in vivo expression of VEGF, it is possible that Bcl-2 affects VEGF expression through modulation of the activity of NF-κB or other transcription factors.
Bcl-2 overexpression increases the metastatic potential of MCF7 ADR breast cancer cell line by inducing cellular invasion, and migration, in vitro and in vivo (Del Bufalo et al., 1997; Ricca et al., 2000). It has also been shown that bcl-2 involves in tumorigenicity, invasion, migration, and metastasis of different tumors (Takaoka et al., 1997; Wick et al., 1998). In glioma cell lines, bcl-2 expression has been shown to correlate with matrix metalloproteinase-2 (MMP-2) therefore the invasiveness (Wick et al., 1998). On the other hand, the in vivo aggressiveness of tumors derived from cells overexpressing Bcl-2 is much more than cells which do not. It has been attributed to the anti-apoptotic properties of Bcl-2 (Fernandez et al., 2001). Zuo et al. (Zuo et al.) demonstrated a decrease in epithelial markers such as desmoglein-3, zonula occluding-1, cytokeratin and E-Cadherin and a increase in mesenchymal markers such as N-Cadherin, vimentin, fibronectin and also a transition from a cobblestone to a scattered appearance with increased bcl-2 expression. Therefore, they suggested that bcl-2 overexpression induced epithelial to mesenchymal transition and enhanced mobility and invasive character of HSC-3 human squamous carcinoma cells by promoting persistent ERK signaling and elevating MMP-9 production. Wang et al. have shown that a bcl-2 small inhibitor, TW-37, led to increased apoptosis, decreased MMP-9 and VEGF gene transcriptions and their activities consequently inhibited tumor growth in a pancreatic cancer model (Wang et al., 2008). It has been shown that bcl-2 upregulation in tumor associated endothelial cells was sufficient to enhance tumor progression in vivo (Nor et al., 2001). The same group also showed that bcl-2 expression was significantly elevated in tumor blood vessels from head and neck cancer patients as compared to control samples and when they compared bcl-2 expression in tumor blood vessels from lymph node-positive cancer patients with lymph-node negative patients, they found that lymph node-positive cancer patients had significantly higher number of bcl-2 positive blood vessels (Kumar et al., 2008). They showed in human head and neck cancer specimens that bcl-2 expression in tumor associated endothelial cells was directly linked to metastasis, they further found in an in vivo SCID mouse model that tumors with bcl-2 expressing endothelial cells showed significant increase in lung metastasis suggesting bcl-2 expression mediated metastasis through increase in angiogenesis, tumor cell invasion and blood vessel leakiness (Kumar et al., 2008).

4. Bcl-2 as a candidate for targeted therapy in breast cancers

Bcl-2 anti-apoptotic and anti-autophagic protein has been proposed as an excellent therapeutic target in various cancers to overcome resistance to conventional therapies and enhance the effects of these therapies. Previous studies suggested that downregulation of bcl-2 by ASO enhances their sensitivity to chemotherapeutic drugs, such as doxorubicin, pactitaxel, mitomycin C and cyclophosphamide in breast cancer experimental models, suggesting a downregulation of Bcl-2 may be a useful strategy to prevent drug resistance and enhance-chemosensitivity (Emi et al., 2005; Tanabe et al., 2003). Bcl-2 specific ASO (Oblimersen) in clinical studies have ended up somewhat disappointing results and tocixity (Tanabe et al, 2003). SiRNA has been shown to be 10 to 100-fold more potent than ASO and causes its degradation, leading to shut down protein expression (Bertrand et al, 2002). *In vivo* efficient delivery of the siRNA-based therapeutics into tumors , remains a great challenge. Traditionally cationic (positively charged) liposomes have been used as nonviral delivery systems for oligonucleotides (e.g., plasmid DNA, ASO, and siRNA). However, their effectiveness as potential carriers for siRNA has been limited due to the toxicity. We recently developed non-toxic, neutrally charged 1,2-dioleoyl-*sn*-glycero-3-phosphatidylcholine (DOPC)-based nanoliposomes (mean size 65nM) leading to significant and robust target gene knock down in human tumors animal models (Landen et al, 2005). We found that liposomal siRNA targeting Bcl-2 led to 73 % and 61 % inhibition in Bcl-2 target protein expression on 4 day and day 6, respectively in MDA-MB-231 tumors in mice (Tekedereli et al, in press), indicating that Bcl-2 siRNA therapeutics can be used successfully inhibit overexpressed proteins in *in vivo* therapeutic modality in cancer.

4.1 Bcl-2 expression in prognosis of breast cancer patients

Overexpression of Bcl-2 occurs in about 40 to 80% of human breast tumors (Doglioni et al., 1994; Hellemans et al., 1995; Joensuu et al., 1994) and confers drug resistance, an aggressive clinical course, and poor survival in patients (Reed, 1995). Recently, Buchholz et al, found that 61% of breast cancer patients are Bcl-2 positive and patients with positive Bcl-2 expression had a poor response to chemotherapy compared to those had less Bcl-2 expression (Buchholz et al., 2005). Because most Bcl-2 positive breast cancers express estrogen and/or progesterone receptors and respond hormonal therapy, Bcl-2 does not seem to be an independent prognostic marker in short-term (5 year) follow up (Joensuu et al., 1994). However, Bcl-2 fails to maintain its prognostic relationship in breast cancer when considered in multivariate analysis and long-term follow up studies (Daidone et al., 1999; Joensuu et al., 1994). Lack of Bcl-2 expression was associated with a higher probability of complete pathological response to doxorubicin-based chemotherapy (Pusztai et al., 2004). Antiestrogens such as tamoxifen and ICI 164384 promote apoptosis by downregulating Bcl-2 without affecting Bax, BCl-X_L or p53 (Kumar et al., 2000) and Bcl-2 upregulation plays a role in resistance to estrogens (Teixeira et al., 1995). Overall, these data suggest that tumors with a decreased level of in Bcl-2 had better response to chemotherapy and hormonal therapy, and targeting Bcl-2 is a viable strategy.

5. Concluding remarks

Apoptosis (type I) and Autophagic (type II) programmed cell death play crucial roles in such physiological processes as the development, homeostasis and elimination of unwanted or cancer cells. Autophagy is characterized by the sequestration of cytoplasmic contents through the formation of double-membrane vesicles (autophagosomes). Subsequently, the autophagosomes merge with lysosomes and digest the organelles, leading to cell death if its induced excessively. In contrast to apoptosis, autophagic cell death is caspase-independent and does not involve classic DNA laddering (Ng & Huang, 2005). Targeting autophagy is can be used as a therapeutic strategy where autophagy is induced as a protective mechanism or induction of autophagic cell death can also be used as a therapeutic strategy where apoptosis is defective or anti-apoptotic proteins is overexpressed.

6. References

Akar U, Chaves-Reyez A, Barria M, Tari A, Sanguino A, Kondo Y, Kondo S, Arun B, Lopez-Berestein G and Ozpolat B. (2008). *Autophagy*, 4, 669-79.

Akar U, Ozpolat B, Mehta K, Fok J, Kondo Y and Lopez-Berestein G. (2007). *Mol Cancer Res*, 5, 241-9.

Alvarez RH, Valero V and Hortobagyi GN (2010). *J Clin Oncol*, 28, 3366-79.

Anai S, Goodison S, Shiverick K, Hirao Y, Brown BD and Rosser CJ. (2007). *Mol Cancer Ther*, 6, 101-11.

Bardeesy N and DePinho RA. (2002). *Nat Rev Cancer*, 2, 897-909.

Beau I, Esclatine A and Codogno P. (2008). *Trends Cell Biol*, 18, 311-4.

Belanger S, Cote M, Lane D, L'Esperance S, Rancourt C and Piche A. (2005). *Gynecol Oncol*, 97, 796-806.

Bertrand,J.-R., Pottier,M., Vekris,A., Opolon,P., Maksimenko,A. and Malvy,C. (2002) Comparison of antisense oligonucleotides and siRNAs in cell culture and in vivo. Biochem. *Biophys. Res. Commun.*, 296, 1000–1004"

Biroccio A, Candiloro A, Mottolese M, Sapora O, Albini A, Zupi G and Del Bufalo D. (2000). *Faseb J*, 14, 652-60.

Bishop JM. (1991). *Cell*, 64, 235-48.

Boya P and Kroemer G. (2009). *Oncogene*, 28, 2125-7.

Buchholz TA, Garg AK, Chakravarti N, Aggarwal BB, Esteva FJ, Kuerer HM, Singletary SE, Hortobagyi GN, Pusztai L, Cristofanilli M and Sahin AA. (2005). *Clin Cancer Res*, 11, 8398-402.

Buglioni S, D'Agnano I, Cosimelli M, Vasselli S, D'Angelo C, Tedesco M, Zupi G and Mottolese M. (1999). *Int J Cancer*, 84, 545-52.

Cheng N, Janumyan YM, Didion L, Van Hofwegen C, Yang E and Knudson CM. (2004). *Oncogene*, 23, 3770-80.

Daidone MG, Luisi A, Veneroni S, Benini E and Silvestrini R. (1999). *Endocr Relat Cancer*, 6, 61-8.

Dalby KN, Tekedereli I, Lopez-Berestein G and Ozpolat B. (2010) *Autophagy*, 6, 322-9.

Del Bufalo D, Biroccio A, Leonetti C and Zupi G. (1997). *Faseb J*, 11, 947-53.

Doglioni C, Dei Tos AP, Laurino L, Chiarelli C, Barbareschi M and Viale G. (1994). *Virchows Arch*, 424, 47-51.

Emi M, Kim R, Tanabe K, Uchida Y and Toge T. (2005). *Breast Cancer Res*, 7, R940-52.

Fernandez A, Udagawa T, Schwesinger C, Beecken W, Achilles-Gerte E, McDonnell T and D'Amato R. (2001). *J Natl Cancer Inst*, 93, 208-13.

George J, Banik NL and Ray SK. (2009). *Neurochem Res*, 34, 66-78.

Glick D, Barth S and Macleod KF (2010). *J Pathol*, 221, 3-12.

Gross A, McDonnell JM and Korsmeyer SJ. (1999). *Genes Dev*, 13, 1899-911.

He C and Klionsky DJ. (2009). *Annu Rev Genet*, 43, 67-93.

Hellemans P, van Dam PA, Weyler J, van Oosterom AT, Buytaert P and Van Marck E. (1995). *Br J Cancer*, 72, 354-60.

Holle L, Hicks L, Song W, Holle E, Wagner T and Yu X. (2004). *Int J Oncol*, 24, 615-21.

Huang DC, O'Reilly LA, Strasser A and Cory S. (1997). *Embo J*, 16, 4628-38.

Iervolino A, Trisciuoglio D, Ribatti D, Candiloro A, Biroccio A, Zupi G and Del Bufalo D. (2002). *Faseb J*, 16, 1453-5.

Jemal A, Siegel R, Xu J and Ward E (2010). *CA Cancer J Clin*, 60, 277-300.

Joensuu H, Pylkkanen L and Toikkanen S. (1994). *Am J Pathol*, 145, 1191-8.

Klionsky DJ and Emr SD. (2000). *Science*, 290, 1717-21.

Konopleva M, Tari AM, Estrov Z, Harris D, Xie Z, Zhao S, Lopez-Berestein G and Andreeff M. (2000). *Blood*, 95, 3929-38.
Kumar P, Ning Y and Polverini PJ. (2008). *Lab Invest*, 88, 740-9.
Kumar R, Vadlamudi RK and Adam L. (2000). *Endocr Relat Cancer*, 7, 257-69.
Landen CN, Jr., Chavez-Reyes A, Bucana C, Schmandt R, Deavers MT, Lopez-Berestein G, Sood AK: *Cancer Res* 2005, 65:6910-6918.
Liang XH, Jackson S, Seaman M, Brown K, Kempkes B, Hibshoosh H and Levine B. (1999). *Nature*, 402, 672-6.
Lima RT, Martins LM, Guimaraes JE, Sambade C and Vasconcelos MH. (2004). *Cancer Gene Ther*, 11, 309-16.
Lin JF, Lin YC, Lin YH, Tsai TF, Chou KY, Chen HE and Hwang TI. *J Urol.*
Linette GP, Li Y, Roth K and Korsmeyer SJ. (1996). *Proc Natl Acad Sci U S A*, 93, 9545-52.
Lockshin RA, Zakeri Z. *Cell death in health and disease. J Cell Mol Med. 2007; 11:1214–24.*
Maiuri MC, Criollo A, Tasdemir E, Vicencio JM, Tajeddine N, Hickman JA, Geneste O and Kroemer G. (2007). *Autophagy*, 3, 374-6.
Mathew R, Kongara S, Beaudoin B, Karp CM, Bray K, Degenhardt K, Chen G, Jin S and White E. (2007). *Genes Dev*, 21, 1367-81.
Meterissian SH, Kontogiannea M, Al-Sowaidi M, Linjawi A, Halwani F, Jamison B and Edwardes M. (2001). *Ann Surg Oncol*, 8, 533-7.
Moretti K, Attia, Kim Lu. Autophagy 2007;3(2):142-4.
Nahta R and Esteva FJ. (2003). *Semin Oncol*, 30, 143-9.
Ng G and Huang J. (2005). *Mol Carcinog*, 43, 183-7.
Nor JE, Christensen J, Liu J, Peters M, Mooney DJ, Strieter RM and Polverini PJ. (2001). *Cancer Res*, 61, 2183-8.
Oh S, E X, Ni D, Pirooz SD, Lee JY, Lee D, Zhao Z, Lee S, Lee H, Ku B, Kowalik T, Martin SE, Oh BH, Jung JU and Liang C. *Cell Death Differ*, 18, 452-64.
Ozpolat B, Akar U, Mehta K and Lopez-Berestein G. (2007). *Autophagy*, 3, 480-3.
Ozpolat B, Sood AK, Lopez-Berestein G: *J Intern Med*, 267:44-53
Patel MP, Masood A, Patel PS and Chanan-Khan AA. (2009). *Curr Opin Oncol*, 21, 516-23.
Pattingre S and Levine B. (2006). *Cancer Res*, 66, 2885-8.
Pusztai L, Krishnamurti S, Perez Cardona J, Sneige N, Esteva FJ, Volchenok M, Breitenfelder P, Kau SW, Takayama S, Krajewski S, Reed JC, Bast RC, Jr. and Hortobagyi GN. (2004). *Cancer Invest*, 22, 248-56.
Qu X, Yu J, Bhagat G, Furuya N, Hibshoosh H, Troxel A, Rosen J, Eskelinen EL, Mizushima N, Ohsumi Y, Cattoretti G and Levine B. (2003). *J Clin Invest*, 112, 1809-20.
Reed JC. (1995). *Hematol Oncol Clin North Am*, 9, 451-73.
Ricca A, Biroccio A, Del Bufalo D, Mackay AR, Santoni A and Cippitelli M. (2000). *Int J Cancer*, 86, 188-96.
Scarlatti F, Granata R, Meijer AJ and Codogno P. (2009). *Cell Death Differ*, 16, 12-20.
Shen HM and Codogno P. *Autophagy*, 7.
Shimizu S, Kanaseki T, Mizushima N, Mizuta T, Arakawa-Kobayashi S, Thompson CB and Tsujimoto Y. (2004). *Nat Cell Biol*, 6, 1221-8.
Simoes-Wust AP, Schurpf T, Hall J, Stahel RA and Zangemeister-Wittke U. (2002). *Breast Cancer Res Treat*, 76, 157-66.
Takaoka A, Adachi M, Okuda H, Sato S, Yawata A, Hinoda Y, Takayama S, Reed JC and Imai K. (1997). *Oncogene*, 14, 2971-7.

Tanabe K, Kim R, Inoue H, Emi M, Uchida Y and Toge T. (2003). *Int J Oncol*, 22, 875-81.
Teixeira C, Reed JC and Pratt MA. (1995). *Cancer Res*, 55, 3902-7.
Tormo M, Tari AM, McDonnell TJ, Cabanillas F, Garcia-Conde J and Lopez-Berestein G. (1998). *Leuk Lymphoma*, 30, 367-79.
Wang Z, Song W, Aboukameel A, Mohammad M, Wang G, Banerjee S, Kong D, Wang S, Sarkar FH and Mohammad RM. (2008). *Int J Cancer*, 123, 958-66.
Wick W, Wagner S, Kerkau S, Dichgans J, Tonn JC and Weller M. (1998). *FEBS Lett*, 440, 419-24.
Xue L, Fletcher GC and Tolkovsky AM. (1999). *Mol Cell Neurosci*, 14, 180-98.
Yue Z, Jin S, Yang C, Levine AJ and Heintz N. (2003). *Proc Natl Acad Sci U S A*, 100, 15077-82.
Yousefi S, Perozzo R, Schmid I, Ziemiecki A, Schaffner T, Scapozza L, Brunner T. Nature Cell Biol. 8, 1124–1132 (2006)
Zuo J, Ishikawa T, Boutros S, Xiao Z, Humtsoe JO and Kramer RH. *Mol Cancer Res*, 8, 170-82.

Part 2

New Anti-Cancer Targets

5

The ATF/CREB Family of Transcription Factors in Breast Cancer

Jeremy K. Haakenson, Mark Kester and David X. Liu
Pennsylvania State University College of Medicine, USA

1. Introduction

Transcription factors are proteins that bind DNA and either promote or block gene transcription. The activating transcription factor/cyclic AMP response element binding (ATF/CREB) family of transcription factors are involved in various cellular processes, including cell stress responses, cell survival, and cell growth. In this chapter, we will first give an overview of the transcriptional regulation of oncogenesis, followed by a brief summary of the roles of ATF/CREB family members in breast cancer. After this, we will describe the structure of ATF/CREB family members and then go into detail concerning each ATF/CREB family member that has a function relevant to breast cancer. Finally, we will end the chapter with some forward-looking remarks on ATF/CREB-based breast cancer therapeutics.

2. Transcriptional regulation in breast cancer

Transcription factors play an important role in breast cancer tumorigenesis and progression. For example, ETS1, ELF3, PDEF, PEA3, HIF-1, and MYC are all transcription factors that are overexpressed in breast cancer (Kurpios and others 2003). Overexpression of MYC in MCF7 human non-metastatic breast cancer cells causes those cells to display a metastatic-like phenotype (de Launoit and others 2000). The transcriptional targets of PEA3 include MMP1, MMP3, MMP9, vimentin, and ICAM-1, genes that are involved in breast cancer cell invasion and migration (de Launoit and others 2000). Other transcription factors involved in breast cancer include snail, which blocks E-cadherin transcription (Cano and others 2000); CBP/p300, a transcriptional co-activator involved in HER2 expression (Wang and others 2001); STAT6, which blocks the immune response to breast cancer (Sinha and others 2005); and Fra-1, whose overexpression leads to increased invasion in breast cancer (Mizutani and others 2004). Like PEA3, Runx2 is also involved in breast cancer metastasis, specifically, metastasis to bone (Shore 2005). Its targets include collagenase-3 and BSP, which are upregulated in metastatic breast cancer cells (Shore 2005). Since it is well known that tumors can become hypoxic, it is not surprising that HIF-1 is overexpressed in primary breast tumors (Kimbro and Simons 2006). Its best known target is VEGF, an inducer of angiogenesis (Kimbro and Simons 2006). MYC is amplified and overexpressed in breast cancer (Chen and Olopade 2008). Its amplification is correlated with tumor progression and poor prognosis (Chen and Olopade 2008). MYC binds MAX to form a heterodimer that induces the transcription of genes such as MTA1, which is involved in transformation; PEG10, which plays a role in proliferation; hTERT; and VEGF (Chen and Olopade 2008). In a transgenic mouse model, overexpression of MYC in the mammary epithelium caused breast cancer to develop after eight months (Rose-Hellekant and Sandgren 2000). Similar to MYC, MYB is amplified in hereditary breast cancer (Kauraniemi and others 2000). MYB is involved in ER-dependent breast cancer cell proliferation (Ramsay and Gonda 2008). Its targets are anti-apoptotic genes, such as MYC, cyclin A1, and BCL2 (Ramsay and Gonda 2008).

Several transcription factors are constitutively active in breast cancer, including the aryl hydrocarbon receptor, STAT3, and NF-κB (Pensa, Watson, Poli 2009; Schlezinger and others 2006; Vogel and Matsumura 2009). The aryl hydrocarbon receptor targets CYP1B1, a P450 enzyme (Schlezinger and others 2006). STAT3 is correlated with increased breast cancer cell survival, cytoskeletal reorganization, and migration (Pensa, Watson, Poli 2009). It activates HGF (Elliott and others 2002), cyclin D1, MYC, and bcl-XL (Silva and Shupnik 2007). In addition, it blocks the transcription of p21, which is an inhibitor of cell cycle progression (Silva and Shupnik 2007). Constitutively active NF-κB, which is found in more than 90% of breast cancer (Vogel and Matsumura 2009), leads to breast cancer tumors that are hormone-independent (Wysocki and Wierusz-Wysocka 2010) and drug resistant (Garg and others 2003).

Many transcription factors act as tumor suppressors, including FoxP3, KLF10, p53, and GATA3. FoxP3, an X-linked breast cancer tumor suppressor, blocks HER2 expression (Medema and Burgering 2007). KLF10 is a transcription factor whose expression is inversely correlated with breast cancer stage (Subramaniam and others 2010). Its targets are BARD1 and Smad2, which are tumor suppressors (Subramaniam and others 2010). The tumor suppressor, p53, is mutated in about 26% of all breast cancers (Patocs and others 2007). It transactivates p21 and can also transcriptionally activate Bax1, leading to apoptosis (Ingvarsson 1999). GATA3, the most highly expressed transcription factor in the mammary epithelium (Kouros-Mehr and others 2008), is normally involved in luminal epithelial cell differentiation (Chou, Provot, Werb 2010). However, it is lost during cancer progression (Chou, Provot, Werb 2010). Indeed, decreased GATA3 expression is correlated with a worse prognosis, characterized by less differentiated, ER^- cancer (Chou, Provot, Werb 2010).

The steroid hormone receptors, which are ligand-activated nuclear receptors that act as transcription factors, deserve special mention when it comes to breast cancer. The estrogen receptor (ER) and the progesterone receptor (PR) are overexpressed in many breast cancers. This has led to the development of anti-estrogens and aromatase inhibitors for breast cancer treatment. Besides leading to breast cancer tumorigenesis, ER also induces breast cancer progression (Carroll and Brown 2006), and it is not only overexpression, but mutations and alternative splicing that can cause breast cancer (Toran-Allerand 2004). ER targets include PR, c-jun (Fang, Chen, Weigel 2009), p52/TFF1, MYC, cyclin D1, and BCL2 (Welboren and others 2009). Like ER, PR also contributes to breast cancer. The progesterone receptor causes cells to enter S phase and mediates anchorage-independent growth in response to progestin (Daniel, Knutson, Lange 2009). PR targets include MYC (Lange 2008), p21, EGFR, SGK, Tissue Factor, Muc-1, HB-EGF, and IRS-1 (Daniel, Knutson, Lange 2009). In addition to ER and PR in breast cancer, it is interesting to note that the androgen receptor (AR) protects against breast cancer. AR expression is correlated with a better prognosis (Yeap, Wilce, Leedman 2004), and mutations in the AR DNA-binding domain have been found in male breast cancer (MacLean, Warne, Zajac 1995).

3. ATF/CREB transcription factors in breast cancer

Like the transcription factors described in the previous section, the ATF/CREB family of transcription factors plays a role in breast cancer and may prove to be an effective therapeutic target. Some family members, such as ATF1, are protective against breast cancer, while the roles of others, such as ATF2 and ATF3, remain controversial. Still other family members, such as ATF4, ATF5, and CREB, promote breast cancer pathology (Table 1). These latter may be the most promising targets for intervention, since inhibiting their production or activation could block tumor growth and metastasis. The following sections will focus on the structure and function of individual ATF/CREB transcription factors.

4. Structure of ATF/CREB family members

The ATF/CREB family consists of a group of transcription factors that all contain an N-terminal DNA-binding domain and a C-terminal basic leucine zipper (B-ZIP) domain that binds other B-ZIP transcription factors to form homo- and heterodimers (Vinson and others 2002). ATF and CREB were both originally named in 1987 and were later found to bind to the same consensus sequence (Hai and Hartman 2001). The DNA-binding consensus sequence for this family is GTGACGT A/C A/G, which is found in the promoter region of target genes (Hai and Hartman 2001). Specificity is achieved by homo- and heterodimerization and epigenetic mechanisms, such as DNA methylation (Hai and Hartman 2001). For example, ATF1 forms heterodimers with CREM Ia and CREM IIb (Newman and Keating 2003). Likewise, ATF2, ATF4, and ATF5 all form heterodimers with C/EBPγ (Newman and Keating 2003). Based on the dimers that they form, ATF/CREB transcription factors are able to regulate the transcription of many target genes involved in breast cancer pathology and suppression.

5. ATF1

Several groups have identified ATF1 targets in both mice and humans. For example, Torti's group at Wake Forest found that ATF1 aids in the transcription of H ferritin in mouse fibroblasts (Tsuji, Torti, Torti 1998). Perhaps more relevant to breast cancer, ATF1 increases the transcription of $H\text{-}2D^d$, a major histocompatibility complex (MHC) class I gene (Ishiguro, Brown, Meruelo 1997). The transcription of such a gene could allow the immune system to tag breast cancer cells for destruction. Besides its effects on the immune system, ATF1 may also play a role in breast cancer via its regulation of steroidal hormone synthesis. Clem et al. (Clem, Hudson, Clark 2005) showed that ATF1 binds the steroidal acute regulatory protein (StAR) promoter, although they failed to determine whether this association activates or blocks transcription. Regardless of ATF1's effect, regulation of StAR, an enzyme necessary for estradiol synthesis, may play an important role in preventing breast cancer because a longer time of exposure to estradiol (menarche to menopause) is correlated with increased breast cancer risk. In addition to its actions on $H\text{-}2D^d$ and StAR in mice, ATF1 blocks thrombospondin1 transcription in human thyroid cancer cells (Ghoneim and others 2007). Whether or not this effect translates to breast cancer cells has yet to be confirmed. Most relevant to breast cancer is that BRCA1 activates ATF1 (Houvras and others 2000). BRCA1 and BRCA2 act as tumor suppressor genes, and they often contain mutations in breast cancer. Houvras et al. (Houvras and others 2000) found that wild type (wt) BRCA1 bound ATF1, causing transcription of a luciferase reporter gene. Such a finding strongly suggests

ATF/CREB Family Member	Role in Breast Cancer	Targets
ATF1	Most likely supresses tumor formation	H ferritin (Tsuji, 1998) H-2D^d (Ishiguro, 1997) StAR (Clem, 2005) Thrombospondin 1 (Ghoneim, 2007)
ATF2	Unclear	Collagen, type X, α1 (Tsuchimochi, 2010) MMP13 (Tsuchimochi, 2010) Cyclin A (van Dam, 2001) Aromatase (Deb, 2006) MMP2 (Song, 2006) COX2 (Subbaramaiah, 2002) Cyclin D1 (Lee, 1999) Maspin (Maekawa, 2008) IFNγ (Xue, 2005) FoxP3 (Liu, 2009)
ATF3	Unclear	Fibronectin (Yin, 2010) Snail (Yin, 2010) Twist (Yin, 2010) Slug (Yin, 2010) av integrin (Yin, 2010) β6 integrin (Yin, 2010) E-cadherin (Yin, 2010)
ATF4	Increased malignancy Angiogenesis	Osteocalcin (St-Arnaud, 2007) Type I collagen (Ameri, 2008) TRB3 (Ameri, 2008) E-selectin (Ameri, 2008) Asparagine synthetase (Ameri, 2008) RANKL (Ameri, 2008) VEGF (Ameri, 2008) GADD34 (Fels, 2006) CHOP (Fels, 2006) Gamma-synuclein (Hua, 2009) LAMP3 (Mujcic, 2009)
ATF5	Cell Survival	Phosphoenolpyruvate carboxykinase 2 (Pascual, 2008) Aldolase B (Pascual, 2008) ID1 (Gho, 2008) Egr-1 (Li, 2009; Liu, 2011) Mcl-1 (Sheng, 2010) Bcl-2 (Dluzen, 2011) Hsp27 (Wang, 2008) CYP2B6 (Pascual, 2008)
CREB	Malignancy	Aromatase (Brown, 2010) Bcl-2 (Dong, 1999)

Table 1. The roles of ATF/CREB family members in breast cancer.

that ATF1 protects against breast cancer. The fact that ATF1 associates with BRCA1, activates H-2D^d, and may block StAR synthesis indicates that it acts as a tumor suppressor in breast cancer. On the other hand, its blockage of thrombospondin would suggest that it plays a pro-tumorigenic role. However, the work with thrombospondin has not been verified *in vivo*, and such an effect may only occur in thyroid cancer cells. Unfortunately, very few studies have been performed on the role of ATF1 in breast cancer. Important future studies will elucidate the effects of ATF1 on immunity and hormone synthesis in both normal and neoplastic breast cells, as well as its role in breast cancer *in vivo.*

6. ATF2

The exact role of ATF2 in breast cancer is unclear. Targets for ATF2 have been found in both chickens and mice. One such target, Col10a1 (collagen, type X, α1), mediates chondrocyte differentiation (Tsuchimochi and others 2010). ATF2 also increases the transcription of matrix metalloproteinase 13 (MMP13), which may help facilitate breast cancer metastasis (Tsuchimochi and others 2010). Matrix metalloproteinases degrade the basement membrane during the metastatic cascade. So the fact that ATF2 enhances the transcription of MMP13 indicates that it may increase the likelihood of tumor metastasis. In addition, Jun-ATF2 dimers have been shown to lead to the transcription of cyclin A, which increases cell proliferation (van Dam and Castellazzi 2001), providing further evidence for a possible oncogenic role for ATF2.

In primary human adipose fibroblasts obtained from breast cancer patients, co-culture with malignant epithelial cells increased the levels of phosphorylated ATF2 (pATF2) found at the I.3/II promoter of aromatase, the enzyme responsible for estrogen synthesis (Deb and others 2006). Co-culture with the malignant cells also increased binding of pATF2 to itself, C/EBPβ, and CBP (Deb and others 2006). The fact that ATF2 aids in the transcription of a gene that increases estrogen levels makes it seem pro-tumorigenic. Furthermore, pATF2 has been shown to aid in the transcription of matrix metalloproteinase 2 (MMP2), which increases migration in H-Ras-transformed MCF10A human breast epithelial cells (Song and others 2006). Such activity indicates that ATF2 may play a role in breast cancer metastasis, if not oncogenesis. ATF2 also forms a complex with c-Jun and c-Fos that mediates HER2's induction of cyclooxygenase-2 (COX2), which itself may be carcinogenic (Subbaramaiah and others 2002). The fact that ATF2 is downstream of HER2 lends strong support to the notion that it is involved in some breast cancers. In addition, Lee et al. (Lee and others 1999) found that v-src causes ATF2 and CREB to bind the CRE/ATF site of the cyclin D1 gene, leading to transcription of cyclin D1 in MCF7 human breast cancer cells. Cyclin D1 inactivates the retinoblastoma tumor suppressor (RB), predisposing cells to malignancy (Hunter and Pines 1994; Sherr 1994). So ATF2's role here would again indicate that it acts as an oncogene.

In contrast to the above-mentioned studies, which describe ATF2 as contributing to a malignant phenotype, several groups have characterized it as protective against breast cancer. For instance, Maekawa et al. found that knockout of ATF2 increased cell number, decreased apoptosis, and increased the number of v-K-ras-induced colonies in mouse embryonic fibroblasts (MEF's) (Maekawa and others 2007). Plus, knockdown of ATF2 decreased levels of one of its targets, the breast cancer suppressor, maspin, in the mammary tumors of $ATF2^{+/-}$ mice (Maekawa and others 2007; Maekawa and others 2008). Such findings would support the argument that ATF2 inhibits breast cancer formation. Along those lines, ATF2 has been shown to bind to the proximal element of interferon gamma (IFNγ) in MCF7 cells (Xue, Firestone, Bjeldanes 2005). Increased production and secretion of IFNγ by breast cancer cells could help the immune system destroy malignant cells before they spread, thereby inhibiting tumor growth and preventing metastasis. In a similar vein, decreased ATF2 levels have been shown to diminish the level of FoxP3, a breast cancer tumor suppressor (Liu and others 2009), lending further support to the idea that ATF2 inhibits breast cancer. However, studies in a wide range of human breast cancer cell lines are needed in order to definitively determine ATF2's role in breast cancer.

7. ATF3

Like ATF2, ATF3's role in breast cancer remains poorly delineated, although recent evidence characterizes it as an oncogene that may be involved in metastasis. Yin et al. (Yin and others 2010) found that ATF3 mediates the TGFβ-induced increase in the expression of fibronectin, twist, snail, and slug in MCF10C1a1 human breast cancer cells. In addition, ATF3 overexpression led to an increase in av and β6 integrins, as well as increased migration in MCF10C1a1 cells (Yin and others 2010). Furthermore, ATF3 caused a decrease in E-cadherin expression, as well as other genetic and morphological changes characteristic of the epithelial to mesenchymal transition (EMT) (Yin and others 2010). All of these findings support the idea tha ATF3 mediates EMT and metastasis in breast cancer. In addition, ATF3 also supports oncogenesis, as overexpression of ATF3 in MCF10C1a1 cell that were injected into nude mice increased the incidence of tumor formation (Yin and others 2010). Similarly, overexpression of ATF3 in the mammary gland myoepithelial cells of transgenic mice caused squamous metaplasia in nulliparous females and led to the formation of mammary tumors in animals that had given birth twice (Wang and others 2008). This is perhaps the most convincing evidence that ATF3 acts as an oncogene in breast cancer.

All of the above findings on ATF3 seem to establish it as an oncogene and metastasis promoter, yet some doubt remains. Einbond et al. (Einbond and others 2007) found that actein decreased cell proliferation in mouse embryonic fibroblasts (MEF's) in an ATF3-dependent manner. However, this finding may pertain only to MEF's and not to breast cancer cells. Other groups have found that the anti-neoplastic agents, doxorubicin and gemcitabine, increase ATF3 levels in human breast cancer cell lines (Hernandez-Vargas and others 2007; Mallory and others 2005). However, it remains unclear whether these drugs are acting through ATF3 or ATF3 is upregulated as part of an intracellular compensatory response. The best evidence that we have today suggests that ATF3 acts to promote tumorigenesis and metastasis. However, more studies must be conducted in order to confirm these results.

8. ATF4

Unlike ATF2 and ATF3, ATF4 is clearly pro-tumorigenic in breast cancer. Perhaps most telling, increased ATF4 levels have been found in human tumors compared to normal tissue (Ameri and Harris 2008), and several ATF4 targets indicate an oncogenic phenotype. Targets of ATF4 include osteocalcin (St-Arnaud and Elchaarani 2007), type I collagen, TRB3, E-selectin, and asparagine synthetase (Ameri and Harris 2008). More relevant to cancer, ATF4 acts as an activating transcription factor for RANKL, which activates Akt/PKB, an anti-apoptotic enzyme (Ameri and Harris 2008). Such activity in the breast would favor the formation of cancer. Besides RANKL expression, ATF4 also induces VEGF transcription (Ameri and Harris 2008), which can lead to angiogenesis at the sites of primary and secondary tumors, allowing hypoxic tumors to reach normoxia. In addition, ATF4 likely protects tumor cells form hypoxia by increasing the transcription of GADD34 and CHOP, which protect cells from hypoxic damage (Fels and Koumenis 2006). The center of a tumor often becomes hypoxic, and ATF4 may play a role in preventing hypoxia-induced cancer cell death. Although ATF4 benefits the organism during development, bone formation, and stress, it can also act in a sinister fashion by aiding in tumor formation.

Indeed, several studies have shown a link between ATF4 levels and a more malignant genotype in human breast cancer cells. For instance, decreased ATF4 levels have been shown to cause a decrease in gamma-synuclein levels in T47D breast cancer cells (Hua and others 2009). Such a correlation with gamma-synuclein, which is up-regulated in advanced breast cancer (Bruening and others 2000), may indicate that ATF4 mediates breast tumor progression. Furthermore, hypoxia has been shown to increase LAMP3 levels in MCF7 cells via the action of ATF4 (Mujcic and others 2009). This further implicates ATF4 in tumor progression and metastasis, as LAMP3 has been shown to play a role in metastasis (Mujcic and others 2009). Interestingly, this finding suggests that hypoxic tumors may be more likely to metastasize than those with an adequate blood supply. Finally, ATF4 has been shown to mediate the osteopontin-induced increase in VEGF expression in MDA-MB-231 cells (Chakraborty, Jain, Kundu 2008). Since VEGF secretion leads to the recruitment of endothelial cells as part of the process of angiogenesis, this would suggest that ATF4 is able to help primary and secondary breast tumors survive, at least once osteopontin has activated it. Clearly, overexpression or constitutive activation of ATF4 causes breast cancer cells to become more malignant.

9. ATF5

Like ATF4, ATF5 contributes to a malignant phenotype. Targets of ATF5 include aldolase B (Pascual and others 2008), ID1 (Gho and others 2008), Egr-1 (Li and others 2009; Liu and others 2011), Mcl-1 (Sheng and others 2010), Bcl-2 (Dluzen and others 2011), and phosphoenolpyruvate carboxykinase 2 (PEPCK) (Pascual and others 2008). Up-regulation of PEPCK, a glycolytic enzyme, could indicate that ATF5 plays a role in the Warburg effect, in which cancer cells use aerobic glycolysis to generate ATP rather than oxidative phosphorylation. It is thought that this use of a less efficient means of producing ATP allows proliferating cells to more efficiently produce other needed metabolites, such as acetyl-CoA and NADPH (Vander Heiden, Cantley, Thompson 2009). In addition to increasing PEPCK production, ATF5 activates the transcription of heat shock protein 27 (Hsp27), which blocks apoptosis (Wang, Lin, Zhang 2007). Such an anti-apoptotic mechanism may lead to breast cancer oncogenesis. Furthermore, ATF5 has been shown to increase the level of CYP2B6 in human hepatoma cells (Pascual and others 2008). This P450 enzyme metabolizes cyclophosphamide, which is used to treat breast cancer. Thus, by inducing an enzyme that degrades cyclophosphamide, ATF5 may contribute not only to oncogenesis, but also to drug resistance. Based on the target genes that it up-regulates, such as Hsp27 and CYP2B6, ATF5 should be pro-tumorigenic in breast cancer.

Indeed, our recent studies indicate that ATF5 induces transcription of the pro-mitogenic early growth response factor (Egr-1) gene in MCF7 human breast cancer cells (Li and others 2009; Liu and others 2011). In addition, ATF5 also binds the Bcl-2 P2 promoter and transactivates Bcl-2, an anti-apoptotic gene, leading to breast cancer cell survival (Dluzen and others 2011). In the future, we may see ATF5 inhibitors used to treat breast cancer, as inhibition of ATF5 leads to cell death in breast cancer cells but not human breast epithelial cells (HBEC's) (Dluzen and others 2011). To this end, we have recently found that Hsp70 interacts with the N-terminal of ATF5 and protects ATF5 from both caspase- and proteosome-dependent protein degradation (Li and others, 2011). The next step will involve using *in vivo* studies to determine the efficacy and toxicity of ATF5 inhibitors as treatments for breast cancer.

10. CREB

Similar to ATF5, CREB can contribute to malignancy of the breast. Importantly, CREB induces the transcription of aromatase in breast adipose mesenchymal cells (Brown and Simpson 2010). Increased levels of aromatase will lead to increased estrogen levels, which have been implicated in breast cancer. In fact, aromatase inhibitors, such as exemestane and anastrazole, are currently used to treat breast cancer (Goodman and others 2006). As an example of positive feedback regulation, estrogen causes CREB to bind and activate the cyclin D1 promoter (Castro-Rivera, Samudio, Safe 2001). By activating cyclin D1, which causes cells to progress through the cell cycle, activation of CREB may further contribute to carcinogenesis. In addition, dominant negative CREB has been shown to block the transcription of bcl-2 in MCF7 cells (Dong and others 1999). Since bcl-2 blocks apoptosis, this implicates CREB as being proto-oncogenic. Although good *in vitro* studies have been done on the role of CREB in breast cancer, *in vivo* studies are needed to confirm its status as a transcription factor that supports tumor growth.

11. Conclusions

A host of transcription factors regulate breast cancer, acting as both oncogenes and tumor suppressors. The ATF/CREB family is an example of a group of transcription factors involved in breast cancer development, with some family members leading to breast cancer pathogenesis and some blocking it. Therapeutic approaches that target members that are oncogenic may lead to the next generation of breast cancer therapies. A drug that inhibits those three genes without affecting other members of the ATF/CREB family could be especially powerful because it could block many downstream targets at once. An appropriate drug discovery screen would use luciferase assays of ATF 1-5 and CREB. Compounds that inhibit ATF4, ATF5, and CREB while not affecting ATF1, ATF2, and ATF3 would be considered hits. The screen could initially compare a highly metastatic breast cancer cell line, such as 410.4 cells to a normal mammary epithelial cell line, such as HC11 cells. The screen would then be confirmed in both ER^+ (MCF7) and ER^- (MDA-MB-231) cells. Such a screen could lead to efficacious new breast cancer therapeutics with relatively little toxicity.

12. Acknowledgements

This work was supported in part by NIH grant R01HL076789 and Tobacco Settlement Fund, State of Pennsylvania to M.K. and American Cancer Society Research Scholar Award RSG-08-288-01-GMC and Department of Defense grant BC085617 to D.X.L.

13. Abbreviations

Acetyl-CoA, acetyl coenzyme A; ATF/CREB, activating transcription factor/cyclic AMP response element binding; BARD1, BRCA1 associated RING domain 1; Bcl-2, B-cell

CLL/lymphoma 2; BRCA1, breast cancer 1, early onset; BRCA2, breast cancer 2, early onset; BSP, integrin-binding sialoprotein; C/EBPβ, CCAAT/enhancer binding protein, beta; C/EBPγ, CCAAT/enhancer binding protein, gamma; CHOP, DNA-damage-inducible transcript 3; CREM, cyclic AMP responsive element modulator; CYP1B1, cytochrome P450, family 1, subfamily B, polypeptide 1; CYP2B6, cytochrome P450, family 2, subfamily B, polypeptide 6; EGFR, epidermal growth factor receptor; Egr-1, early growth response 1; ELF3, E74-like factor 3 (ets domain transcription factor, epithelial specific); ER, estrogen receptor; ETS1, v-ets erythroblastosis virus E26 oncogene homolog 1 (avian); GADD34, protein phosphatase 1, regulatory (inhibitor) subunit 15A; GATA3, GATA binding protein 3; HB-EGF, heparin-binding EGF-like growth factor; HER2, v-erb-b2 erythroblastic leukemia viral oncogene homolog 2, neuro/glioblastoma derived oncogene homolog (avian); HIF-1, hypoxia inducible factor 1; Hsp27, heat shock protein 27; Hsp70, heat shock protein 70; hTERT, human telomerase reverse transcriptase; ICAM-1, intercellular adhesion molecule 1; ID1, inhibitor of DNA binding 1, dominant negative helix-loop-helix protein; IRS-1, insulin receptor substrate 1; KLF10, Kruppel-like factor 10; LAMP3, lysosomal-associated membrane protein 3; MAX, MYC associated factor X; Mcl-1, myeloid cell leukemia sequence 1 (BCL2-related); MMP1, matrix metallopeptidase 1 (interstitial collagenase); MMP2, matrix metallopeptidase 2 (gelatinase A, 72 kDa gelatinase, 72 kDa type IV collagenase); MMP3, matrix metallopeptidase 3 (stromelysin 1, progelatinase); MMP9, matrix metallopeptidase 9 (gelatinase B, 92kDa gelatinase, 92kDa type IV collagenase); MTA1, metastasis associated 1; MYB, v-myb myeloblastosis viral oncogene homolog (avian); MYC, v-myc myelocytomatosis viral oncogene homolog (avian); NADPH, nicotinamide adenine dinucleotide phosphate; NF-κB, nuclear factor of kappa light polypeptide gene enhancer in B cells; PDEF, SAM pointed domain containing ets transcription factor; PEA3, ets variant 4; PEG10, paternally expressed 10; RANKL, tumor necrosis factor (ligand) superfamily, member 11; SGK, serum/glucocorticoid regulated kinase; STAT3, signal transducer and activator of transcription 3 (acute-phase response factor); STAT6, signal transducer and activator of transcription 6, interleukin 4-induced; TGFβ, transforming growth factor, beta; TRB3, tribbles homolog 3 (Drosophila); VEGF, vascular endothelial growth factor.

14. References

Ameri K and Harris AL. 2008. Activating transcription factor 4. Int J Biochem Cell Biol 40(1):14-21.

Brown KA and Simpson ER. 2010. Obesity and breast cancer: Progress to understanding the relationship. Cancer Res 70(1):4-7.

Bruening W, Giasson BI, Klein-Szanto AJ, Lee VM, Trojanowski JQ, Godwin AK. 2000. Synucleins are expressed in the majority of breast and ovarian carcinomas and in preneoplastic lesions of the ovary. Cancer 88(9):2154-63.

Cano A, Perez-Moreno MA, Rodrigo I, Locascio A, Blanco MJ, del Barrio MG, Portillo F, Nieto MA. 2000. The transcription factor snail controls epithelial-mesenchymal transitions by repressing E-cadherin expression. Nat Cell Biol 2(2):76-83.

Carroll JS and Brown M. 2006. Estrogen receptor target gene: An evolving concept. Mol Endocrinol 20(8):1707-14.

Castro-Rivera E, Samudio I, Safe S. 2001. Estrogen regulation of cyclin D1 gene expression in ZR-75 breast cancer cells involves multiple enhancer elements. J Biol Chem 276(33):30853-61.

Chakraborty G, Jain S, Kundu GC. 2008. Osteopontin promotes vascular endothelial growth factor-dependent breast tumor growth and angiogenesis via autocrine and paracrine mechanisms. Cancer Res 68(1):152-61.

Chen Y and Olopade OI. 2008. MYC in breast tumor progression. Expert Rev Anticancer Ther 8(10):1689-98.

Chou J, Provot S, Werb Z. 2010. GATA3 in development and cancer differentiation: Cells GATA have it! J Cell Physiol 222(1):42-9.

Clem BF, Hudson EA, Clark BJ. 2005. Cyclic adenosine 3',5'-monophosphate (cAMP) enhances cAMP-responsive element binding (CREB) protein phosphorylation and phospho-CREB interaction with the mouse steroidogenic acute regulatory protein gene promoter. Endocrinology 146(3):1348-56.

Daniel AR, Knutson TP, Lange CA. 2009. Signaling inputs to progesterone receptor gene regulation and promoter selectivity. Mol Cell Endocrinol 308(1-2):47-52.

de Launoit Y, Chotteau-Lelievre A, Beaudoin C, Coutte L, Netzer S, Brenner C, Huvent I, Baert JL. 2000. The PEA3 group of ETS-related transcription factors. role in breast cancer metastasis. Adv Exp Med Biol 480:107-16.

Deb S, Zhou J, Amin SA, Imir AG, Yilmaz MB, Lin Z, Bulun SE. 2006. A novel role of sodium butyrate in the regulation of cancer-associated aromatase promoters I.3 and II by disrupting a transcriptional complex in breast adipose fibroblasts. J Biol Chem 281(5):2585-97.

Dluzen D, Li G, Tacelosky D, Moreau M, Liu DX. 2011. BCL-2 is a downstream target of ATF5 that mediates the prosurvival function of ATF5 in a cell type-dependent manner. J Biol Chem 286(9):7705-13.

Dong L, Wang W, Wang F, Stoner M, Reed JC, Harigai M, Samudio I, Kladde MP, Vyhlidal C, Safe S. 1999. Mechanisms of transcriptional activation of bcl-2 gene expression by 17beta-estradiol in breast cancer cells. J Biol Chem 274(45):32099-107.

Einbond LS, Su T, Wu HA, Friedman R, Wang X, Ramirez A, Kronenberg F, Weinstein IB. 2007. The growth inhibitory effect of actein on human breast cancer cells is associated with activation of stress response pathways. Int J Cancer 121(9):2073-83.

Elliott BE, Hung WL, Boag AH, Tuck AB. 2002. The role of hepatocyte growth factor (scatter factor) in epithelial-mesenchymal transition and breast cancer. Can J Physiol Pharmacol 80(2):91-102.

Fang SH, Chen Y, Weigel RJ. 2009. GATA-3 as a marker of hormone response in breast cancer. J Surg Res 157(2):290-5.

Fels DR and Koumenis C. 2006. The PERK/eIF2alpha/ATF4 module of the UPR in hypoxia resistance and tumor growth. Cancer Biol Ther 5(7):723-8.

Garg AK, Hortobagyi GN, Aggarwal BB, Sahin AA, Buchholz TA. 2003. Nuclear factor-kappa B as a predictor of treatment response in breast cancer. Curr Opin Oncol 15(6):405-11.

Gho JW, Ip WK, Chan KY, Law PT, Lai PB, Wong N. 2008. Re-expression of transcription factor ATF5 in hepatocellular carcinoma induces G2-M arrest. Cancer Res 68(16):6743-51.

Ghoneim C, Soula-Rothhut M, Blanchevoye C, Martiny L, Antonicelli F, Rothhut B. 2007. Activating transcription factor-1-mediated hepatocyte growth factor-induced down-regulation of thrombospondin-1 expression leads to thyroid cancer cell invasion. J Biol Chem 282(21):15490-7.

Goodman LS, Gilman A, Brunton LL, Lazo JS, Parker KL. 2006. Goodman & gilman's the pharmacological basis of therapeutics. 11th ed. New York: McGraw-Hill.

Hai T and Hartman MG. 2001. The molecular biology and nomenclature of the activating transcription factor/cAMP responsive element binding family of transcription factors: Activating transcription factor proteins and homeostasis. Gene 273(1):1-11.

Hernandez-Vargas H, Rodriguez-Pinilla SM, Julian-Tendero M, Sanchez-Rovira P, Cuevas C, Anton A, Rios MJ, Palacios J, Moreno-Bueno G. 2007. Gene expression profiling of breast cancer cells in response to gemcitabine: NF-kappaB pathway activation as a potential mechanism of resistance. Breast Cancer Res Treat 102(2):157-72.

Houvras Y, Benezra M, Zhang H, Manfredi JJ, Weber BL, Licht JD. 2000. BRCA1 physically and functionally interacts with ATF1. J Biol Chem 275(46):36230-7.

Hua H, Xu L, Wang J, Jing J, Luo T, Jiang Y. 2009. Up-regulation of gamma-synuclein contributes to cancer cell survival under endoplasmic reticulum stress. J Pathol 217(4):507-15.

Hunter T and Pines J. 1994. Cyclins and cancer. II: Cyclin D and CDK inhibitors come of age. Cell 79(4):573-82.

Ingvarsson S. 1999. Molecular genetics of breast cancer progression. Semin Cancer Biol 9(4):277-88.

Ishiguro N, Brown GD, Meruelo D. 1997. Activation transcription factor 1 involvement in the regulation of murine H-2Dd expression. J Biol Chem 272(25):15993-6001.

Kauraniemi P, Hedenfalk I, Persson K, Duggan DJ, Tanner M, Johannsson O, Olsson H, Trent JM, Isola J, Borg A. 2000. MYB oncogene amplification in hereditary BRCA1 breast cancer. Cancer Res 60(19):5323-8.

Kimbro KS and Simons JW. 2006. Hypoxia-inducible factor-1 in human breast and prostate cancer. Endocr Relat Cancer 13(3):739-49.

Kouros-Mehr H, Kim JW, Bechis SK, Werb Z. 2008. GATA-3 and the regulation of the mammary luminal cell fate. Curr Opin Cell Biol 20(2):164-70.

Kurpios NA, Sabolic NA, Shepherd TG, Fidalgo GM, Hassell JA. 2003. Function of PEA3 ets transcription factors in mammary gland development and oncogenesis. J Mammary Gland Biol Neoplasia 8(2):177-90.

Lange CA. 2008. Integration of progesterone receptor action with rapid signaling events in breast cancer models. J Steroid Biochem Mol Biol 108(3-5):203-12.

Lee RJ, Albanese C, Stenger RJ, Watanabe G, Inghirami G, Haines GK,3rd, Webster M, Muller WJ, Brugge JS, Davis RJ, et al. 1999. pp60(v-src) induction of cyclin D1 requires collaborative interactions between the extracellular signal-regulated kinase, p38, and jun kinase pathways. A role for cAMP response element-binding protein and activating transcription factor-2 in pp60(v-src) signaling in breast cancer cells. J Biol Chem 274(11):7341-50.

Li G, Li W, Angelastro JM, Greene LA, Liu DX. 2009. Identification of a novel DNA binding site and a transcriptional target for activating transcription factor 5 in c6 glioma and mcf-7 breast cancer cells. Mol Cancer Res 7(6):933-43.

Li G, Xu Y, Guan D, Liu Z, Liu DX. 2011. HSP70 protein promotes survival of C6 and U87 glioma cells by inhibition of ATF5 degradation. J Biol Chem 286(23):20251-9.

Liu DX, Qian D, Wang B, Yang JM, Lu Z. 2011. p300-dependent ATF5 acetylation is essential for Egr-1 gene activation and cell proliferation and survival. Mol Cell Biol 31(18):3906-16.

Liu Y, Wang Y, Li W, Zheng P, Liu Y. 2009. Activating transcription factor 2 and c-jun-mediated induction of FoxP3 for experimental therapy of mammary tumor in the mouse. Cancer Res 69(14):5954-60.

MacLean HE, Warne GL, Zajac JD. 1995. Defects of androgen receptor function: From sex reversal to motor neurone disease. Mol Cell Endocrinol 112(2):133-41.

Maekawa T, Sano Y, Shinagawa T, Rahman Z, Sakuma T, Nomura S, Licht JD, Ishii S. 2008. ATF-2 controls transcription of maspin and GADD45 alpha genes independently from p53 to suppress mammary tumors. Oncogene 27(8):1045-54.

Maekawa T, Shinagawa T, Sano Y, Sakuma T, Nomura S, Nagasaki K, Miki Y, Saito-Ohara F, Inazawa J, Kohno T, et al. 2007. Reduced levels of ATF-2 predispose mice to mammary tumors. Mol Cell Biol 27(5):1730-44.

Mallory JC, Crudden G, Oliva A, Saunders C, Stromberg A, Craven RJ. 2005. A novel group of genes regulates susceptibility to antineoplastic drugs in highly tumorigenic breast cancer cells. Mol Pharmacol 68(6):1747-56.

Medema RH and Burgering BM. 2007. The X factor: Skewing X inactivation towards cancer. Cell 129(7):1253-4.

Mizutani N, Luo Y, Mizutani M, Reisfeld RA, Xiang R. 2004. DNA vaccines suppress angiogenesis and protect against growth of breast cancer metastases. Breast Dis 20:81-91.

Mujcic H, Rzymski T, Rouschop KM, Koritzinsky M, Milani M, Harris AL, Wouters BG. 2009. Hypoxic activation of the unfolded protein response (UPR) induces expression of the metastasis-associated gene LAMP3. Radiother Oncol 92(3):450-9.

Newman JR and Keating AE. 2003. Comprehensive identification of human bZIP interactions with coiled-coil arrays. Science 300(5628):2097-101.

Pascual M, Gomez-Lechon MJ, Castell JV, Jover R. 2008. ATF5 is a highly abundant liver-enriched transcription factor that cooperates with constitutive androstane receptor in the transactivation of CYP2B6: Implications in hepatic stress responses. Drug Metab Dispos 36(6):1063-72.

Patocs A, Zhang L, Xu Y, Weber F, Caldes T, Mutter GL, Platzer P, Eng C. 2007. Breast-cancer stromal cells with TP53 mutations and nodal metastases. N Engl J Med 357(25):2543-51.

Pensa S, Watson CJ, Poli V. 2009. Stat3 and the inflammation/acute phase response in involution and breast cancer. J Mammary Gland Biol Neoplasia 14(2):121-9.

Ramsay RG and Gonda TJ. 2008. MYB function in normal and cancer cells. Nat Rev Cancer 8(7):523-34.

Rose-Hellekant TA and Sandgren EP. 2000. Transforming growth factor alpha- and c-myc-induced mammary carcinogenesis in transgenic mice. Oncogene 19(8):1092-6.

Schlezinger JJ, Liu D, Farago M, Seldin DC, Belguise K, Sonenshein GE, Sherr DH. 2006. A role for the aryl hydrocarbon receptor in mammary gland tumorigenesis. Biol Chem 387(9):1175-87.

Sheng Z, Li L, Zhu LJ, Smith TW, Demers A, Ross AH, Moser RP, Green MR. 2010. A genome-wide RNA interference screen reveals an essential CREB3L2-ATF5-MCL1 survival pathway in malignant glioma with therapeutic implications. Nat Med 16(6):671-7.

Sherr CJ. 1994. The ins and outs of RB: Coupling gene expression to the cell cycle clock. Trends Cell Biol 4(1):15-8.

Shore P. 2005. A role for Runx2 in normal mammary gland and breast cancer bone metastasis. J Cell Biochem 96(3):484-9.

Silva CM and Shupnik MA. 2007. Integration of steroid and growth factor pathways in breast cancer: Focus on signal transducers and activators of transcription and their potential role in resistance. Mol Endocrinol 21(7):1499-512.

Sinha P, Clements VK, Miller S, Ostrand-Rosenberg S. 2005. Tumor immunity: A balancing act between T cell activation, macrophage activation and tumor-induced immune suppression. Cancer Immunol Immunother 54(11):1137-42.

Song H, Ki SH, Kim SG, Moon A. 2006. Activating transcription factor 2 mediates matrix metalloproteinase-2 transcriptional activation induced by p38 in breast epithelial cells. Cancer Res 66(21):10487-96.

St-Arnaud R and Elchaarani B. 2007. Identification of additional dimerization partners of FIAT, the factor inhibiting ATF4-mediated transcription. Ann N Y Acad Sci 1116:208-15.

Subbaramaiah K, Norton L, Gerald W, Dannenberg AJ. 2002. Cyclooxygenase-2 is overexpressed in HER-2/neu-positive breast cancer: Evidence for involvement of AP-1 and PEA3. J Biol Chem 277(21):18649-57.

Subramaniam M, Hawse JR, Rajamannan NM, Ingle JN, Spelsberg TC. 2010. Functional role of KLF10 in multiple disease processes. Biofactors 36(1):8-18.

Toran-Allerand CD. 2004. Minireview: A plethora of estrogen receptors in the brain: Where will it end? Endocrinology 145(3):1069-74.

Tsuchimochi K, Otero M, Dragomir CL, Plumb DA, Zerbini LF, Libermann TA, Marcu KB, Komiya S, Ijiri K, Goldring MB. 2010. GADD45beta enhances Col10a1 transcription via the MTK1/MKK3/6/p38 axis and activation of C/EBPbeta-TAD4 in terminally differentiating chondrocytes. J Biol Chem 285(11):8395-407.

Tsuji Y, Torti SV, Torti FM. 1998. Activation of the ferritin H enhancer, FER-1, by the cooperative action of members of the AP1 and Sp1 transcription factor families. J Biol Chem 273(5):2984-92.

van Dam H and Castellazzi M. 2001. Distinct roles of jun : Fos and jun : ATF dimers in oncogenesis. Oncogene 20(19):2453-64.

Vander Heiden MG, Cantley LC, Thompson CB. 2009. Understanding the warburg effect: The metabolic requirements of cell proliferation. Science 324(5930):1029-33.

Vinson C, Myakishev M, Acharya A, Mir AA, Moll JR, Bonovich M. 2002. Classification of human B-ZIP proteins based on dimerization properties. Mol Cell Biol 22(18):6321-35.

Vogel CF and Matsumura F. 2009. A new cross-talk between the aryl hydrocarbon receptor and RelB, a member of the NF-kappaB family. Biochem Pharmacol 77(4):734-45.

Wang A, Arantes S, Yan L, Kiguchi K, McArthur MJ, Sahin A, Thames HD, Aldaz CM, Macleod MC. 2008. The transcription factor ATF3 acts as an oncogene in mouse mammary tumorigenesis. BMC Cancer 8:268.

Wang H, Lin G, Zhang Z. 2007. ATF5 promotes cell survival through transcriptional activation of Hsp27 in H9c2 cells. Cell Biol Int 31(11):1309-15.

Wang SC, Zhang L, Hortobagyi GN, Hung MC. 2001. Targeting HER2: Recent developments and future directions for breast cancer patients. Semin Oncol 28(6 Suppl 18):21-9.

Welboren WJ, Sweep FC, Span PN, Stunnenberg HG. 2009. Genomic actions of estrogen receptor alpha: What are the targets and how are they regulated? Endocr Relat Cancer 16(4):1073-89.

Wysocki PJ and Wierusz-Wysocka B. 2010. Obesity, hyperinsulinemia and breast cancer: Novel targets and a novel role for metformin. Expert Rev Mol Diagn 10(4):509-19.

Xue L, Firestone GL, Bjeldanes LF. 2005. DIM stimulates IFNgamma gene expression in human breast cancer cells via the specific activation of JNK and p38 pathways. Oncogene 24(14):2343-53.

Yeap BB, Wilce JA, Leedman PJ. 2004. The androgen receptor mRNA. Bioessays 26(6):672-82.

Yin X, Wolford CC, Chang YS, McConoughey SJ, Ramsey SA, Aderem A, Hai T. 2010. ATF3, an adaptive-response gene, enhances TGF{beta} signaling and cancer-initiating cell features in breast cancer cells. J Cell Sci 123(Pt 20):3558-65.

6

Newly-Recognized Small Molecule Receptors on Human Breast Cancer Cell Integrin αvβ3 that Affect Tumor Cell Behavior

Hung-Yun Lin[1], Faith B. Davis[1], Mary K. Luidens[1,2], Aleck Hercbergs[3], Shaker A. Mousa[4], Dhruba J. Bharali[4] and Paul J. Davis[1,2]

[1]Signal Transduction Laboratory, Ordway Research Institute, Albany, NY,
[2]Albany Medical College, Albany, NY,
[3]Cleveland Clinic, Cleveland, OH,
[4]Pharmaceutical Research Institute,
Albany College of Pharmacy, Albany, NY,
USA

1. Introduction

Hormonal regulation of the growth of breast cancer cells has been largely seen to result from interactions of estrogen and progestins with nuclear receptors for these steroids that may reside, unliganded, in cytoplasm or be transcriptionally active as steroid-protein nuclear receptor complexes. Receptors for nonpeptide hormones exist in the plasma membrane, however, and when activated may stimulate breast cancer cell proliferation. For example, the functional classical estrogen receptor-α (ERα) is found in the cell membrane. Recently, the identification has been made of a novel receptor for thyroid hormone and for dihydrotestosterone (DHT) on the plasma membrane of cells; this receptor is the αvβ3 integrin, which promotes proliferation of human breast cancer cells by these two hormones. Integrins are heterodimeric structural proteins of the plasma membrane whose primary functions are to interact with extracellular matrix proteins and growth factors. One integrin, αvβ3, bears discrete receptors for thyroid hormone (L-thyroxine, T4; 3, 5, 3′-triiodo-L-thyronine, T3) and for DHT. A receptor for the polyalcohol, resveratrol, also exists on this integrin in breast cancer cells, mediating the anti-proliferative, pro-apoptotic action of this compound. Resveratrol has certain structural features that are estrogen-like. Disparate actions of T4, T3, DHT and resveratrol that are initiated at the integrin depend downstream upon stimulation of the activity of mitogen-activated protein kinase (MAPK), suggesting the existence of distinct, function-specific pools of MAPK within the cell. Tetraiodothyroacetic acid (tetrac) is a model specific inhibitor of hormone actions on the thyroid hormone integrin receptor. Tetrac and a nanoparticulate formulation of tetrac block stimulation by thyroid hormone analogues of cancer cell proliferation and of angiogenesis. Interestingly, tetrac also acts in the absence of T4 and T3 to block the tumor-relevant angiogenic responses to vascular growth factors, e.g., vascular endothelial growth factor (VEGF), basic fibroblast growth factor (bFGF) and other growth factors. Tetrac and nanoparticulate tetrac also disable expressions of families of genes important to cancer cell survival pathways. This chapter reviews the functions of the several nonpeptide hormone receptors on integrin $\alpha v\beta 3$.

The possibility that the hormone-directed biology of the breast cancer cell might be in part regulated from the cell surface was first suggested by the identification of estrogen receptor protein in the plasma membrane (Levin, 1999). Discrete receptors on the plasma membrane $\alpha v\beta 3$ integrin of breast cancer cells have also recently been described for thyroid hormone (Bergh *et al.*, 2005; Cheng *et al.*, 2010; Davis, P. *et al.*, 2011), for dihydrotestosterone (DHT) (Lin, H. *et al.*, 2009b) and for resveratrol (Lin, H. *et al.*, 2006). The several functions of these membrane receptors include modulation of cancer cell proliferation and, in the case of thyroid hormone, of tumor-relevant angiogenesis (Cheng *et al.*, 2010; Mousa *et al.*, 2009). Expression of integrin $\alpha v\beta 3$ is concentrated in tumor cells and rapidly-dividing endothelial and vascular smooth muscle cells, so that receptors for these hormones—and resveratrol is a polyalcohol with estrogen-like structural features—may be considered targets for manipulation of breast cancer. In the present review we will describe the features of these receptors in the breast cancer cell, and will also propose clinical therapeutic applications that are based on inhibition of these small molecule plasma membrane receptors.

2. Thyroid hormone stimulates human breast cancer cell proliferation via plasma membraneilntegrin $\alpha v\beta 3$

In the absence of estrogen, thyroid hormone (L-thyroxine [T_4]) was shown in 2004 to enhance proliferation of human estrogen receptor-α (ERα)-positive breast cancer cells (Tang *et al.*, 2004). The thyroid hormone effect required extracellular-regulated kinases 1 and 2 (ERK1/2)-dependent phosphorylation of Ser-118 of ERα, precisely mimicking the action of estradiol (Kato *et al.*, 1995) on breast cancer cell proliferation. The nuclear estrogen receptor inhibitor ICI 182,780 (Fulvestrant®) blocked this action of thyroid hormone (Lin H. , unpublished), as did tetraiodothyroacetic acid (tetrac), an analogue of T_4 in which the alanine side chain of T_4 is converted to acetic acid (Tang *et al.*, 2004). Tetrac is an inhibitor of actions of T_4 and T_3 that are initiated at the thyroid hormone receptor site on integrin $\alpha v\beta 3$ (Bergh *et al.*, 2005; Yalcin *et al.*, 2010a; Yalcin *et al.*, 2010b; Davis, F. *et al.*, 2006). Studied *in vitro*, T_4 and T_3 are anti-apoptotic in breast cancer cells (Tang *et al.*, 2004) and other tumor cells (Lin *et al.*, 2008a), at least in part via a mechanism that blocks effectiveness of the oncogene suppressor protein and pro-apoptotic factor, p53 (Lin *et al.*, 2011).

Acting via the plasma membrane integrin receptor, agonist thyroid hormone analogues T_4 and T_3 are also pro-angiogenic (Mousa *et al.*, 2009; Davis, P. *et al.*, 2009; Luidens *et al.*, 2010). In the absence of tumor cells and in the setting of tissue ischemia, stimulation of neovascularization by T_4 and T_3 may be desirable (Tomanek *et al.*, 1998; Chen *et al.*, 2010). In the setting of cancer, however, these agents appear to enhance tumor-related angiogenesis. The mechanism of angiogenesis is complex and involves the release by endothelial cells of vascular growth factors (Tomanek *et al.*, 1998) and the resulting autocrine effects of such factors. T_4 and T_3 may also enhance the actions of vascular growth factors (Davis, F. *et al.*, 2004).

The effectiveness of tetrac as an inhibitor of actions of T_4 and T_3 on the plasma membrane of cancer cells caused us to study tetrac as an anti-cancer and anti-angiogenic agent. We found that unmodified tetrac as well as tetrac re-formulated as a nanoparticulate, in which it is covalently bound to poly-lactic-co-glycolic acid (PLGA), have anti-proliferative effects in tumor cells. These actions reflect the ability of tetrac and nanoparticulate tetrac to 1) antagonize the pro-proliferative, anti-apoptotic actions of T_4 and T_3; 2) to disable, in the absence or presence of T_4 and T_3, the expression of a number of survival pathway genes (Glinsky *et al.*, 2004); and 3) to *suppress* the *death-from-cancer* gene signature of a number of cancer cell lines (Glinsky *et al.*, 2005). This 11-gene signature is a predictor of aggressiveness of cancer cells as demonstrated by shortened "time-to-tumor recurrence", the presence of distant metastasis, and death after tumor therapy. The PLGA formulation of tetrac acts exclusively at the integrin receptor for thyroid hormone; in contrast, unmodified tetrac acts at the integrin, but also gains access to the interior of the cell and may mimic actions of T_4 (Moreno *et al.*, 2008).

Actions of nanoparticulate tetrac on gene expression in human breast cancer cells are coherent (Glinskii *et al.*, 2009). While the expression of a number of cyclin genes is suppressed and *anti*-apoptotic gene expression is decreased, *pro*-apoptotic gene expression is enhanced. Fairly remarkably, the expression of *thrombospondin 1* (*TBSP1*) is increased. The TBSP1 protein is anti-angiogenic and the protein rarely accumulates in cancer cells. Nanoparticulate tetrac can also suppress expression of the *epidermal growth factor receptor* (*EGFR*) whose gene product supports cancer growth and angiogenesis and whose receptor is an oncologic target (Glinskii *et al.*, 2009). In the same study, however, while unmodified tetrac blocked expression of cyclin genes and certain genes relevant to apoptosis, this unmodified form of tetrac did *not* affect *EGFR* expression. Thus, the fit of the nanoparticulate formulation into its receptor on integrin αvβ3 appears to be distinct from that of tetrac, itself. Nanoparticulate tetrac is also 10- to 100-fold more potent than unmodified tetrac, depending on the particular cell line studied (Glinskii *et al.*, 2009; Yalcin *et al.*, 2010a; Yalcin *et al.*, 2010b).

These observations on the two formulations of tetrac are consistent with the complexity of the receptor for thyroid hormone on the integrin (Cody *et al.*, 2007) and with the ability of the integrin to generate a spectrum of intracellular actions via several signal-transducing kinase pathways, including MAPK (extracellular-regulated kinases 1/2, or ERK1/2) and phosphatidyl-inositol 3-kinase (PI3K). Studied in human glioma cells by mathematical modeling of the kinetics of binding, the receptor site appears to contain two thyroid hormone-binding domains, one that recognizes only T_3 and a second that transduces both the T_4 and T_3 signals (Lin *et al.*, 2009c). Recent computer graphics analysis of the interactions of T_3 and T_4 with the integrin (V. Cody, unpublished observations) is consistent with the existence of two hormone-binding domains in the receptor. While tetrac and nanotetrac interact with both domains, they do so differently, as the resulting gene expression profiles obtained in breast cancer cells indicate (Glinskii *et al.*, 2009).

It is important to note that the integrin-mediated anti-angiogenic activity of tetrac and nanotetrac transcend the inhibition of the pro-angiogenic thyroid hormone agonists, T_4 and T_3. That is, in the absence of agonist thyroid hormone, tetrac can block the actions of vascular endothelial growth factor (VEGF) (Mousa *et al.* , 2008), bFGF (FGF2) (Mousa *et al.* , 2008), platelet-derived growth factor (PDGF) (SA Mousa: unpublished observations) and, as mentioned above, EGF. Because tumor cells can secrete multiple vascular growth factors to support their needs, it is desirable to identify potential therapeutic agents that antagonize the actions of more than one such growth factor.

It is clear from the foregoing that the actions of tetrac formulations at the cell surface integrin and of T_4 and T_3 at αvβ3 generate complex downstream events. However, it is also apparent that the hormone receptor on the integrin can also engage in crosstalk with growth factors on the plasma membrane. Interference by tetrac formulations with the actions of VEGF, bFGF and other growth factors imply this, since such growth factors include Arg-Gly-Asp (RGD) sequences that are validated by the RGD recognition site on the integrin before each growth factor can activate its growth factor-specific receptor clustered with the integrin (Davis, P. *et al.*, 2011). The αvβ3-vascular growth factor receptor interaction, e.g., with VEGF (Sarmishtha *et al.*, 2005) and bFGF (Sahni and Francis, 2004), have been described in other studies that did not include thyroid hormone. The integrin receptor for agonist thyroid hormone analogues and for tetrac, however, influences other local cell membrane events. For example, activity of the Na^+/H^+ exchanger (NHE1) is regulated by thyroid hormone analogues and this action is blocked by tetrac (Incerpi *et al.*, 2003). The insertion of Na, K-ATPase protein into the plasma membrane and activity of the ATPase (sodium pump) are also affected nongenomically by a MAPK- and PI3K-dependent mechanism (Lei *et al.*, 2007).

Such observations caused us to examine in doxorubicin-resistant human breast cancer cells (MCF-7) whether the state of resistance, in part determined by the expression and activity of the P-glycoprotein (MDR) pump (Dönmez *et al.*, 2010), may be affected by tetrac. Treatment of such breast cancer cells with tetrac reversed chemoresistance of the cells and resulted in increased intracellular residence time of radiolabeled doxorubicin (Rebbaa *et* al., 2008). Such *in vitro* studies suggest that the combination of tetrac and doxorubicin should be tested in xenografts of doxorubicin-resistant MCF-7 cells. The mechanism of this particular action of tetrac has not been established. While it is possible that the function of the P-glycoprotein is affected by crosstalk with the tetrac-occupied hormone receptor on the integrin, we have also suggested that the action of tetrac on the NHE may be involved (Incerpi *et al.*, 2003). That is, inhibition of the NHE and a resultant intracellular decrease in pH may affect P-glycoprotein function because of the pH optimum of the MDR pump.

We would also point out that tetrac radiosensitizes tumor cells (Hercbergs *et al.*, 2009) by interfering with repair of DNA double-strand breaks (Hercbergs *et al.*, 2011). However, this has been studied to-date only in murine and human glioma cells and whether the agent affects DNA repair in breast cancer cells is not yet known.

A final consideration with regard to thyroid hormone is the recently described effect of the hormone on the abundance of integrin αvβ3 on the tumor cell plasma membrane. Agonist thyroid hormone analogues have a modest effect on the expression of the αvβ3 gene (Yonkers *et al.*, 2009) and may also increase the internalization of the αv, but not the β3 component (Lin *et al.*, 2009). The disparate distribution of the αv and β3 monomers within the cell is also conditioned by thyroid hormone, including import of αv into the cell nucleus (Lin *et al.*, 2007).

3. Actions of resveratrol and the integrin receptor on the biology of breast cancer cells

Resveratrol is an extensively-studied, naturally-occurring alcohol with desirable properties in several biologic models. These activities include extension of lifespan in *C. elegans* (Zarse *et al.*, 2010) and remarkable anti-cancer properties (Pezzuto *et al.*, 2011; Hsieh *et al.*, 2011; Lin, C *et al.*, 2011). Substantial attention has been devoted to the metabolism of this agent because of its rapid disappearance from the circulation post-administration to intact animals and its cellular uptake and chemical modification (Delmas *et al.*, 2011). The half-life of the parent compound is sufficiently short to promote speculation about the nature of the active biologic material.

We recently described a cell surface receptor for resveratrol on breast cancer cells which, like the thyroid hormone receptor on tumor cells (Bergh *et al.*, 2005), is on integrin αvβ3 (Lin *et al.*, 2006). The existence of such a receptor and its ability to transduce the plasma membrane resveratrol signal into MAPK activity and downstream into pro-apoptotic action suggested that the parent compound has substantial bioactivity. Integrins have been widely-viewed to bear receptors or binding sites only for large molecules—extracellular matrix proteins and growth factors (Plow *et al.*, 2000)—and thus it was surprising to find apparent biologically relevant binding sites for two small molecules on this integrin. It was also remarkable that the receptors for thyroid hormone and for resveratrol did not appear to interact functionally with one another. That is, both agents activated intracellular pools of MAPK (ERK1/2), but resveratrol was pro-apoptotic (Lin H *et al.*, 2008a; Lin C *et al.*, 2011) whereas thyroid hormones (T_4, T_3) were anti-apoptotic (Lin H *et al.*, 2008b), as noted above. Such observations suggested that the results of any efficacy testing of resveratrol as a chemotherapeutic agent in the presence of physiologic concentrations of thyroid hormone *in vitro* or in the intact animal with a normal pituitary-thyroid axis may be difficult to interpret (see below). An Arg-Gly-Asp (RGD) peptide prevents both the pro-apoptotic activity of resveratrol and the anti-apoptotic activity of thyroid hormone, indicating that the receptor is near the RGD recognition site on the integrin that was mentioned above (see section on *Thyroid Hormone Action*). The interactions of tetrac with either T_4 or resveratrol, however, indicate that the two integrin binding sites are distinct, in that while tetrac inhibits the proliferative action of T_4 in cancer cells, tetrac does not inhibit the pro-apoptotic actions of resveratrol (Lin C *et al.*, 2011).

Our own studies of the mechanism by which resveratrol may act to induce apoptosis in tumor cells have revealed several unexpected findings. First, resveratrol is able to induce p53-related apoptosis in cancer cells expressing certain mutations in p53. What is required in p53 for expression of resveratrol's apoptotic activity is that the Ser-15 be intact, as it is a target of phosphorylation by resveratrol-activated MAPK (Lin H *et al.*, 2002). Second, one of the actions of resveratrol in tumor cells is to induce a nuclear pool of cyclooxygenase-2 (COX-2) (Lin C *et al.*, 2011; Lin H *et al.*, 2009a). Chronic accumulation of COX-2 in cytoplasm is a marker of tumor cell aggressiveness (Schmitz *et al.*, 2006; Perdiki *et al.*, 2007) and long-term pharmacologic inhibition of the enzymatic activity of COX-2—the product of which is prostaglandins—appears to improve clinical outcomes or prevent emergence of certain cancers, such as that of the colon (Galalmb *et al.*, 2010).

Inducible COX-2 in the nucleus, however, is a wholly different biologic product. It is pro-apoptotic, can interact with Ser-15-phosphorylated p53 and can even bind to DNA (Lin H *et al.*, 2008b). The latter observation raises the possibility that COX-2 can be a co-activator and, indeed, resveratrol-induced nuclear COX-2 co-localizes with p300, a coactivator for p53 (Song *et al.*, 2010), as well as for proteins in the superfamily of nuclear hormone receptors (Kalkhoven, 2004). Activation of MAPK is required for formation of the complex of p53, p300 and COX-2, since that complex is not obtained in resveratrol-treated cells in the presence of the MEK-MAPK inhibitor, PD 98059 (Tang *et al.*, 2006). In contrast, inhibition of the enzymatic activity of COX-2 with indomethacin does not affect the pro-apoptotic activity of COX-2 (Tang *et al.*, 2006).

Third, a thyroid hormone analogue such as T_4 prevents or disrupts the formation of the nuclear p53-COX-2 complex in cells treated with resveratrol (Lin *et al.*, 2008a, b). It is thought that this hormonal effect explains the blunting of the pro-apoptotic action of resveratrol in the presence of thyroid hormone. Competition between thyroid hormone and resveratrol for binding to the αvβ3 integrin is thought to be responsible for this inhibition. Not unexpectedly, in a tumor cell system that includes resveratrol and a physiologic concentration of T_4, the addition of tetrac protects the pro-apoptotic action of resveratrol from the anti-apoptotic effect of thyroid hormone (Lin *et al.*, 2008b). All of these actions compete at the αvβ3 integrin receptor. In the absence of T_4, the induction of apoptosis by resveratrol is not affected by the addition of tetrac (Lin *et al.*, 2008b).

The antecedent review suggests that further testing of resveratrol as a cancer chemotherapeutic agent might be pursued in two ways. First, the combination of nanotetrac and resveratrol may be evaluated against breast tumor cells *in vitro* or *in vivo* in the nude mouse xenograft model. Second, the potential manufacture of a nanoparticulate formulation of resveratrol in which the polyalcohol is covalently bound to the nanoparticle may be desirable, so as to permit biologic activity but restrict that effect of resveratrol to the integrin receptor. This formulation would prevent cellular uptake and subsequent metabolism/degradation of the nanoparticulate compound.

There is another implication with regard to the dependence of the pro-apoptotic action of resveratrol on an inducible pool of nuclear COX-2. New pharmacologic inhibitors of the enzymatic function of cyclooxygenase-2 should be examined for their ability to block the action of resveratrol, and perhaps of other polyalcohols as model inducers of nuclear COX-2. For example, NS398 is an experimental inhibitor of COX-2 that has been shown to prevent induction of COX-2 by resveratrol (Tang *et al.*, 2006).

4. Dihydrotestosterone (DHT) acts via integrin αvβ3 to induce proliferation of human breast cancer cells

Although androgens may have an inhibitory effect on the proliferation of breast cancer cells, the actions of these steroids on such cells are variable. When we examined the action of dihydrotestosterone (DHT) on ERα-positive MCF-7 and ERα-negative MDA-MB-231 human breast cancer cells, we found that the androgen promoted proliferation in both cell lines (Lin *et al.*, 2009b). Integrin αvβ3 antibody inhibited the action of DHT in MDA-MB-231 cells, but was ineffective in MCF-7 cells (Lin *et al.*, 2009b). On the other hand, ICI 182,780 treatment and siRNA knockdown of ERα blocked the proliferative effect of DHT in MCF-7 cells, but not in the MDA-MB-231 cells. Thus, the mechanisms of DHT action differ in the two cell lines, and only in the ER-negative cells was there evidence for the existence of a DHT receptor on integrin αvβ3. In neither breast cancer cell line could participation of a classical androgen receptor be implicated in the action of DHT. Tetrac did not affect the action of DHT (HY Lin: unpublished observations), indicating that these two small molecule receptors on the integrin function independently of one another.

It is not yet clear what the clinical significance may be of the DHT receptor on the breast cancer cell surface. We speculate, however, that in the patient with a recurrent ERα-positive tumor and taking tamoxifen or an aromatase inhibitor, residual circulating androgen may be promoting cancer cell proliferation. Useful information relevant to this possibility will come from determination of the androgen analogue-specificity of the receptor for DHT, and of a possible contribution of DHT to breast cancer cell growth. In the case of the ER-negative human breast cancer cell, we have already demonstrated its susceptibility to DHT-stimulation (Lin *et al.*, 2009b).

It will also be important to analyze solid tumors beyond breast cancer for the presence of DHT-induced growth stimulation, including cancer cell growth as well as angiogenesis. In a recent report, Sieveking *et al.* (2010) have reported that androgen treatment of male endothelial cells *in vitro* enhanced angiogenesis; in contrast, gene knockdown of the androgen receptor (AR) in these cells caused unresponsiveness of these cells to androgen treatment. Female endothelial cells lacking AR did not respond to androgen treatment, but overexpression of the androgen receptor in female endothelial cells caused angiogenesis to occur.

5. Discussion and conclusions

Modulation of the proliferation of breast cancer cells is largely viewed as a function of the presence or absence of estrogen in ER-positive tumor cells and the presence of polypeptide growth factors that are autocrine or systemic. The emphasis on ER-mediated actions has grown from a broad understanding, emerging from a number of laboratories, of the molecular functions of ER in the cell nucleus and genomic actions of estrogens. Management of breast cancer—beyond surgery, tumor irradiation and chemotherapeutic agents—specifically emphasizes suppression of the action of endogenous estrogen with tamoxifen or inhibition of estrogen synthesis with aromatase inhibition. That estrogen may support breast tumor growth nongenomically is now under consideration (Silva & Shupnik, 2007), perhaps involving nuclear ERα insinuated into the plasma membrane or ER-like proteins in the membrane (Levin, 2011).

The concept that thyroid hormone may be a growth factor for breast cancer has been advanced by various investigators (Goodman *et al.*, 1980; Borek *et al.*, 1983; Cristofanilli *et al.*, 2005). That thyroid hormone could nongenomically support ER-positive human breast cancer cell proliferation and to be estrogen-like was shown when T_4 caused MAPK-dependent specific serine phosphorylation of nuclear ER, mimicking estradiol upon which depended stimulation of proliferation by the iodothyronine. This work led to the subsequent identification of a thyroid hormone receptor on plasma membrane integrin αvβ3 at which a variety of effects of thyroid hormone are initiated that are nongenomic in mechanism (Tang *et al.*, 2004). The integrin (and, therefore, the receptor) is expressed primarily on cancer cells of various types and on rapidly-dividing blood vessel cells (Dijkgraaf *et al.*, 2009; Wei *et al.*,2009; Dimastromatteo *et al.*, 2010).

An interesting inhibitor of this receptor target exists. This is tetraiodothyroacetic acid (tetrac), a deaminated analogue of T_4 that blocks binding of T_4 and T_3 to the integrin, but also has novel anti-cancer activities at the αvβ3 hormone-binding site in the absence of T_4 and T_3. These actions, initiated at the cell surface, are on expression of specific genes and the actions are inimical to tumor cell survival and on angiogenesis (Glinskii, A. *et al.*, 2009), including that initiated by several vascular growth factors. The hormone receptor on the integrin also disables or garbles crosstalk between the integrin and growth factor receptors that are clustered with αvβ3 (Davis, F. *et al.*, 2004; Mousa S. *et al.*, 2008).

Tetrac has been re-formulated as a nanoparticle in which the outer ring hydroxyl group is stably covalently bonded through a linker to the nanoparticle. This formulation does not enter the cell and its actions are limited to the tetrac/thyroid hormone receptor on integrin αvβ3 (Bergh J. *et al.*, 2005). The agent has been shown to suppress growth of a variety of human cancer cell xenografts and to be anti-angiogenic at the tumor site (Davis F. *et al.*, 2004; Davis F. *et al.*, 2006; Glinskii A. *et al.*, 2009; Davis P. *et al.*, 2011). This hormone target on the integrin is fairly remarkable, in that as a single target, it has a relatively large number of downstream actions on cancer cells that emphasize vulnerability of such cells.

Recognition and characterization of the thyroid hormone receptor on integrin αvβ3 were premonitory to the identification of other small molecule binding sites—now understood to be receptors in that, when occupied, they cause predictable downstream cellular events. These receptors appear to be quite independent of one another and of the thyroid hormone binding domain. Identification of the resveratrol receptor on the integrin of breast cancer cells and other solid tumor cells may provide useful insights into the actions of this stilbene. The rapid cellular uptake and metabolism of resveratrol (Kroon *et al.*, 2010)—leading to pharmacokinetic and pharmacodynamic speculation about the relative bioactivity of resveratrol analogues—is less puzzling if, in fact, the parent compound (resveratrol) can act on the outside of the cell. That is, resveratrol binds to the integrin and rapidly initiates a MAPK-requiring, p53-dependent apoptotic process, regardless of uptake of the compound and chemical processing. What was somewhat surprising was the observation that resveratrol-induced apoptosis was blocked by thyroid hormone, but by a mechanism that begins at a different domain on the integrin and utilizes MAPK, but is effected by interruption of a resveratrol-induced phosphorylation sequence in the cancer cell nucleus that involves p53 and other nucleoproteins. The outcomes of a recent pharmaceutical industry-sponsored clinical trial of resveratrol as an anti-cancer agent were disappointing (McBride, 2010). Where there may be multiple explanations for these results, we can speculate that in the setting of normal thyroid function that the anti-cancer activity of resveratrol may be wholly suppressed by the hormone.

A third small molecule receptor on the integrin of breast cancer cells was recently described and this is a site that responds to the androgen, dihydrotestosterone (DHT) (Lin, H. *et al.*, 2009b). It was not wholly unexpected that an authentic steroid was found to act at the integrin, since resveratrol, while not a steroid, has certain structural features and functional activities that are estrogen-like. Acting via integrin αvβ3, DHT is a trophic agent for breast cancer cells. Of some interest is that the mechanisms by which DHT acts *in vitro* differ in ERα-negative and ERα-positive cells. The cell surface integrin receptor for DHT is required for the proliferative effect of the androgen in ERα-negative cells, but is irrelevant in ER-positive cells, where the estrogen receptor protein, itself, is needed for DHT action. In neither type of cell is the authentic nuclear androgen receptor a part of the mechanism by which DHT recognizes the existence of a receptor on integrin αvβ3 in ERα-negative breast cancer cells. As we have pointed out above, recognition of the existence of the androgen receptor on αvβ3 in ERα-negative breast cancer may help to explain recurrences of tumor in postmenopausal women in whom some effect of circulating androgen, now apparent in the absence of estrogen, may be seen.

6. Acknowledgment

An endowment at Ordway Research Institute supported by M. Frank Rudy and Margaret Domiter Rudy supported a significant portion of the work described here.

7. References

Bergh, J.J., Lin, H.Y., Lansing, L., Mohamed, S.N., Davis, F.B., Mousa, S., & Davis, P.J. Integrin alphaVbeta3 contains a cell surface receptor site for thyroid hormone that is linked to activation of mitogen-activated protein kinase and induction of angiogenesis. *Endocrinology*. 2005;146:2864-71.

Borek, C., Guernsey, D.L., Ong, A., & Edelman, I.S. Critical role played by thyroid hormone in induction of neoplastic transformation by chemical carcinogens in tissue culture. *Proc. Natl. Acad. Sci. USA*. 1983; 80:5749-5752.

Chen, Y.F., Redetzke, R.A., Said, S., Beyer, A.J., & Gerdes, A.M. Changes in left ventricular function and remodeling after myocardial infarction in hypothyroid rats. *Am J Physiol Heart Circ Physiol*. 2010 Jan; 298(1):H259-62.

Cheng, S.Y., Leonard, J.L., & Davis, P.J. Molecular aspects of thyroid hormone actions. *Endocr. Rev*. 2010; 31:139-70.

Cody, V., Davis, P.J., & Davis, F.B. Molecular modeling of the thyroid hormone interactions with alpha v beta 3 integrin. *Steroids*. 2007; Feb;72(2):165-70.

Cristofanilli, M., Yamamura, Y., Kau, S.W., Bevers, T., Strom, S., Patangan, M., Krishnamurthy, S., Theriault, R.L., & Hortobagyi, G.N. Thyroid hormone and breast carcinoma. Primary hypothyroidism is associated with a reduced incidence of breast carcinoma. *Cancer*. 2005; 103:1122-1128.

Davis, F.B., Mousa, S.A., O'Connor, L., Mohamed, S., Lin, H.Y., Cao, H.J., & Davis, P.J. Proangiogenic action of thyroid hormone is fibroblast growth factor-dependent and is initiated at the cell surface. *Circ Res*. 2004 Jun; 94(11):1500-6.

Davis, F.B., Tang, H.Y., Shih, A., Keating, T., Lansing, L., Hercbergs, A., Fenstermaker, R.A., Mousa, A., Mousa, S.A., Davis, P.J., & Lin, H.Y. Acting via a cell surface receptor, thyroid hormone is a growth factor for glioma cells. *Cancer Res*. 2006 Jul 15;66(14):7270-5.

Davis, P.J., Davis, F.B., Mousa, S.A., Luidens, M.K., & Lin, H.Y. Membrane receptor for thyroid hormone: physiologic and pharmacologic implications. *Annu. Rev. Pharmacol. Toxicol*. 2011;51:99-115.

Davis, P.J., Davis, F.B., & Mousa, S.A. Thyroid hormone-induced angiogenesis. *Curr Cardiol Rev*. 2009 Jan; 5(1):12-16.

De, S, Razorenova, O, McCabe, NP, O'Toole, T, Qin, J & Byzova, TV. VEGF-integrin interplay controls tumor growth and vascularization. *Proc. Natl. Acad. Sci. USA* 2005; 102:7589-7594.

Delmas, D., Aires, V., Limagne, E., Dutartre, P., Mazué, F., Ghiringhelli, F., & Latruffe, N. Transport, stability, and biological activity of resveratrol. *Ann. N Y Acad. Sci*. 2011 Jan; 1215(1):48-59.

Dijkgraaf, I., Beer, A.J., Wester, H.J., Application of RGD-containing peptides as imaging probes for alphavbeta3 expression. *Front. Biosci*. 2009; 14:887-899.

Dimastromatteo, J., Riou, L.M., Ahmadi, M., Pons, G., Pellegrini, E., Broisat, A., Sancey, L., Gavrilina, T., Boturyn, D., Dumy, P., Fagret, D., & Ghezzi, C. In vivo molecular imaging of myocardial angiogenesis using the alpha(v)beta3 integrin-targeted tracer 99m Tc-RAFT-RGD. *J. Nucl. Cardiol*. 2010; 17:435-443.

Dönmez, Y., & Gündüz, U. Reversal of multidrug resistance by small interfering RNA (siRNA) in doxorubicin-resistant MCF-7 breast cancer cells. *Biomed Pharmacother*. 2011, *in press*.

Galamb, O., Spisák, S., Sipos, F., Tóth, K., Solymosi, N., Wichmann, B., Krenács, T., Valcz, G., Tulassay, Z., & Molnár, B. Reversal of gene expression changes in the colorectal normal-adenoma pathway by NS398 selective COX2 inhibitor. *Br. J. Cancer.* 2010 Feb 16;102(4): 765-73.

Glinskii, A.B., Glinsky, G.V., Lin, H.Y., Tang, H.Y., Sun, M., Davis, F.B., Luidens, M.K., Mousa, S.A., Hercbergs, A.H., & Davis, P.J. Modification of survival pathway gene expression in human breast cancer cells by tetraiodothyroacetic acid (tetrac). *Cell Cycle.* 2009 Nov; 8(21): 3554-62.

Glinsky, G.V., Glinskii, A.B., Stephenson, A.J., Hoffman, R.M., & Gerald, W.L. Gene expression profiling predicts clinical outcome of prostate cancer. *J Clin Invest.* 2004 Mar;113(6): 913-23.

Glinsky, G.V., Berezovska, O., & Glinskii, A.B. Microarray analysis identifies a death-from-cancer signature predicting therapy failure in patients with multiple types of cancer. *J Clin Invest.* 2005 Jun;115(6):1503-21.

Goodman, A.D., Hoekstra, S.J., & Marsh, P.S. Effects of hypothyroidism on the induction and growth of mammary cancer induced by 7,12-dimethylbenz(a)anthracene in the rat. *Cancer Res.* 1980; 40:2336-2342.

Hercbergs, A., Davis, P.J., Davis, F.B., Ciesielski, M.J., & Leith, J.T. Radiosensitization of GL261 glioma cells by tetraiodothyroacetic acid (tetrac). *Cell Cycle.* 2009 Aug 15;8(16):2586-91.

Hercbergs, A.H., Lin, H.Y., Davis, F.B., Davis, P.J., & Leith, J.T. Radiosensitization and production of DNA double-strand breaks in U87MG brain tumor cells induced by tetraiodothyroacetic acid (tetrac). *Cell Cycle.* 2011 Jan 15;10(2):352-7.

Hsieh, T.C., Wong, C., Bennett, D.J., & Wu, J.M. Regulation of p53 and cell proliferation by resveratrol and its derivatives in breast cancer cells: an *in silico* and biochemical approach targeting integrin αvβ3. *Int. J. Cancer.* In press, 2011.

Incerpi, S., D'Arezzo, S., Marino, M., Musanti, R., Pallottini, V., Pascolini, A., & Trentalance, A. Short-term activation by low 17beta-estradiol concentrations of the Na+/H+ exchanger in rat aortic smooth muscle cells: physiopathological implications. *Endocrinology.* 2003 Oct;144(10):4315-24.

Kalkhoven E. CBP and p300: HATs for different occasions. *Biochem. Pharmacol.* 2004 Sep 15;68(6):1145-55.

Kato, S., Endoh, H., Masuhiro, Y., Kitamoto, T., Uchiyama, S., Sasaki, H., Masushige, S., Gotoh, Y., Nishida, E., Kawashima, H., Metzger, D., & Chambon, P. Activation of the estrogen receptor through phosphorylation by mitogen-activated protein kinase. *Science* 1995; 270:1491-4.

Kroon, P.A., Iyeer, A., Chunduri, P., Chan, V., & Brown, L. The cardiovascular nutrapharmacology of resdveratrol: pharmacokinetics, molecular mechanisms and therapeutic potential. *Curr. Med. Chem.* 2010; 17:2442-2455.

Lei, J., Wendt, C.H., Fan, D., Mariash, C.N., & Ingbar, D.H. Developmental acquisition of T3-sensitive Na-K-ATPase stimulation by rat alveolar epithelial cells. *Am. J. Physiol. Lung Cell Mol. Physiol.* 2007 Jan; 292(1):L6-14.

Levin, E.R. Cellular Functions of the Plasma Membrane Estrogen Receptor. *Trends Endocrinol. Metab.* 1999 Nov;10(9): 374-377.

Lin, C., Crawford, D.R., Lin, S., Hwang, J., Sebuyira, A., Meng, R., Westfall, J.E., Tang, H.Y., Lin, S., Yu, P.Y., Davis, P.J., & Lin, H.Y. Inducible COX-2-dependent apoptosis in human ovarian cancer cells. *Carcinogenesis.* 2011 Jan;32(1): 19-26.

Lin, H.Y., Davis, P.J., Tang, H.Y., Mousa, S.A., Luidens, M.K., Hercbergs, A.H., & Davis, F.B. The pro-apoptotic action of stilbene-induced COX-2 in cancer cells: convergence with the anti-apoptotic effect of thyroid hormone. *Cell Cycle.* 2009a Jun 15;8(12): 1877-82.

Lin, H.Y., Lansing, L., Merillon, J.M., Davis, F.B., Tang, H.Y., Shih, A., Vitrac, X., Krisa, S., Keating, T., Cao, H.J., Bergh, J., Quackenbush, S., & Davis, P.J. Integrin alphaVbeta3 contains a receptor site for resveratrol. *FASEB J.* 2006; 20:1742-4.

Lin, H.Y., Shih, A., Davis, F.B., Tang, H.Y., Martino, L.J., Bennett, J.A., & Davis, P.J. Resveratrol-induced serine phosphorylation of p53 causes apoptosis in a mutant p53 prostate cancer cell line. J. Urol. 2002 Aug; 168(2): 748-55.

Lin, H.Y., Sun, M., Lin, C., Tang, H.Y., London, D., Shih, A., Davis, F.B., & Davis, P.J. Androgen-induced human breast cancer cell proliferation is mediated by discrete mechanisms in estrogen receptor-alpha-positive and -negative breast cancer cells. *J. Steroid Biochem. Mol. Biol.* 2009b Feb; 113(3-5): 182-8.

Lin, H.Y., Sun, M., Tang, H.Y., Lin, C., Luidens, M.K., Mousa, S.A., Incerpi, S., Drusano, G.L., Davis, F.B., & Davis, P.J. L-Thyroxine vs. 3,5,3'-triiodo-L-thyronine and cell proliferation: activation of mitogen-activated protein kinase and phosphatidylinositol 3-kinase. *Am J Physiol Cell Physiol.* 2009c May;296(5): C980-91.

Lin, H.Y., Sun, M., Tang, H.Y., Simone, T.M., Wu, Y.H., Grandis, J.R., Cao, H.J., Davis, P.J., & Davis, F.B. Resveratrol causes COX-2- and p53-dependent apoptosis in head and neck squamous cell cancer cells. *J. Cell. Biochem.* 2008a Aug 15;104(6): 2131-42.

Lin, H.Y., Tang, H.Y., Davis, F.B., & Davis, P.J. Resveratrol and apoptosis. *Ann N Y Acad Sci.* 2011 Jan;1215(1): 79-88.

Lin, H.Y., Tang, H.Y., Lin, C., Davis, F.B., & Davis, P.J. Thyroid hormone induces nuclear accumulation of monomeric integrin αv and formation of integrin-nucleoprotein complexes. *Thyroid* 2007 Oct;17(Suppl. 1): abstr. 261.

Lin, H.Y., Tang, H.Y., Keating, T., Wu, Y.H., Shih, A., Hammond, D., Sun, M., Hercbergs, A., Davis, F.B., & Davis, P.J. Resveratrol is pro-apoptotic and thyroid hormone is anti-apoptotic in glioma cells: both actions are integrin- and ERK-mediated. *Carcinogenesis* 2008b Jan; 29(1): 62-9.

Luidens, M.K., Mousa, S.A., Davis, F.B., Lin, H.Y., & Davis, P.J. Thyroid hormone and angiogenesis. *Vascul. Pharmacol.* 2010 Mar-Apr; 52(3-4):142-5.

McBride, R. Glaxo ends resveratrol drug study. *Xconomy/Boston* 2010; 12/01

Moreno, M., de Lange, P., Lombardi, A., Silvestri, E., Lanni, A., & Goglia, F. Metabolic effects of thyroid hormone derivatives. *Thyroid.* 2008 Feb;18(2):239-53.

Mousa, S.A., Bergh, J.J., Dier, E., Rebbaa, A., O'Connor, L.J., Yalcin, M., Aljada, A., Dyskin, E., Davis, F.B., Lin, H.Y., & Davis, P.J. Tetraiodothyroacetic acid, a small molecule integrin ligand, blocks angiogenesis induced by vascular endothelial growth factor and basic fibroblast growth factor. *Angiogenesis.* 2008;11(2):183-90.

Mousa, S.A., Davis, F.B., & Davis, P.J. Hormone-Integrin Cross Talk and Angiogenesis Modulation. *Immunology, Endocrine & Metabolic Agents in Medicinal Chemistry* 2009; 9:75-83.

Perdiki, M., Korkolopoulou, P., Thymara, I., Agrogiannis, G., Piperi, C., Boviatsis, E., Kotsiakis, X., Angelidakis, D., Diamantopoulou, K., Thomas-Tsagli, E., & Patsouris, E. Cyclooxygenase-2 expression in astrocytomas. Relationship with microvascular parameters, angiogenic factors expression and survival. *Mol. Cell. Biochem.* 2007 Jan; 295 (1-2):75-83.

Pervaiz, S., & Holme, A.L. Resveratrol: its biological targets and functional activity. *Antioxidants & Redox Signaling*. 2009 Oct 15; 11(11):2851-97.

Pezzuto, J.M. The phenomenon of resveratrol: redefining the virtues of promiscuity. *Ann. N.Y. Acad. Sci.* 2011 Jan; 1215(1):123-30.

Plow, E.F., Haas, T.A., Zhang, L., Loftus, J., & Smith, J.W. Ligand binding to integrins. *J. Biol. Chem.* 2000 Jul 21; 275(29):21785-8.

Rebbaa, A., Chu, F., Davis, F.B., Davis, P.J., & Mousa, S.A. Novel function of the thyroid hormone analog tetraiodothyroacetic acid: a cancer chemosensitizing and anti-cancer agent. *Angiogenesis.* 2008 Nov; 11(3):269-76.

Sahni, A, & Francis, CW. Stimulation of endothelial cell proliferation by FGF-2 in the presence of fibrinogen requires αvβ3. *Blood.* 2004; 104:3635-3641.

Schmitz, K.J., Callies, R., Wohlschlaeger, J., Kimmig, R., Otterbach, F., Bohr, J., Lee, H.S., Takeda, A., Schmid, K.W., & Baba, H.A. Overexpression of cyclo-oxygenase-2 is an independent predictor of unfavourable outcome in node-negative breast cancer, but is not associated with protein kinase B (Akt) and mitogen-activated protein kinase (ERK1/2, p38) activation or with Her-2/neu signaling pathways. *J. Clin. Pathol.* 2006 Jul; 59(7):685-91.

Sieveking, D.P., Lim, P., Chow, R.W., Dunn, L.L., Bao, S., McGrath, K.C., Heather, A.K., Handelsman, D.J., Celermajer, D.S., & Ng, M.K. A sex-specific role for androgens in angiogenesis. *J. Exp. Med.* 2010 Feb 15; 207(2):345-52.

Song, L., Gao, M., Dong, W., Hu, M., Li, J., Shi, X., Hao, Y., Li, Y., & Huang, C. p85α mediates p53 K370 acetylation by p300 and regulates its promoter-specific transactivity in the cellular UVB response. *Oncogene* 2011, in press.

Tang, H.Y., Lin, H.Y., Zhang, S., Davis, F.B., & Davis, P.J. Thyroid hormone causes mitogen-activated protein kinase-dependent phosphorylation of the nuclear estrogen receptor. *Endocrinology* 2004 July; 145(7):3265-72.

Tang, H.Y., Shih, A., Cao, H.J., Davis, F.B., Davis, P.J., & Lin, H.Y. Resveratrol-induced cyclooxygenase-2 facilitates p53-dependent apoptosis in human breast cancer cells. *Mol. Cancer Ther.* 2006 Aug; 5(8):2034-42.

Tomanek, R.J., Doty, M.K., & Sandra, A. Early coronary angiogenesis in response to thyroxine: growth characteristics and upregulation of basic fibroblast growth factor. *Circ. Res.* 1998 Mar; 82(5):587-93.

Wei, L, Ye, Y., Wadas, T.J., Lewis, J.S., Welch, M.J., Achilefu, S, & Anderson, C.J. (64)Cu-labeled CB-TE2A and diamsar-conjugated RGD peptide analogs for targeting angiogenesis: comparison of their biological activity. *Nucl. Med. Biol.* 2009; 36:277-285.

Yalcin, M., Bharali, D.J., Lansing, L., Dyskin, E., Mousa, S.S., Davis, F.B., Davis, P.J., & Mousa, S.A. Tetraiodothyroacetic acid (tetrac) and tetrac nanoparticles inhibit growth of human renal cell carcinoma. *Anticancer Res.* 2009 Oct; 29(10):3825-31.

Yalcin, M., Dyskin, E., Lansing, L., Bharali, D.J., Mousa, S.S., Bridoux, A., Hercbergs, A.H., Lin, H.Y., Davis, F.B., Glinsky, G.V., Glinskii, A., Ma, J., Davis, P.J., & Mousa, S.A. Tetraiodothyroacetic acid (tetrac) and nanoparticulate tetrac arrest growth of medullary carcinoma of the thyroid. *J. Clin. Endocrinol. Metab.* 2010b Apr;95(4):1972-80.

Yonkers, M.A., & Ribera, A.B. Molecular components underlying nongenomic thyroid hormone signaling in embryonic zebrafish neurons. *Neural Dev.* 2009 Jun; 4:20.

Zarse, K., Schmeisser, S., Birringer, M., Falk, E., Schmoll, D., & Ristow, M. Differential effects of resveratrol and SRT1720 on lifespan of adult *Caenorhabditis elegans*. *Horm. Metab. Res.* 2010 Nov; 42(12):837-9.

7

DNA Damage Response and Breast Cancer: An Overview

Leila J. Green and Shiaw-Yih Lin
Department of Systems Biology,
The University of Texas M. D. Anderson Cancer Center, Houston, Texas,
USA

1. Introduction

The cells throughout the human body are constantly subjected to both internal forces and external insults that cause damage to their DNA. This damage to the DNA can be harmful to the overall integrity of the cell and the ability for replication. Accurate transmission of genetic information from one cell to its progeny is dependent upon mechanisms within the cell to monitor any defects within its genome and to repair these deficiencies so as not to pass them to subsequent generations. These mechanisms are mainly mediated through an array of DNA damage response proteins including DNA damage sensors, signal transducers and effectors. Sensors, such as ATM (ataxia telangiectasia mutated) and ATR (ATM-Rad3-related), have the ability to recognize areas of damage and activate signal transducers, which either activate or inactivate effectors. Effector proteins trigger cell cycle checkpoint and the cell may successfully repair the damage or proceed towards apoptosis if these damages are irreparable. These molecules are not only necessary for surveillance of occasional non-lethal DNA damage, but are also important for the survival of the cell and the organism. Moreover, mutations to these DNA damage response proteins may contribute to an unstable genome and the development of cancer.

In this chapter we will briefly review the cell cycle and relevant checkpoint proteins. We will also discuss in detail the DNA damage response signal transduction pathway and associated proteins: ATM, ATR, ChK1, Chk2, p53, BRCA-1, PARP-1, and BRIT-1,. Finally, we will discuss the future strategy in targeting the defects of these proteins in the treatment of breast cancer.

Key Words: DNA Damage Response, ATM, ATR, p53, BRCA-1, BRIT-1, PARP-1, PARP inhibitors, Triple Negative Breast Cancer

2. The cell cycle: A brief overview

The cell cycle, first described in 1979, has been accepted as the central dogma of cell replication and contains two main phases; Interphase and the Mitotic phase (Fig. 1.)

The G1 (Gap 1) phase of the cycle is the period in which the cell may grow and function normally. New proteins are synthesized and organelles that the daughter cells will need are created. The synthesis or S phase of the cell cycle follows the G1 phase and is the period of the cell cycle in which the genetic material of the cell is replicated. As stated before, accurate

DNA replication is needed to prevent genetic aberrations that may lead to cell death. The regulatory pathways and proteins that govern this event are highly conserved in eukaryotic cells.

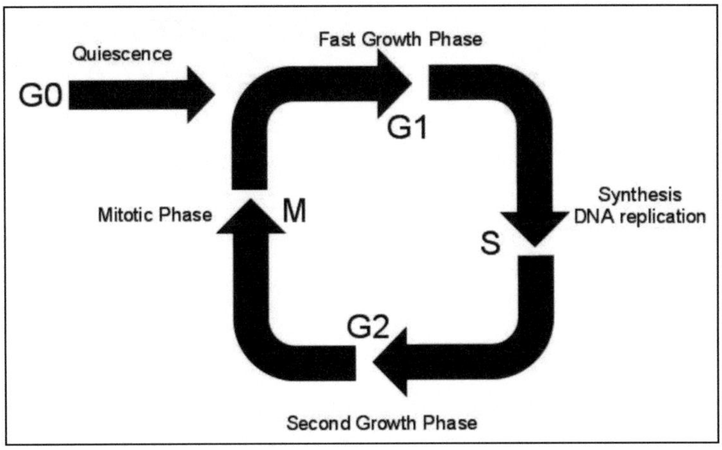

Fig. 1. The Cell Cycle

The G1/S phase transition is a major checkpoint in the cell cycle. The checkpoint response to DNA damage at the G1 phase is mediated by the ATM(ATR)/Chk2(Chk1)—p53/MDM1-p21 pathway, which will be discussed later in this chapter. Expression of ATM and Chk2 are relatively constant during the cell cycle while the concentrations of ATR and Chk1 increase closer to the G1/S transition (Kastan & Bartek, 2004). The end of the G1 Phase consists of the induction of Cyclin E and A, and CDC25A phosphatase, the activator of Cyclin E (A)/CDK2 kinase. In the event of DNA damage, Chk1 down-regulates CDC25A and in effect inhibits Cyclin E (A)/CDK2 kinase which stalls the transition from G1 to S. During the S phase of the cell cycle as the genome is replicated, intra S phase checkpoint networks can also be activated as a result of genotoxic insult. The two parallel branches of this checkpoint, controlled by the ATM/ATR signaling mechanism, will also be further discussed in the chapter.

Arguably, the most important phase of the cell cycle is the Synthesis and G2 phases. The G2 phase of interphase is the second growth period as the cell prepares for mitosis. Using a large number of highly conserved proteins, the G2/M checkpoint prevents cells from entering the mitosis should they experience DNA damage after the S phase, or if they should progress through G1-S-G2 with damage having occurred in previous phases that had been heretofore unrepaired (Kuntz & O'Connell, 2009). All forms of DNA damage, as well as incomplete replication, activate the checkpoint. The mitosis promoting Cyclin B/CDK1 kinase activity is a critical target of the G2 checkpoint. Cyclin B/CDK1 kinase is inhibited by the actions of ATM(ATR)/Chk2(Chk1) and/or p38 kinase mediated subcellular sequestration, degradation and inhibition of CDC25 family of phosphatases that normally activate CDK1 (Kastan & Bartek, 2004). The G2 checkpoint also relies on checkpoint mediators BRCA-1 and p53 which lead to the upregulation of cell cycle inhibitors p21 and GADD45a.

The G0 (Gap zero) phase of the cell cycle in which the cells enter a quiescent state. It can be viewed as an extended G1 phase or as a separate phase outside of the cell cycle. It is separate from apoptosis or senescence in that the cell is metabolically active may enter the G1 phase and carry out the rest of the replicative cell cycle if needed. Should the cell complete interphase and not be ushered towards G0 or apoptosis the cell is allowed to enter the much shorter Mitotic phase consisting of Prophase, Metaphase, Anaphase and Telophase, the details of which will not be discussed in this chapter.

3. DNA damage

Sources of DNA damage may be endogenous or environmental. Reactive oxygen and nitrogen compounds are produced by macrophages and neutrophils at sites of inflammation and infection. These reactive species can attack DNA which leads to adducts that impair baseparing and/or block DNA replication and transcription, base loss, or cause DNA single strand breaks. Spontaneous alterations in DNA base chemistry and errors in the replication of DNA in the S phase may also contribute to endogenous DNA damage. The most pervasive environmental DNA-damaging agent is ultraviolet radiation. Ultraviolet A and B in strong sunlight can induce ~100,000 lesions per exposed cell per hour (Jackson & Bartek, 2009). Ionizing radiation can also generate various forms of DNA damage, and double strand DNA breaks (DSBs). Most environmental carcinogens operate by generating DNA damage and causing mutation. DSBs can also form in a programmed manner during development including meiosis (germ cell generation) and immunoglobin rearrangement.

DNA strand breaks occur after topoisomerase activity is aborted. Topoisomerase I and II are enzymes that unwind and wind DNA to control the synthesis of proteins and facilitate replication and damage repair. This action is targeted by chemotherapies such as Etoposide, which works by forming a complex with the Topoisomerase II enzyme preventing the re-ligation of the DNA Strands causing errors in DNA synthesis and promotes cell apoptosis.

DNA Mismatches occur via physiological processes such as DNA replication and are strand specific. They are recognized by DNA Mismatch repair proteins MSH1 and MLH2 and when theses proteins are deficient or mutated this may lead to micro satellite instability as seen in hereditary nonpolyposis colorectal cancers and Muir-Torre Syndrome.

4. DNA damage repair

A complex network of proteins and enzymes are designated to detect, signal the presence of, and repair DNA damage. This highly conserved DNA Damage Repair (DDR) signal transduction pathway (figure 2.) allows the cell to survive and maintain the integrity of the genome prior to replication or directs a cell with an overwhelming number of genomic defects towards apoptosis.

4.1 Non Homologous End Joining and Homologous Recombination

Non Homologous End Joining (NHEJ) seen in the repair of DSBs that are induced by radiation. Double strand breaks are recognized by the Ku protein, which then binds to and activates the protein kinase DNA pKcs. This leads to the recruitment and activation of end processing enzymes, polymerases, and DNA Ligase IV. While this mechanism is error prone, it has the advantage of the ability to occur in any phase of the cell cycle. Homologous recombination (HR) results in fewer errors as it uses sister chromatid sequences as the template to mediate faithful repair. HR is initiated by DSBs, stalled replication forks and single strand DNA (ssDNA), and is restricted to the S and G2 phases of the cell cycle. Single strand DNA recruited by RAD51, BRCA-1 and BRCA-2 invades the damaged DNA template. DNA ligation occurs with nucleases, polymerases, and helicases. HR restart stalled replication forks and requires Fanconi Anemia Protein complex (FANC) to repair interstrand DNA crosslinks.

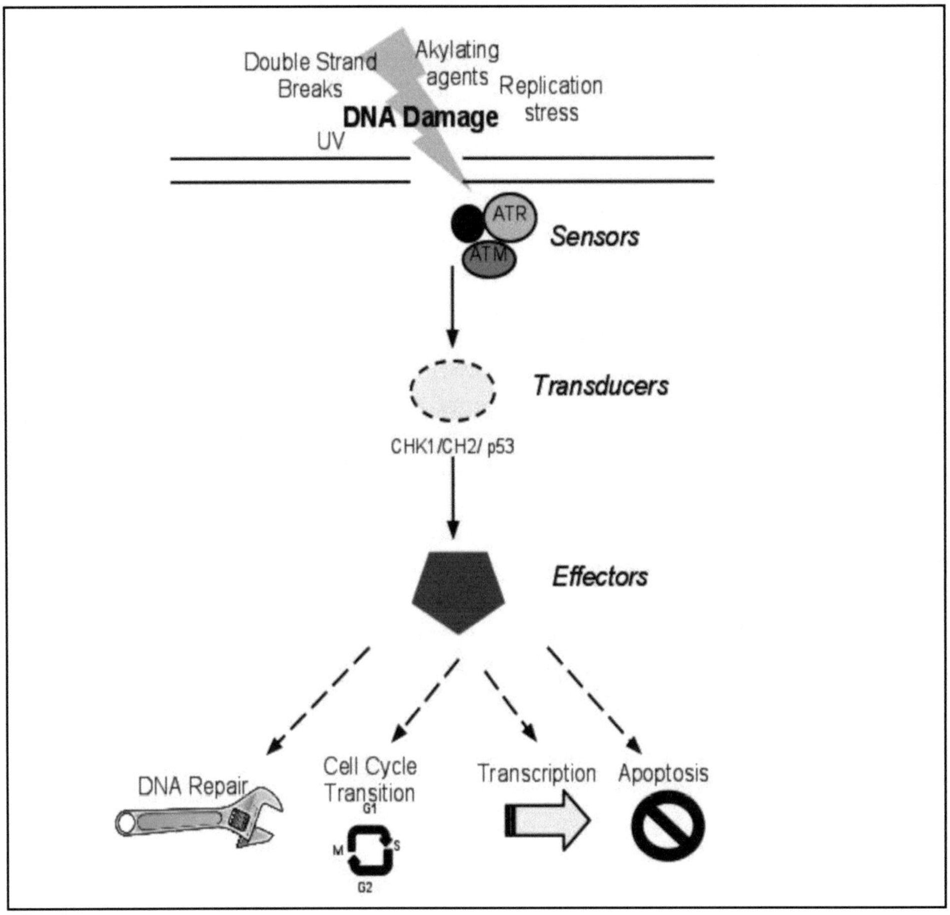

Fig. 2. The DNA Damage Response

4.2 The role of ATM and ATR

Two phosphatidylinositide-3-related kinases, Ataxia telangiectasia mutated (ATM) and ATM-rad3 related (ATR), are sensors integral to the DNA damage response. Their recruitment to DNA lesions is highly conserved and is required for PIKK-dependent DNA damage signalling (Falck et al., 2005). ATM responds to double strand breaks created by ionizing radiation, controlling the initial phosphorylation of several proteins including p53, Mdm2, BRCA-1, Chk2 and Nbs1. While ATR responds to stalled replication forks, ssDNA and DNA damage induced by UV damage. ATR also diminishes the G2/M checkpoint response induced by γ-radiation (Zhou & Elledge, 2000).

ATM and ATR are recruited to and activated by DSBs and replication protein A (RPA) coated ssDNA. ATM-ATR complexes with DNA dependent protein kinases, which phosphorylate Serine 139 on H2AX, a histone variant. Phosphorylated H2AX is referred to

as γH2Ax and recruits DDR factors and relaxes the chromatin actively marking the sites of DNA damage. The resulting immunostainable nuclear foci dubbed IRIFs (irradiation-induced foci) serve as a platform where checkpoint and DNA repair proteins accumulate to promote propagation of the damage signals and repair (Peng & Lin, 2008).
Effector protein kinases, Chk1 and Chk2, are the most understood targets of ATM and ATR respectively. They are serine/threonine kinases that are structurally unrelated but share overlapping substrate specificity (Zhou & Elledge, 2000). Chk2 is the homologue of yeast Rad53 and Cds1, and is phosphorylated in response to ionizing radiation in an ATR dependent fashion. Chk1 is phosphorylated on Ser 345 in response to hydroxyurea and ultraviolet light. The complex of ATM/ATR and Chk1/Chk2 leads to the reduction of Cyclin Dependent Kinases which, as previously described, slows/arrests the cell cycle at G1-S, intra S and G2-M check points, allowing for time to repair the damaged DNA prior to replication (Jackson & Bartek, 2009; Falck et al. 2001; Zhou & Elledge, 2000). Mutations of Chk2 alleles in irradiated cells are unable to undergo phosphorylation and fail to inhibit DNA synthesis after damage, making Chk2 a candidate tumor suppressor (Falck et al., 2001).
ATM and ATR also enhance DDR repair by inducing the DNA-repair proteins by modulating their phosphorylation, acetylation, ubiqutylation or SUMOylation (Jackson & Bartek, 2009). After cell cycle arrest, if the DSB gets repaired via NHEJ or HR, the DDR is inactivated and the cell is able to complete mitosis. If the DNA is unable to be repaired, chronic DDR signaling triggers cell death by apoptosis or cellular senescence.

4.3 p53

TP53 is a tumor suppressor gene that is known as the custodian of the genome. Ironically, it is also the most frequently mutated gene in human cancer. The p53 gene encodes a nuclear phosphoprotein that normally activates G1 cell cycle arrest in response to DNA damage (Fan et al. 1995). This arrest extends the time available before S phase entry. Cells with mutant p53 fail to arrest in G1, but rather accumulate in the G2 phase. P53 can also activate an apoptotic response to DNA damage, especially in hematopoetic and lymphoid cells. In breast carcinomas, 15-40% of tumors present an altered TP53 gene and are associated with aggressive disease and poor overall survival. Although p53 mutations are less frequent in hormone expressing tumors, the prognostic value of TP53 function is relevant in determining the patient's response to chemotherapy.
Focal adhesion kinase, FAK/PTK, is a tyrosine kinase that is over expressed in a variety of human cancers. FAK is a regulator of adhesion and motility and its upregulation is associated with increased metastatic potential. FAK has been shown to contain p53 responsive elements that are down regulated by DNA damage in a p53 dependent manner. When p53 is defective in estrogen receptor positive breast cancer cell lines, loss of FAK down-regulation is associated with increased proliferation and invasion when these cells are exposed to estradiol (Anaganti, 2011). This suggests that the loss of p53 function not only promotes tumorigenesis but also contributes to the metastatic potential of estrogen-responsive tumors.

4.4 BRCA-1 and BRCA-2

The breast cancer genes, BRCA-1 and BRCA-2, encode a nuclear phosphoprotein that acts as a tumor suppressor and plays a role in maintaining genomic stability and are located on chromosome 17 and 13 respectively. The *BRCA-1* gene was identified in 1994 as a cause of hereditary breast cancer and has since been shown to function in the complex HR pathway of DNA repair. The encoded protein combines with other tumor suppressors, DNA damage sensors, and signal transducers to form a large multi-subunit protein complex known as the BRCA-1-associated genome surveillance complex (BASC). BRCA-1 promotes cell cycle arrest with p53 and associates with DSBs marked by RAD51 foci. ATM and BRCA-2 gather with BRCA-1 and RAD51 at the sites of double-strand DNA damage. BRCA-2 does not seem to play as important a role in the cell cycle checkpoint responses to DNA damage as BRCA-1, however it has been implicated in the mitotic spindle checkpoint, homologous recombination, and chromatin remodeling.

Mutations in breast cancer genes are responsible for approximately 40% of sporadic breast cancers and more than 80% of inherited breast and ovarian cancers. In the case of BRCA-1 and BRCA-2, heterozygous BRCA-1 mutation carriers have a high lifetime risk of breast and ovarian cancer, and patients with a BRCA-2 mutation will also have a high lifetime risk, though with later onset. The majority of pathogenic BRCA-1 and BRCA-2 mutations are small insertions, deletions or nonsense mutations that result in premature stop codons and a shortened, non-functional BRCA protein.

Women carrying a heterozygous deleterious mutation in the *BRCA-1* gene carry a 57% cumulative risk of developing breast cancer by the age of 70 years and a 40% risk of developing ovarian cancer (Annunziata & Bates, 2010). In cells lacking functional BRCA-1 or BRCA-2, HR is deficient and DDR may proceed through more error-prone NHEJ. This, when applied with a PARP inhibitor, may lead to further propagation of DNA damage and the death of the cell as will be detailed below. It is unclear why breast or ovarian epithelial cells are more susceptible to the oncogenic outcome of BRCA deficiency.

4.5 PARP-1 and PARP inhibitors

Poly (ADP-Ribose) polymerase is an abundant nuclear protein and is a key regulator of base excision repair process. PARP1 detects single strand breaks arising from reactive oxygen species and is also involved in the repair of DSBs. The poly ADP ribose activates histones, transcription factors, and signalers (NFkB, DNAPk, Laminin B) and has an N-terminal DNA binding domain that contains two zinc fingers, which bind to both SSBs and DSBs. PARP activates itself to recruit other component of SSB repair. When PARP-1 is inhibited, normal cells proceed towards homologous recombination repair of the DNA damage. As stated above, when BRCA-1 and BRCA-2 is mutated, cells are unable to proceed towards HR. When PARP-inhibitors are applied, the cell cannot repair the DNA damage and becomes apoptotic, leaving the normal cells unaffected (Liang et al. 2009) as seen in figure 3. This inhibition of PARP-1 also sensitizes tumor cells to chemotherapy and radiation in vitro. Currently, clinical trails are being conducted to assess the efficacy of PARP-1 inhibitors, such as Olaparib, in the treatment of patients with breast and ovarian cancer with BRCA-1/BRCA-2 mutations and triple negative receptor breast cancers (Annunziata & Bates, 2010).

4.6 BRIT-1

The BRCT-Repeat Inhibitor or hTET expression/Microcephalin or BRIT-1 gene is located on chromosome 8 (8p23.1) and is a damage response protein that is physically recruited to sites of damaged DNA. The most distinct role of BRIT-1 is to stop the G2-M transition in the cell cycle of damaged cells. ATM and ATR act on BRIT, However, BRIT is NOT required to phosphorylate ATM but is needed to recruit pATM to the damaged DNA and also positively regulates CHK1 and BRCA-1 expression. BRIT binds to chromatin and forms nuclear foci after exposure to ionizing radiation or UV rays as short as 2 minutes after the radiation occurs (Chaplet et al., 2006). This chromosome region is frequently deleted in breast, ovarian and prostate cancers. Microarray data from a public database show that BRIT1 mRNA levels are markedly decreased in 19 of 30 cases; 63% of ovarian cancer specimens relative benign ovarian tissue specimens and 72% or the 54 breast cancer cell lines tested also showed a decrease in the BRIT1 gene copy number (Lin et al. 2010).

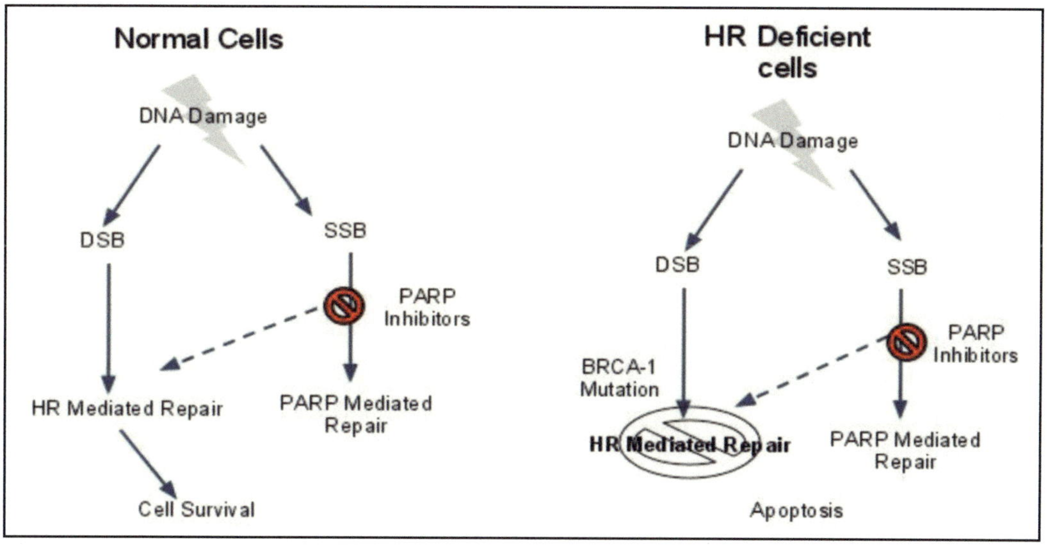

Fig. 3. Action of PARP-inhibitors in HR deficient cells.

When wild type and BRIT knock down cells are irradiated, BRIT deficient cells continue to enter mitosis at a greater rate than the wild types cells (Chaplet et al., 2006). This supposes that the DNA damage that was created during irradiation is not being sufficiently repaired in the BRIT1- group and thus genome mutations are propagated through subsequent generations. BRIT1 has also been clearly demonstrated to be crucial for maintaining genomic stability *in vivo*. Using gene targeting technology to create BRIT1 knock out mice, the BRIT-/- mice were able to survive to adulthood but they were growth retarded and hypersensitive to IR when compared to wild type and heterozygous mice (Liang et al., 2010). Our data suggest that breast tumors can be induced in the mammary glands of mice with conditional BRIT1 deficiency via irradiation, but not in the control littermates. BRIT knock down cells also show reduced expression of BRCA-1 and Chk1 (Lin et al. 2005). The next step will be to investigate if, and to what extent, BRIT1 deficiency may contribute to the initiation and progression of cancer with the existence of oncogenic or genotoxic stress.

5. DNA damage repair and triple negative breast cancer

5.1 Breast cancer epidemiology

Breast cancer is the most common female malignancy and second to lung cancer in terms of mortality. It is the leading cause of death among women aged 40 to 50 years. According to the Surveillance Epidemiology and End Results (SEER) Program of the National Cancer Institute, based on rates from 2005-2007, 12.15% of women born in the United States today will be diagnosed with cancer of the breast at some time during their lifetime. The estimated new cases of breast cancer in 2010 were 207,090 (female); 1,970 (male) and deaths were 39,840 (female); 390 (male) (Altekruse et al., 2010). The SEER data also show that from 2003-2007, the median age at diagnosis for cancer of the breast was 61 years of age with 0.0% were diagnosed under age 20; 1.9% between 20 and 34; 10.5% between 35 and 44; 22.6% between 45 and 54; 24.1% between 55 and 64; 19.5% between 65 and 74; 15.8% between 75 and 84; and 5.6% 85+ years of age The age-adjusted incidence rate was 122.9 per 100,000 women per year. These rates are based on cases diagnosed in 2003-2007 from 17 SEER geographic areas. (Altekruse et al., 2010).

5.2 Breast cancer risk factors

The most important risk factor for the development of breast cancer is gender with the female to male ratio being 100:1. Further risk factors for breast cancer and relative risks as elegantly described by Singletary in 2003 are shown in table 1. A personal history of breast cancer is a significant risk factor for the development of contralateral breast cancer with an incidence of 0.5%-1.0% per year. As stated previously in the chapter, exposure to ionizing radiation, such as for the treatment of Hodgkin's Lymphoma, has been associated with an increased risk of breast cancer, especially if it occurs prior to age 30, however the risk is less in the first 15 years after treatment than after 15 years (Zager et al, 2006).

Risk Factors	Category at Risk	Relative Risk
Alcohol Intake	2 drinks per Day	1.2
Body Mass Index	80th percentile, age 55 or older	1.2
Hormone replacement therapy with estrogen AND progesterone	Current user for at least 5 Years	1.3
Ionizing radiation exposure	Treatment for Hodgkin's Disease	5.2
Age at first Childbirth	Nulliparous or 1st Child after 30	1.7-1.9
Current age	65 or older	5.8
Past History of Breast Cancer	Invasive Breast Cancer	6.8
Family History	First Degree relative with premenopausal breast cancer	3.3
	First Degree relative with postmenopausal breast cancer	1.8
Germline Mutation	Heterozygous for BRCA1 age <40	200
	Heterozygous for BRCA1 age 60-69	15

Table 1. Risk Factors for Breast cancer (Singletary, 2003).

Breast diseases such as adenosis, fibroadenomas, apocrine changes, duct ectasias and mild hyperplasias carry no increased risk for breast cancer as they are non-proliferative. However, proliferative diseases, such as atypical ductal or lobular hyperplasias do carry an increased risk. Hormone replacement therapy used for the treatment of postmenopausal symptoms have been shown to increase a woman's risk of developing breast cancer, yet patients may weigh this risk with the benefits of hormone therapy such as a decrease in postmenopausal symptoms and increased bone density.

The age of the patient is also a risk factor for breast cancer. For women who experience menopause after the age of 55 the risk of breast cancer is twice that of women who enter menopause before age 44. Women who experience regular ovulatory cycles prior to age 13 have a 4 fold increased risk of breast cancer than women who had up to a 5 year delay in the development of regular cycles. Women who menstruate for more than 30 years are also at a greater risk for developing breast cancer than women who menstruate for less than 30 years (Zager et al. 2006).

Family history of breast cancer is very important in determining the risk of breast and other cancers. Though the majority of breast cancers are of the sporadic type, the highest risk is seen in patients with a young (premenopausal) first-degree relative with bilateral breast cancer (Zager et al. 2006). Overall risk is determined by the number of relatives with cancer, their ages at diagnosis and laterality of their disease (unilateral or bilateral). The above risk factors have been used in the Gail breast cancer risk model, which will be discussed later in this chapter.

Genetic abnormalities have also been seen to predispose individuals to breast and ovarian cancers. Autosomal dominant mutations such as Li-fraumeni syndrome, Muir-torre Syndrome and, of course, BRCA-1 and BRCA-2 mutations which predispose patients to breast cancer have been well described and are diagrammed in table 2. As seen in the previous table, heterozygosity for BRAC-1 germline mutation carries a relative risk of 200 for the development of breast cancer.

Syndrome	Site of Mutation	Increased Malignancies of:
BRCA-1	Chromosome 17q	Breast, Ovarian, Prostate, Colon
BRCA-2	Chromosome 13q	Breast (including male), Ovaries, Prostate, larynx, pancreas
Li- Fraumeni	p53 gene on chromosome 17p	Breast, brain, adrenal glands, soft tissue sarcomas
Muir-Torre	DNA Mismatch repair genes hMLH1 and hMSH2 on chromosome 2p	Breast, gastrointestinal tract, genitourinary tract, sebaceous tumors, keratoacanthomas
Cowden Disease	PTEN gene on chromosome 10q	Breast, Colon, Uterus, thyroid, lung, bladder. Hamartomatous polyps in the GI tract.
Peutz-Jegers	STK11 gene on chromosome 19p	Breast, Pancreas, mucocutaneous melanin deposition Hamartomatous polyps in the GI tract.

Table 2. Autosomal dominant mutations and syndromes associated with increased risk for breast cancer (Zager et al, 2006).

5.3 Luminal and basal sub-typing

Breast cancers are often described in terms of luminal and basal subtypes corresponding to their likely origin based on hormone receptor status. The luminal subtypes A and B are characterized by estrogen receptor (ER+) expression and expression of genes associated with luminal epithelial cells. Luminal A tumors are often low grade while luminal B tumors are often high grade. Human epidermal growth factor Receptor 2 receptor positive tumors (also known as HER2/neu or ERBB2) encode a member of the epidermal growth factor (EGF) receptor family of receptor tyrosine kinases. These tumors respond to trastuzumab, a monoclonal antibody that binds to the domain IV of the extracellular segment of the HER2/neu receptor causing arrest during the G1 phase of the cell cycle. While the HER2 phenotype is aggressive, this response to trastuzumab makes for a favorable prognosis.

The basal-like subtype is characterized by the expression of basal keratins 5 and 17, laminin and fatty acid binding protein 7. Large portions of basal subtype tumors are also lacking expression of ER, Progesterone Receptor (PR) and HER2. These tumors are termed triple negative breast cancer due to their lack of the three receptors (Jaspers et al. 2009).

5.4 Triple negative breast cancer

Triple negative breast cancers (TNBC) show the poorest survival of all US groups and are larger than and show a higher rate of node positivity at the time of diagnosis. Triple negative breast cancers have a high prevalence in young, obese women; and pre-menopausal African-American women, compared to post menopausal African-American and non-African-American women. They also present as interval cancer with a weak association between tumor size and lymph node involvement. TNBCs have a high risk of early recurrence with a peak recurrence rate seen between the first and third years after diagnosis with metastasis rarely preceded by local recurrence and most mortalities occurring in within the first 5 years, further highlighting the need for close clinical follow-up (Chacón & Constanzo, 2010).

Like basal subtype tumors, TNBC patients have significantly higher rates of pathological complete response following neoadjuvant chemotherapy, with increased frequency of distant metastasis formation but not local relapse (Jaspers et al. 2009). The majority of BRCA-1-related breast tumors share phenotypic features with TNBCs and basal- like tumors as they mostly lack expression of ER and HER2, and have epidermal growth factor over-expression and p53 mutations. These similarities suggest that basal-like breast cancers arise through common genetic pathways as BRCA-1 mutated cancers. Recently, an unselected cohort of patients with TNBC was found to have a 19.5% incidence of BRCA mutations with 12.6% in BRCA-1 and 3.9% in BRCA-2 (Gonzalez-Angulo et al., 2011). This suggests that TNBC and basal- like breast cancers may be similar to BRCA-1 mutated tumors in their pathogenesis and that they may be susceptible to PARP-1 inhibitors and other chemotoxins that are designed for BRCA-1 mutated tumors. These findings also suggest that genetic counseling may be indicated in patients presenting with triple receptor negative breast cancer.

6. Targeting DNA damage repair defects in the treatment of breast cancer

6.1 Development of new treatment modalities

For patients with breast cancer, treatment consists of surgery, radiation, hormonal and chemotherapy. Commonly, clinicians employ a combination of all of these modalities to prevent loco-regional recurrence or to treat distant metastasis. Radiation and some chemotherapeutics rely on the inherent DDR impairment of tumor cells to induce apoptosis. Cancer cells, which proliferate more rapidly than most normal cells, are thought to be especially vulnerable DNA damage exposure, which occurs during S phase of the cell cycle. Chemotherapeutics that induce DDR inhibition might enhance the effectiveness of radiotherapies and DNA damaging chemotherapies.

The status of DNA damage repair proteins may also allow for the prediction of breast cancer sensitivity to neoadjuvant chemotherapy. In a recently published study (Asakawa et al. 2010) sixty patients with primary breast invasive ductal carcinoma consecutively underwent neoadjuvant chemotherapy with Epirubicin and Cyclophosphamide (EC), two chemotherapies that induce DSBs, followed by treatment with docetaxel. The investigators were able to correlate focus formation of BRCA-1, γH2AX, and RAD51 prior to treatment and RAD51 focus formation after treatment with mean tumor volume reduction and tumor response rate. When cells showed a high percentage of DDR nuclear foci staining shortly after the first EC treatment, they showed poor tumor response when evaluated for mean tumor volume reduction, which, in breast cancer, is a major goal of neoadjuvant chemotherapy. These findings may lead to the possibility of using DDR status clinically to determine which patients will respond to chemotherapy.

Targeting specific DDR proteins to inhibit is another way to develop tailored treatment modalities. As stated prior in the case of PARP-1 inhibitors, breast and ovarian cancer patients with BRCA-1 and BRCA-2 mutations may be more likely to respond favorably than those patients with functioning BRCA-1. This could be a great breakthrough for these patients as they generally have more aggressive disease with high rates of loco-regional recurrence, elevated risk of contralateral breast cancer formation and are notoriously resistant to the chemotherapeutics available today. We can further these efforts to investigate patients with deficiencies in other DDR associated proteins.

DDR targeted cancer therapies currently in clinical trails include those targeting the Chk1 and Chk2 proteins. The inherent resistance to radiation of cancer stem cells is another challenge to overcome and inhibiting the Chk1 auto phosphorylation may increase the toxicity of DNA damaging agents that are currently in use and may improve radiosensitvity. In the case of p53, which is functionally reduced in 50% of cancers, efforts have been made to restore the wild type p53 activity via recombinant adenovirus encoding p53 or by using small compounds and short peptides to restore the function. (Bolderson et al. 2009)

6.2 Development of new cancer screening modalities and risk assessments

As stated previously, women who have BRCA-1 germline mutations have a higher risk of developing breast cancer than the general population, and the cancer that they develop is exceedingly aggressive with a high rate of recurrence, development of contralateral disease and resistance to current chemotherapies. Genetic testing is now being used to identify patients with the genetic predispositions to develop tumors. This testing allows clinicians to better define a patient's effective risk and to allow for preventive treatment strategies such as prophylactic surgery or hormonal therapies. In the case of multiple family members presenting with breast cancer, genetic counseling should be offered to the patient affected with the disease first to determine what type of mutation is being expressed before testing any unaffected relatives for the disease. In the case of BRCA-1 and BRCA-2 mutation screening, commonly used methods their advantages and disadvantages were described in the 2006 paper by Palma and is reproduced here in table 3. These methods include: Direct Sequencing (DS); Single Strand Conformation Polymorphism Analysis (SSCA); Heteroduplex Analysis (HAD); Denaturing Gradient Gel Electrophoresis (DGGE); Chemical Cleavage Mismatch (CCM); Protein Truncation Test (PTT); and Denaturing High Performance Liquid Chromatography (DHPLC).

Technique	Principle for Detection	Advantages/Disadvantages
DS	Direct sequencing of DNA fragments	Best sensitivity ~100%, Exact location and nature of deletion . Labor intensive and expensive
DHPLC	Detects heteroduplex through their chromographic elution profiles	High sensitivity ≤ 100%, rapid and precise Initial investment in equipment is high. However, low cost single analysis
PTT	Detects pre-terminal in vitro synthesized protein products	98% sensitive, gives approximate location of pathogenetic mutations in large fragments. Only detects sequence alterations responsible for truncated proteins. Cannot analyze small exons.
CCM	Detects heteroduplex through chemical cleavage at the site of DNA mismatch	Good sensitivity (>95%) Scans large fragments. Approximates location of damage. Time consuming and labor intensive.
DGGE	Altered Electrophilic mobility of heteroduplex based on their melting behavior (denaturing)	Rapid and easy after initial planning. Low detection rate. Difficult to set up technique.
HAD	Altered Electrophilic mobility of heteroduplex (non-denaturing)	Rapid and easy to carry out, Detects insertion/ deletion mutations in large fragments. Low detection rate (80%) poor for point mutations
SSCA	Altered Electrophilic mobility of single stranded DNA	Rapid and easy to carry out Low detection rate (70-80%) scans short fragments.

Table 3. Commonly used methods for BRCA1 / 2 mutational screening in descending order of sensitivity. (Palma et al., 2006)

In the interpretation of these genetic tests, patients who test negative and have a known affected relative who is positive for a specific mutation are thought of as "real negatives" and have a risk of that of the general population. "Non informative" tests are from patients who test negative but who do not have a previously identified familial BRCA-1 or BRCA-2 alteration. There may be a mutation in another gene or a low penetrance gene. The subsequent treatment of family members who test positive for a BRCA-1 or BRCA-2 mutation depends on the age of the patient and the desire of child bearing. Prophylactic bilateral mastectomies reduce the risk of breast cancer by up to 90%, and while the risk of ovarian cancer is lower than the risk for breast cancer in the context of BRCA mutation, the absence of early detection screening for ovarian cancer has increased the necessity for prophylactic oophorectomy (Palma et al., 2006).

DNA damage repair protein function may be another useful tool to incorporate into our risk stratification models. The Gail Breast Cancer Risk Assessment model has been in use since 1989 (Gail, et al. 1989). This model, adopted by the National Cancer Institute, uses individual risk factors of age; family breast cancer history (amongst first degree relatives); age of first menarche and first live birth; personal medical history including number of previous breast biopsies and confirmed atypical hyperplasia; and race. A 5-year risk estimate and lifetime risk are calculated via logistic regression of the risk factors and converted into absolute risk based on epidemiological data for breast cancer incidence and other risks. A Gail 5-year risk score greater than or equal to 1.66% has been seen to be an important tool to identify women who have an increased risk for developing breast cancer.

This method is not without shortcomings, including having a lower sensitivity for women of color, having been based on a cohort of Caucasian women, and has been challenged in the use of patients younger than age 40 (MacKarem et al., 2001). However when these clinical features of the Gail model are combined with genetic information they may increase the power of the test. Single-nucleotide polymorphisms (SNPs) are reproducibly associated with breast cancer risk in women of European and other racial or ethnic backgrounds. Investigators located seven SNPs associated with breast cancer risk from the literature and genotyped in white non-Hispanic women in a nested case- control cohort of 1664 case patients and 1636 control patients within the Women's Health Initiative Clinical Trail. SNP risk scores were calculated and combined with Gail risk estimates. These investigators found that the SNP risk score was nearly independent of Gail risk with good agreement between predicted and observed SNP relative risks. Combining validated genetic risks factors with clinical risk factors modestly improved classification of breast cancer risk in these women (Mealiffe et al., 2010). This may be able to be extrapolated to other genetic mutations further combining what we know to be absolute clinical risk factors with DNA damage repair gene germline mutations to create a more inclusive model for the prediction of breast cancer development.

7. Conclusion

The cells throughout the human body are constantly subjected to both internal forces and external insults that cause damage to their DNA. Understanding the DNA damage response pathway is key to the understanding breast cancer tumorigenesis and to the creation of superior chemotherapeutics.

8. Acknowledgements

We would like to acknowledge the Systems Biology and Surgical Oncology Departments at the M. D. Anderson Cancer Center and also the Ruth L. Kirschstein National Research Service Award from the National Institute of Health for providing the funding to support the research for this chapter.

9. References

Altekruse, SF., Kosary, CL., Krapcho, M. et al. (eds) (2010). SEER Cancer Statistics Review, 1975-2007, National Cancer Institute. Bethesda, MD, http://seer.cancer.gov/csr/1975_2007/, based on November 2009 SEER data submission, posted to the SEER web site, 2010.

Anaganti, S., Fernández-Cuesta, L., Langerød, A. et al. (2011), p53 -Dependent repression of focal adhesion kinase in response to estradiol in breast cancer cell lines, *Cancer Letters*, Vol. 300, Issue 2 (Jan 2011), pp 215-224.

Annunziata, C; Bates, SE. (2010), PARP inhibitors in BRCA-1/BRCA-2 germline mutation carriers with ovarian and breast cancer, *Biology Reports,*Vol 2 issue 10 (Feb 2010) retrieved from http://f1000.com/reports/b/2/10.

Askawa, H., Koizumi, H., Koike,A. et al. (2010), Prediction of breast cancer sensitivity of neoadjuvant chemotherapy based on status of DNA damage repair proteins, *Breast Cancer Research,* Vol. 12 Issue 2 (March 2010) retrieved from http://breast-cancer-research.com/content/12/2/R17.

Bolderson, E., Richard, DJ., Zhou, BS., et al. (2009), Recent Advances in Cancer Therapy Targeting proteins Involved in DNA Double-Strand Break repair. *Clincial Cancer Research,* Vol. 15, Issue 20, (October 2009) pp.6314-6320.

Chacón, RD., Constanzo, MV. (2010) Triple Negative Breast Cancer, *Breast Cancer Research,* Vol. 12, Supplement 2 (October 2010) retrieved from http://breast-cancer-research.com/supplements/12/52/53.

Chaplet, M., Rai,R., Jackson-Bernitsas, D., et al. (2006), BRIT1/MCPH1 A guardian of the Genome and an Enemy of Tumors, *Cell Cycle,* Vol. 5, Issue 22, (November 2006) pp. 2579-2583.

Falck, J., Coates, J., Jackson, S. (2005), Conserved modes of recruitment of ATM, ATR andDNA-PKcs to sites of DNA Damage, *Nature,* Vol. 434, Issue31 (March 2005) pp. 605-611.

Falck, J., Mailand, N., Syljuåsen, R., et al. (2001) Letters to Nature: The ATM-Chk2-Cdc25A Checkpoint pathway guards against radioresistant DNA synthesis, *Nature,* Vol. 410, Issue 12 (April 2001), pp. 842-847.

Fan, S., Smith, M., Rivet II, D., et al. (1995), Disruption of p53 function Sensitizes Breast Cancer MCF-7 cells to cisplatin and pentoxifylline, *Cancer Research,* Vol. 55, (April 1995) pp. 1629-1654.

Gail, MH. Brinton, LA., Byar, DP. et al. (1989), Projection individualized Probabilities of developing breast cancer for White Females who are being examined annually, *Journal of the National Cancer Institute,* Vol. 81, Issue 24 (December 1989) pp. 1879-1886.

Gonzalez-Angulo, AM., Timms, KM., Liu, S. et al., (2011), Incidence and outcome of BRCA Mutations in unselected patients with triple receptor negative breast cancer, *Clinical Cancer Research,* Vol. 17, Issue 5 (March 2011) pp. 1082-1089.

Jackson, SP., Bartek, J. (2009), The DNA-Damage response in human biology and disease, *Nature,* Vol. 461, Issue 22, (October 2009), pp. 1071-1078.

Jaspers, JE., Rottenberg, S., Jonkers, J. (2009) Therapeutic options for triple negative breast cancers with defective homologous recombination, *Biochemica et Biophysica Acta.* Vol. 1796, Issue 2 (December 2009) pp. 266-280.

Kastan, MB., Bartek, J. (2004), Cell-cycle checkpoints and cancer, *Nature,* Vol. 432, Issue 18 (November 2004) pp. 316-323.

Kuntz, K., O'Connell, MJ. (2009), The G2 DNA Damage Checkpoint, *Cell Biology and Therapy,* Vol. 8, Issue 15 (August 2009), pp.1433-1439

Liang, Y., Gao, H., Lin, SY., et al. (2010), BRIT1/MCPH1 is Essential for Mitotic and Meiotic Recombination DNA Repair and Maintaining Genomic Stability in Mice, *PLOS Genetics,* Vol. 6, Issue 1 (January 2010) retrieved from http://www.plosgenetics.org/article/info%3Adoi%2F10.1371%2Fjournal.pgen.1000826

Liang, Y., Lin, SY., Brunicardi, FC., et al. (2009), DNA Damage Response Pathways in Tumor Suppression and Treatment, *World Journal of Surgery* Vol. 33, Issue 4 (April 2009) pp. 661-666.

Lin, SY, Liang, Y., Li, K. (2010), Multiple Roles of BRIT1/MCPH1 in DNA Damage Response, DNA Repair, and Cancer suppression, *Yonsei Medical Journal,* Vol. 51, Issue 3, (May 2010), pp. 295-301.

Lin, SY., Rai, R., Li, K., et al. (2005), BRIT1/MCPH1 is a DNA Damage responsive protein that regulates the BRCA-1-Chk1 pathway, implicating checkpoint dysfunction in microcehpaly. *PNAS,* Vol. 102, Issue 42, (October 2005), 15105-15109.

MacKarem, G., Roche, CA., Hughes, KS. (2001), The effectiveness of the Gail model in estimating risk for development of breast cancer in women under 40 years of age, *Breast Journal,* Vol. 7, Issue 1(January-February 2001) pp. 34-39.

Mealiffe, ME., Stokowski, RP., Rhees, BK. et al. (2010) Assessment and clinical validity of a breast cancer risk model combining genetic and clinical information, *Journal of the National Cancer Institute,* Vol. 102, Issue 21 (November 2010), pp. 1618-1627.

Miyoshi, Y., Murase, K., Oh, K. (2008) Basal-like Subtype and BRCA1 Dysfunction in Breast Cancers, *International Journal of Clinical Oncology,* Vol. 13, Issue 5 (October 2008) pp. 395-400.

Palma, M., Risorti,E., Ricevuto, E., et al. (2006), BRCA-1 and BRCA-2: The genetic testing and the current management options for mutation carriers, *Critical Reviews in Oncology/Hematology,* Vol. 57, Issue 1 (January 2006) pp. 1-23.

Peng, G., Lin, SY. (2008)., BRIT1, a Novel DNA Damage Responsive Protein Dysfunctioned in Primary Microcephaly and Cancer, In: *New Research on DNA Damage,* Honoka Kimura and Aoi Suzuki, Editors, pp. 99-112, Nova Science Publishers, Inc., ISBN: 978-1-60456-581-2 New York.

Singletary, SE. (2003). Rating the Risk Factors for Breast Cancer, *Annals of Surgery,* Vol. 237, Issue 4 (April 2003) pp. 474-482

Zager, JS., Colorzano, CC., Thomas, E., et al. (2006). Invasive Breast Cancer, In: *The M. D. Anderson Surgical Oncology Handbook,4th Ed.,* Barry W. Feig, David H. Berger, George M. Fuhrman Editors, pp. 23-59, Lippincott Williams & Wilkins Publishers, ISBN 978-0-7817-5643-3, Philadelphia, PA.

Zhou, BS., Elledge, SJ. (2000), The DNA damage response: putting checkpoints in perspective, *Nature,* Vol. 408, Issue 23 (November 2000) pp. 433-439.

8

Cell Cycle Regulatory Proteins in Breast Cancer: Molecular Determinants of Drug Resistance and Targets for Anticancer Therapies

Aamir Ahmad, Zhiwei Wang, Raza Ali, Bassam Bitar, Farah T. Logna, Main Y. Maitah, Bin Bao, Shadan Ali, Dejuan Kong, Yiwei Li and Fazlul H. Sarkar
Karmanos Cancer Institute, Wayne State University, Detroit, MI, USA

1. Introduction

Deregulation of cell-cycle is a distinguishing hallmark of tumor cells (Stewart *et al*, 2003). Regulation of cell cycle is a key mechanism for the maintenance of homeostasis of normal cell growth and viability, and this is a very tightly regulated process. However, deregulation of cell cycle is well known to contribute to tumor development (Maya-Mendoza *et al*, 2009). Normal cells possess an ability to arrest cell-cycle after DNA damage in an attempt to maintain genome integrity whereas tumor-initiating cells are characterized by deregulated cell-cycle whereby the DNA-damaged cells proceed to undergo DNA synthesis and cell division, which leads to the development of tumor mass. Since cancer cells, including breast cancer cells, are known to exhibit uncontrolled cell growth and proliferation, one parameter to judge the efficacy of anti-cancer therapies is through their ability to arrest cell cycle. Therefore, it is not surprising that the acquisition of drug-resistance in cancer cells is often linked with defects in cell cycle regulation. Cell cycle arrest involves down-regulation of cyclins and cyclin-dependent kinases (CDKs), and up-regulation of inhibitory p21 and p27. Several investigations, including those from our own laboratory, have revealed that cell-cycle arrest is an important mechanism responsible for apoptosis-inducing ability of cancer therapeutic agents in breast cancer cells. In particular, functional loss of G1-checkpoint inhibitors, p21 and p27, is believed to be important during the progression of many human malignancies, and most therapeutic agents function via induction of these tumor suppressor proteins. Loss of p21 and p27 has also been implicated in the acquisition of drug-resistance phenotype, and conversely, their up-regulation has the ability to re-sensitize cancer cells to conventional therapeutics. This chapter attempts to update the state-of-our understanding of several key cell cycle proteins that play a crucial role in breast cancer tumorigenesis. We will review modulation of such key players by conventional therapeutics, which eventually results in the induction of apoptotic cell death in the context of cell cycle regulation and drug resistance. In addition to the clinically relevant drugs, we will also introduce readers to the potential utility of natural agents as cell cycle regulators.

2. Cell cycle: An overview

The two main events/phases of the cell cycle are - Interphase and Mitosis (Figure 1). Interphase is the phase of cell cycle in which cell performs the majority of its purposes, including preparation for the division of cell. Mitosis is that phase of the cell cycle when cell prepares for and actually completes cell division. Interphase serves as the checkpoint to ensure that the cell is ready to enter into mitosis. Since the cell cycle is a "cycle", cells are continually entering and exiting the various phases of this dynamic cycle. Cells spend a majority of their time in interphase and this phase has three distinct stages - G1, S and G2.

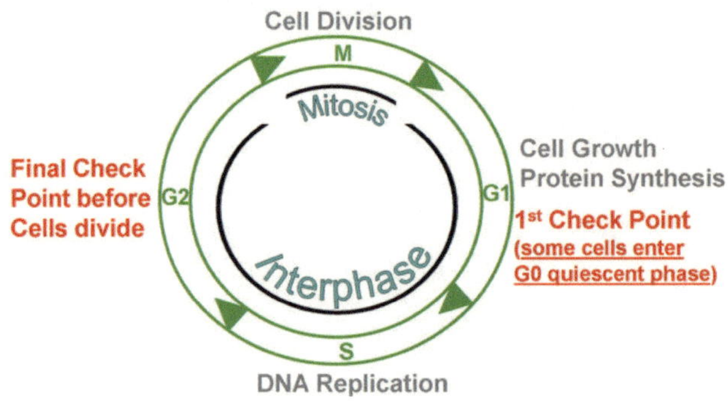

Fig. 1. An overview of cell cycle.

2.1 G1 phase

G1 is the phase of cell cycle immediately following a round of cell division and occupies the time between mitosis and the beginning of DNA replication during S phase. In the G1 phase, cells grow and function normally. Prior to another round of cell division, cell has to make sure that it is completely ready for division. G1 is the phase when this monitoring takes place and if the cell is not ready yet to divide, it will continue to remain in this phase. Cells are even known to enter a phase called G0 if they are not ready to continue in the cell cycle. G0 can last for days, weeks, or even years. However, if cell decides to divide, it grows in size during G1 phase, more cell organelles are synthesized, protein synthesis occurs and cell prepares itself for DNA replication.

2.2 S phase

Immediately following G1 phase is the S (synthesis) phase. It is the phase when DNA replication takes place. This phase represents a particular sensitive point in cell cycle because fidelity of DNA replication is required to ensure that the resulting daughter cells will have exactly the same genetic make-up as the dividing mother cell. Most of the events that occur during S phase are related to DNA replication and this phase is marked by synthesis of proteins/enzymes that are involved in DNA replication machinery. At the end of S phase, cells contain twice the normal number of chromosomes.

2.3 G2 phase

S phase is followed by G2 phase. This phase is marked by further growth of cell in anticipation of mitosis. Since this phase occurs after the duplication of DNA and just before the commencement of cell division in mitosis, it represents another checkpoint in the cell cycle and a final chance for the cells to make sure that their DNA and other cellular components have been properly duplicated.

3. Regulation of cell cycle

3.1 Cyclins

Cyclins are so named because they undergo a constant 'cycle' of synthesis and degradation during cell division. There are now several recognized classes or types of cyclins, active in different stages of the cell cycle. The D- and E-type cyclins are associated with the G1-S phase transition of the cell cycle (Sherr, 1994). Cyclins are proteins that play important roles in the functioning of CDKs.

3.2 Cyclin-dependent kinases

CDKs, as their names suggest, are kinases that depend on cyclins for their kinase activity i.e. their ability to phosphorylate other molecules. A number of CDKs were discovered independently before their cell cycle regulatory function was recognized, and consequently, the nomenclature of these proteins was not uniform and was often confusing. Based on the outcome of a meeting at Cold Spring Harbor in 1991, the CDK series was born with many of the pre-recognized cell cycle regulators named CDK1, CDK2, CDK3 and so on (Abukhdeir & Park, 2008). CDKs were classified as kinases based on the observation that the total amount of phosphorylated proteins increased following injection of CDKs into the oocytes of a variety of different organisms (Abukhdeir & Park, 2008). A number of CDKs have now been characterized. Cyclins bind to CDKs to form a cyclin-CDK complex (Figure 2). This complex, along with the various phosphorylated targets, acts as a signal for the cell to pass to the next cell cycle phase. Cyclins and CDKs are, therefore, positive modulators of cell cycle. Synthesis of cyclins and CDKs marks the readiness of cells to divide. At the time when cell no longer wants to divide, cyclins are degraded resulting in deactivation of CDKs and arresting the cell cycle.

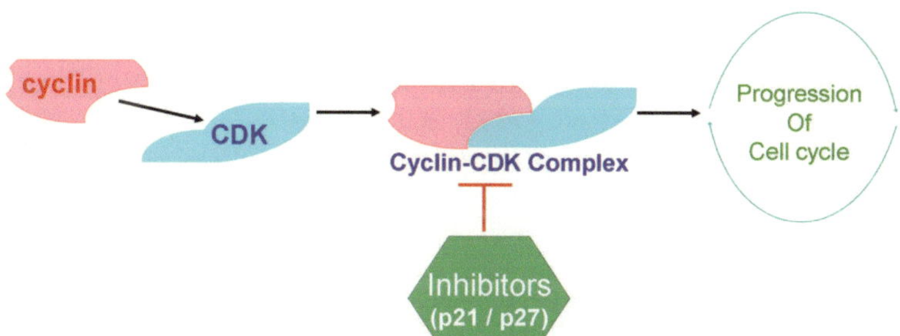

Fig. 2. Role of cyclins, cyclin-dependent kinases (CDKs) and inhibitors in progression of cell cycle.

3.3 Inhibitors of cyclin-dependent kinases

Since CDKs are involved in the progression of cell cycle, molecules that inhibit CDKs are negative regulators of cell cycle and function to induce cell cycle arrest (Figure 2). Cyclin-CDK complexes typically activate their downstream targets by phosphorylation; therefore, inhibitors of cyclin-CDKs modulate cell cycle by preventing or limiting cyclin-CDKs' ability to phosphorylate their targets. There are two classes of CDK inhibitors. Members of the first class specifically bind to CDK4 and CDK6 and inhibit their association with D-type cyclins. Members of the second class, also known as kinase inhibitor proteins (KIPs) and include p21, p27 and p57, are inhibitors of cyclin A-CDK, cyclin D-CDK and cyclin E-CDK complexes (Abukhdeir & Park, 2008). Similar to existence of many CDKs, many inhibitors of CDKs are also known but we will limit our discussion on two such inhibitors - p21 and p27, to keep our discussion more focused.

3.3.1 p21 (cyclin-dependent kinase inhibitor 1)/WAF1

The p21 is coded by human gene *CDKN1A* and belongs to the *Cip/Kip* family of CDK inhibitor proteins. Two research groups, working independently, published the cloning of its gene in 1993 simultaneously. Using a subtractive hybridization approach, el-Deiry et al. (el-Deiry *et al*, 1993) identified a gene whose expression was directly induced by p53 and it was found to be an important mediator of p53-dependent tumor growth suppression in human brain tumor cells. This gene was named WAF1. Using an improved two-hybrid system, Harper et al. (Harper *et al*, 1993) isolated a 21 kDa protein that regulated CDK2 activity. This protein was found to inhibit phosphorylation of retinoblastoma (Rb) by cyclin A-CDK2, cyclin E-CDK2, cyclin D1-CDK4 and cyclin D2-CDK4 complexes. This gene was named CIP1 (CDK-interacting protein 1). In view of the simultaneous discovery of the same protein by two independent groups, thus p21 is also referred to as $p21^{CIP1/WAF1}$.

A number of biological effects of p21 are mediated by its binding to and inhibition of cyclin-dependent kinases (CDKs) (Abbas & Dutta, 2009). Since these cyclin-CDK complexes play a role in the progression through G1 phase, p21 regulates the cell cycle progression at G1 phase of the cell cycle. It has been suggested that the ability to mediate p53-dependent gene repression might be a mechanism by which p21 induces cell cycle inhibition (Abbas & Dutta, 2009). This is based on the knowledge that p21 is important for p53-dependent repression of several genes that are involved in cell cycle progression. While p21 might be important for p53 functions in most cases, there is evidence suggesting that p53 can function in a p21-independent manner as well (Xia *et al*, 2011). Also, p21 binds to proliferating cell nuclear antigen (PCNA), and through binding to PCNA, p21 competes for PCNA binding with DNA polymerase-δ and other key factors involved in DNA synthesis leading to the inhibition of DNA synthesis (Moldovan *et al*, 2007;Abbas & Dutta, 2009). Such modulation of PCNA appears to be one of the regulatory roles of p21 in S phase DNA replication and DNA damage repair. Because of its inhibitory action on cell cycle progression, p21 is widely regarded as a tumor suppressor factor. However, there are reports in the literature which suggest its direct role as an oncogene (Roninson, 2002). Mice genetically engineered to lack p21 develop normally and such mice do not exhibit increased susceptibility to cancer. Thus, while the important role of p21 in the regulation of cell cycle is known, its biological functions are far from being clearly understood.

3.3.2 p27 (cyclin-dependent kinase inhibitor 1B) / KIP

The p27 is coded by human gene *CDKN1B* and, like p21, belongs to the *Cip/Kip* family of CDK inhibitor proteins. Similar to the simultaneous identification and characterization of p21 by two independent research groups, p27 was also cloned simultaneously by two independent research groups. Polyak et al. (Polyak *et al*, 1994) cloned p27Kip1 and reported its ability to inhibit cyclin E-Cdk2 complexes leading to obstruction of entry of cells into S phase. It was found to have a region of sequence similarity to p21Cip1/WAF1 and it inhibited Rb phosphorylation by cyclin E-CDK2, cyclin A-CDK2, and cyclin D2-CDK4 complexes. Using a yeast interaction screen to search for proteins that interacted with cyclin D1-CDK4, Toyoshima et al. (Toyoshima & Hunter, 1994) identified a 27 kDa protein that interacted strongly with D-type cyclins and CDK4. It was identified as a negative regulator of G1 progression.

P27 binds to and prevents the activation of Cyclin A-Cdk2/cyclin E-CDK2/cyclin D-CDK4 complexes. Since these cyclin-CDK complexes also play role in the progression through G1 phase, p27 regulates the cell cycle progression at G1 phase of cell cycle. For the inhibition of cyclin A-CDK2 complex, p27 binds the complex as an extended structure wherein it interacts with both cyclin A and CDK2. In cyclin A, p27 binds within a groove formed by conserved cyclin box residues while to CDK2, it mimics ATP and inserts into the catalytic cleft (Russo *et al*, 1996). Similar to p21, tumor promoting activities have been reported for p27 as well (Besson *et al*, 2007;Blagosklonny, 2002;Lee & Kim, 2009). Despite the dual nature of p27, as a tumor suppressor and tumor promoter, its ability to inhibit CDK complexes is still considered very important Moreover, in a meta-analysis, reduced p27 has been recognized as an independent prognostic factor for poor overall and disease-free survival breast cancer patients (Guan *et al*, 2010), suggesting that agents that could activate p27 would have clinical utility.

4. Drug resistance

The problem of drug-resistance is a major concern for researchers and clinicians because it is a big hindrance in the successful management of cancer patients. In case of breast cancer, a number of targeted therapies are available for cancer subtypes that are marked by the expression of estrogen receptor (ER), progesterone receptor (PR) and overexpression of Her2/neu. Some cancers do not respond to the therapy at all, right from the beginning, and such phenomenon is called *de novo* drug resistance. However, many cancers actually respond to the targeted therapy initially but with the passage of time and continued administration of therapeutic agent, they eventually develop resistance to that therapeutic agent, and this process is called acquired drug resistance. While *de novo* drug resistance is itself challenging, acquired drug resistance is clinically an even bigger problem. The cancers that have acquired drug resistance are usually far more aggressive and difficult to treat. They are invariably linked to poor prognosis as well as overall poor survival. In the few sub-sections to follow, we will discuss the problem of drug-resistance as observed in breast cancer patients, and the role that dysregulated cell cycle plays in the development of drug resistant phenotype.

4.1 Cell cycle regulation in tamoxifen resistant breast cancers

For the management of breast cancers that express ER, tamoxifen is the drug of choice for targeted personalized therapy. Tamoxifen can significantly lower the chances of developing recurrent breast cancer and can be very effective in women who initially present with metastatic disease. It remains the primary therapeutic agent for the management of ER- and/or PR-expressing breast cancers, particularly in premenopausal women without or with conventional chemotherapeutic agents. A number of reports have implicated modulation of cell cycle and cell cycle regulatory proteins as prognostic/predictive markers of progression of ER- positive breast cancers during the acquisition of tamoxifen resistance.

In an early attempt (Rostagno *et al*, 1996) to understand the interaction between ER and cell cycle regulators, ER was found to be induced during the G0/G1-phase in MCF-7 cells, the breast cancer cells that are characterized by expression of ER. Increased expression of ER during the G0/G1-phase was followed by a decrease during the S-phase until the late S-phase where a rapid increase was noted. From these observations, it was concluded that estrogens are involved in DNA synthesis since ER was found to be expressed at a maximal level during late G1. A tamoxifen resistant phenotype was developed by long term exposure of MCF-7 xenografts to tamoxifen and this resulted in an altered profile of ER during the G0/G1 phase. This provided an indication for the relevance of cell cycle regulation in tamoxifen resistance of breast cancers *in vivo*. As a molecular signature, it has been shown that tamoxifen-resistant MCF-7 cells express higher levels of cell cycle regulators cyclin E1 and CDK2, compared to parental cells (Louie *et al*, 2010). Further, cell cycle regulatory proteins have also been shown to be differentially expressed in ER-negative vs. ER-positive breast cancer cells. The ER-negative cells have increased expression of cyclin B1, cyclin D1 as well as cyclin E (Skog *et al*, 2004).

In a report suggesting a role for cyclins, specifically cyclin D1, in tamoxifen resistance of ER-expressing breast cancer cells T47D and MCF-7, it was reported that ectopic expression of cyclin D1 was sufficient to reverse the growth inhibitory effect of tamoxifen as well as steroidal anti-estrogens (Wilcken *et al*, 1997). Such ectopic cyclin D1 induction resulted in activation of cyclin D1-CDK4 complexes and entry of cells into S phase of cells indicating a reversal of cell cycle arrest. Later, it was shown that cyclin D1 was not endogenously up-regulated in tamoxifen-resistant MCF-7 cells, compared to parental MCF-7 cells (Kilker *et al*, 2004). It was up-regulated only on exposure to physiological levels of tamoxifen, suggesting a dependence of cyclin D1 expression on ER. The same research group later reported that cyclin D1 expression is necessary for proliferation of tamoxifen-resistant cells and for tamoxifen-induced cell cycle progression (Kilker & Planas-Silva, 2006). The role of cyclin D1 in tamoxifen resistance was further validated by Stendahl et al. (Stendahl *et al*, 2004) using tissue samples from 167 postmenopausal breast cancers arranged in a tissue array. It was reported that in 55 ER-over-expressing samples, with moderate or low cyclin D1 levels, patients responded well to tamoxifen treatment. However, in 46 patients with ER – over-expression as well as cyclin D1 over-expression, there was no difference in survival between tamoxifen compared to no tamoxifen group. This clearly suggests that the expression of cyclin D1 is related to the overall response of patients to tamoxifen treatment because the patients with cyclin D1 over-expression were found to be associated with tamoxifen resistant phenotype.

In addition to a positive correlation between cyclin D1 expression and aggressive cancers, as documented above, there is evidence to suggest otherwise as well. For example, a study using microarray analysis of cyclin D1 expression identified high cyclin D1 expression as a low risk factor for local recurrence of breast cancer (Jirstrom *et al*, 2003). Low expression of cyclin D1 expression was, conversely, associated with high risk of cancer recurrence. Thus, overexpression of cyclin D1 was reported to be actually beneficial for breast cancer survival, associated with inverse tumor grade, smaller tumor size, and improved relapse-free and overall survival of breast cancer patients (Ishii *et al*, 2008). As a mechanism for such counter-intuitive function, it has been proposed that cyclin D1 represses the activity of signal transducer and activator of transcription 3 (STAT3) (Ishii *et al*, 2006). Since STAT3 is a potent inducer of cell proliferation and survival, its down-regulation might explain the observed reduced aggressiveness of breast cancer.

Based on a recent report which evaluated p27 expression in 328 primary stage II breast cancers from premenopausal patients, it has been suggested that patients with p27-

overexpressing tumors benefit from tamoxifen treatment, which underscores the role of p27 in predicting response to therapy (Stendahl *et al*, 2010). However no association was found between p27 and recurrence-free survival, suggesting that p27 is not a prognostic marker. There is evidence to suggest the involvement of p21 in tamoxifen resistance as well, and the loss of p21 function has been shown to be associated with a tamoxifen-resistant phenotype (Abukhdeir *et al*, 2008). Studies using immortalized human breast epithelial cells with somatic deletion of the p21 gene showed a growth proliferative response to tamoxifen because absence of p21 enabled cyclin-CDK complexes to aberrantly phosphorylate ER when bound to tamoxifen, resulting in a growth-stimulatory phenotype. On the other hand, p21 wild-type cells demonstrated growth inhibition upon tamoxifen exposure.

4.2 Cell cycle regulation in adriamycin resistant breast cancers

Adriamycin (doxorubicin) is another chemotherapeutic drug that is routinely used in the clinic for the management of breast cancer patients. It is used to treat early-stage or node-positive breast cancers, HER2/neu-positive breast cancers as well as metastatic breast cancers. It primarily interferes with the DNA replication machinery leading to inhibition of cancer cell growth. Since DNA replication is crucial to the progression of cell cycle, its inhibition by adriamycin indicates the involvement of cell cycle regulatory proteins associated with the anticancer action of this drug. Moreover, a number of investigations have actually reported modulation of cell cycle as a mechanism of adriamycin action. Similar to tamoxifen, breast cancers that are managed well by adriamycin initially, eventually develop resistance to adriamycin, which is also a major clinical problem.

While earlier investigations found no correlation between p21 and adriamycin resistant phenotype (Staalesen *et al*, 2004), it was later reported that pre-treatment of adriamycin resistant MCF-7 cells with tumor necrosis factor-alpha (TNF-α), followed by adriamycin treatment, was an efficient way for enhancing the cytotoxic effects of adriamycin (Cao *et al*, 2006). Since TNF- α was earlier shown to down-regulate p21 leading to enhanced killing by adriamycin (Cao *et al*, 2005), these studies provided an evidence for the involvement of inhibitory p21 in resistance of breast cancer cells to adriamycin. A role of p21 in adriamycin-induced, twist-1-mediated induction of epithelial-mesenchymal transition has also been suggested (Li *et al*, 2009). In a study profiling the changes induced by prolonged exposure to adriamycin, it was found that long term culture of MCF-7 cells with adriamycin resulted in inhibition of cyclin D1 and increased expression of p21 (Lukyanova *et al*, 2009). Differential expression of p21 in adriamycin resistant MCF-7 cells has also been reported (Saleh *et al*, 2009) further confirming an involvement of p21 in development of adriamycin resistant phenotype. A role of p27 in adriamycin sensitivity was also suggested when 56 out of a total of 119 breast cancer patients demonstrated p27 overexpression and it was found that the susceptibility of adriamycin in tumors with high expression of p27 was significantly higher than in tumors with low expression (Yang *et al*, 2000). In a later investigation, p27 was found to be a good prognostic marker for disease free and overall survival of breast cancer patients in the context of resistance to preoperative doxorubicin-based chemotherapy in primary breast cancer (Davidovich *et al*, 2008).

4.3 Cell cycle regulation in herceptin resistant breast cancers

The Her2/neu (ErbB2) gene encodes an epidermal growth factor receptor (EGFR) family tyrosine kinase that is overexpressed in about 20-30% of invasive breast cancers. Herceptin

(Trastuzumab) is a humanized monoclonal antibody that targets Her2. It is now utilized in the clinic for the management of breast cancers that over-express Her2/neu. Increased expression of Her2/neu provides a proliferative advantage leading to uncontrolled cell division and growth. Treatment with herceptin effectively blocks the signaling through Her2/neu leading to the inhibition of uncontrolled tumor growth. Herceptin treatment is a very effective way to treat patients with Her2/neu overexpression; however, the phenomenon of resistance to this drug is also seen in a lot of patients who stop responding to the treatment. It is believed that a majority of patients with metastatic breast cancer who initially respond to herceptin/trastuzumab, demonstrate disease progression within 1 year of treatment initiation (Nahta *et al*, 2006) indicating progression to drug resistant phenotype. Similar to the resistance to other drugs documented above, resistance to herceptin also involves modulations in cell cycle regulatory proteins. Cyclin D1 and the inhibitory p27, in particular, have been investigated for their role in herceptin resistance. A number of reports that have detailed the modulation of a specific signaling pathway/molecule, resulting in re-sensitizing herceptin resistant cells to herceptin treatment, have indicated a role of these cell cycle regulators. Herceptin is known to induce the expression of p27 (Lu *et al*, 2004). Induction of p27 ensures its association with its target CDK leading to the inhibition of cyclin-CDK complex, resulting in cell cycle arrest. It will, therefore, be logical to expect down-regulation of p27 in herceptin-resistant cells which will attenuate the ability of this inhibitory protein to induce cell cycle arrest. Indeed, this was observed in a cell line model when herceptin-resistant variant of Her-2 over-expressing breast cancer cell line, SKBR3, was actually found to harbor significantly reduced expression of p27 (Nahta *et al*, 2004).
In addition to induction of p27, herceptin also functions via down-regulation of cyclins (Wu *et al*, 2010). Both of these events - increased p27 and decreased cyclins - ensure an effective arrest of cell cycle progression in response to herceptin treatment. A similar role of CDKs in mechanism of anticancer drugs has also been reported. For example, PD 0332991, a highly selective inhibitor of the CDK4 as well as CDK6, was reported to increase the efficacy of tamoxifen in ER-positive cells and that of herceptin in Her-2 over-expressing cells (Finn *et al*, 2009). In this study, an analysis of 47 human breast cancer cell lines revealed that Rb phosphorylation is blocked only in drug-sensitive cells but not in drug-resistant cells. Since Rb phosphorylation is a measure of CDK activity, an effective inhibition of CDKs by drugs such as tamoxifen and herceptin in sensitive cells results in reduced Rb phosphorylation. The resistant cells become refractory to such CDK inhibitory action implying that CDK inhibition can potentially be beneficial for the management of drug-resistant breast cancers (Sutherland & Musgrove, 2009).

5. Cell signaling crosstalk in drug resistant phenotype: Role of cell cycle regulators

The progression of cancer and the development of drug resistant phenotype is particularly challenging because of the excessive cross-talk between multiple signaling molecules and pathways. Regulation of cell cycle proteins plays a crucial role in most of these processes as well. For instance, tamoxifen treatment is known to result in up-regulation of inhibitory p21 and p27 (Cariou *et al*, 2000). The development of tamoxifen resistance, therefore, involves down-regulation of these cell cycle regulatory proteins (Cariou *et al*, 2000). Since cancer cells are known to evade processes that may tend to slow down their progress, tamoxifen treatment is often marked by up-regulation of other signaling pathways that may work to overcome the effects caused by tamoxifen treatment. Over-expression of EGFR (Nicholson *et al*, 1990) and Her2/neu (De Placido *et al*, 1998) are often observed in ER-positive cells that have been exposed to tamoxifen. This activation of alternate cell proliferation pathways represents a mechanism by which ER-positive cells respond to anti-estrogen treatment. As a further proof, it has been reported that ectopic expression of Her2/neu results in reduced sensitivity to tamoxifen treatment (Benz *et al*, 1992). Since tamoxifen therapy results in induced expression of EGFR and Her2/neu, a treatment regimen combining tamoxifen with inhibitors of EGFR and Her2/neu might be a better strategy. This was tested by Chu et al. (Chu *et al*, 2005) who combined lapatinib (a dual EGFR and Her2/neu inhibitor) with tamoxifen for the treatment of ER-positive breast cancer cell lines. It was found that a combination of these two drugs caused cell cycle arrest more effectively than treatment with either drug alone. This enhanced combinational effect was found to be dependent on increased down-regulation of cyclin D1, cyclin E-CDK2 and marked increase in p27. This study provided clear evidence in support of combinational treatments. When a therapeutic agent suppresses the growth of cancer cells by targeting a specific cell cycle regulatory pathway, the cancer cells look for alternate pathways to overcome this regulation. In the process, alternate pathways are activated to derepress the regulation of cell cycle. In such a scenario, it is necessary to simultaneously target these multiple signaling pathways so as to ensure a sustained blockage of cell cycle progression.

In support of a clinical significance of cell cycle regulatory proteins in cell survival pathways cross-talk, it has been reported that the prognostic importance of Her2/neu is significantly better for breast cancer patients whose tumors overexpress cyclin D1 (Ahnstrom *et al*, 2005). In patients with overexpression of cyclin D1, Her2/neu overexpression strongly correlates with increased risk of recurrence and mortality. Further, in ER-positive patients, tamoxifen treatment was reported to be particularly beneficial in patients with moderate cyclin D1. Another mechanism by which cancer cells can evade tamoxifen is through oncogenic kinase Src. Signaling through EGFR and/or Her2 can lead to increased Src activity (Ishizawar & Parsons, 2004) and overexpression of Src results in repression of p27 (Chu *et al*, 2007). Src represses the inhibitory action of p27 on cyclin-CDK complexes and accelerates p27 proteolysis by phosphorylating it at tyrosine residues 74 and 88. Therefore, it appears that tamoxifen therapy leads to the induction of p27. It also leads to the activation of alternate EGFR and Her2/neu pathways which, in turn, lead to the activation of Src and reverse the induction of p27 via its increased degradation. In this context, Src inhibition increased p27 levels in tamoxifen resistant breast cancer cells (Chu *et al*, 2007) indicating that a combination of Src inhibitors with tamoxifen might also be a good strategy for an effective regulation of cell cycle progression leading to desired inhibitory effects on cancer progression.

There is some evidence to support the role of STAT3 signaling in tamoxifen resistant phenotype. In relation to the role of cyclin D1 in the prognosis of recurrent breast cancers, it was reported that repression of STAT3 by cyclin D1 resulted in reduced cell growth, and treatment with tamoxifen abolished such cyclin D1-mediated repression of STAT3 and resulting effects on cell cycle and growth (Ishii *et al*, 2008). Tamoxifen induced the redistribution of cyclin D1 from STAT3 to the ER, resulting in an efficient activation of STAT3 as well as ER. In another study focusing on another STAT, STAT5b, it was reported that STAT5b is required for estrogen-induced proliferation of ER-positive breast cancer cells (Fox *et al*, 2008). Inhibition of STAT5b, using specific siRNA, showed reduced proliferation mediated through reduced expression of cyclin D1. This study also identified a role of EGFR and Src kinase in estrogen-induced cyclin D1 expression and cell growth, and thus indicating a cross-talk between ER, Src, EGFR and STAT5b in ER-positive breast cancer cells. Cyclin D1 interacts with a number of different CDKs as well as p27, an inhibitor of cyclin-CDK complexes. Given the detailed investigations on the role of cyclin D1 in drug resistant phenotype, as discussed above, it may make some sense to investigate whether there is a direct role of CDKs, if any, in drug resistant and aggressive phenotype of breast cancer cells. To that end, Johnson et al. (Johnson *et al*, 2010) studied the therapeutic potential of inhibiting CDK2 and CDK1 in relation to anti-estrogen resistance. It was observed that CDK2 knock-down results in the accumulation of cells in G1 phase. Knock-down of CDK1, however, resulted in G2-M slowing, and simultaneous knock-down of CDK1 and CDK2 caused further accumulation of cells in G2-M phase transition. This was also accompanied by increased cell death, thus confirming the role of CDK2 and CDK1 as targets for breast cancer therapy.

In yet another demonstration of signaling cross-talk, the role of met receptor in herceptin resistance has been reported (Shattuck *et al*, 2008). This Study stemmed from the observation that met receptor is frequently expressed in breast cancer cells that also exhibit Her2 over-expression. Interestingly, Her2 over-expressing cells tend to up-regulate the expression of met in response to herceptin treatment. This might be a way for them to overcome the proliferation inhibition that they are subjected to, post herceptin-treatment. The study (Shattuck *et al*, 2008) observed that the simultaneous inhibition of met might help to overcome resistance to herceptin. This was based on the finding that inhibition of met led to re-sensitization of herceptin resistant cells to herceptin treatment. In this context, the role of cell cycle regulator p27 has been proposed because met-mediated down-regulation of p27 was found to be a significant event that was crucial to the development of herceptin resistant phenotype. Similar to inhibition of met, inhibition of proteasome has also been reported to increase the efficacy of herceptin (Cardoso *et al*, 2006). An effective down-regulation of p27 by the combination treatment, along with down-regulation of NF-κB, was proposed as the mechanism for the observed results.

A further complex cross-talk between signaling pathways, leading to herceptin resistance, has also been reported. This involves a cross-talk between Her2, Her3 and insulin-like growth factor-I receptor (IGF-IR) pathways (Huang *et al*, 2010). This study reported interactions between the three signaling pathways that were observed exclusively in herceptin resistant breast cancer cells, which suggested a cross-talk that might be important for the progression to as well as sustenance of a herceptin resistant phenotype. Down-regulation of Her3 or IGF-IR was found to result in an efficient induction of p27. Since p27 is an inhibitor of cell cycle, such increased p27 levels were correlated with re-sensitization of previously herceptin resistant cells to herceptin. This study again demonstrated how modulation of cell cycle regulatory protein p27 can play a central role in overcoming drug resistant phenotype.

In summary (as schematically shown in Figure 3), anticancer drugs such as tamoxifen, adriamycin and herceptin act via down-regulation of their cellular targets to induce an efficient cell cycle arrest. This is followed, in many cases, by activation of alternate cell proliferation pathways, which function to restore cell cycle and lead to cancer progression.

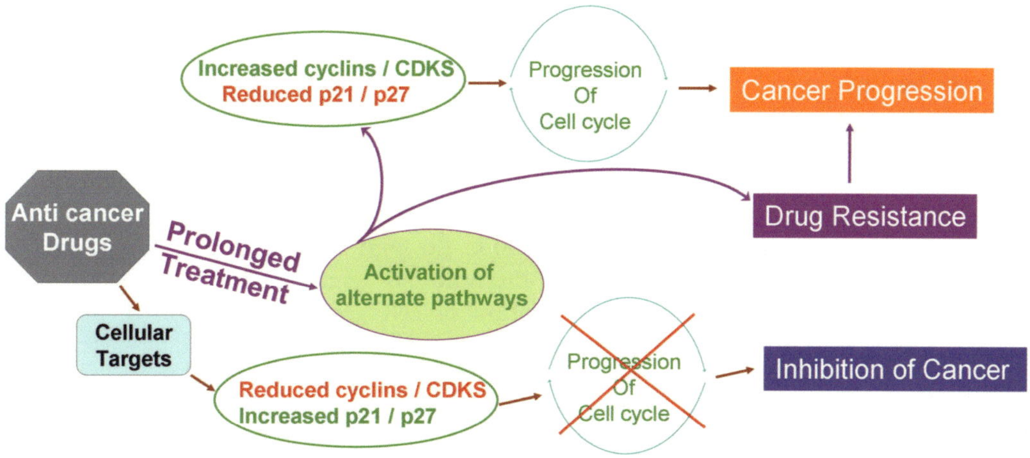

Fig. 3. Complex role of cell cycle regulators in progression of cancer, efficacy of anticancer treatments and development of drug resistant phenotype.

6. Cell cycle regulation by natural compounds: Basis for their apoptosis-inducing and anticancer activity

In addition to various anticancer drugs that are in use for the clinical management of breast cancer patients, a lot of research has been done on plant-derived natural compounds to evaluate their putative role in prevention and progression of cancer. A number of such compounds have shown promise in preclinical studies (Gullett *et al*, 2010). These compounds are potent inducers of apoptosis (Hail, Jr. & Lotan, 2009;Shu *et al*, 2010), and cell cycle arrest is one of the mechanism through which these compounds are able to exert their biological effects (Sarkar & Li, 2004). Cell cycle can be transiently arrested by chemopreventive agents at damage checkpoints which allows for DNA repair, or activation of pathways leading to apoptosis if the damage is irreparable. Our own studies have shown that soy isoflavone genistein can cause G2-M arrest, leading to apoptosis induction, more efficiently in malignant breast cancer cell lines (MCF10CA1a and MDA-MB-231) compared to normal breast epithelial cells (MCF10A and MCF12A) (Upadhyay *et al*, 2001). We found a significant up-regulation of p21 at mRNA as well as protein level in the normal cells. Down-regulation of p21 sensitized normal as well as malignant breast cancer cells to genistein-induced G2-M arrest, suggesting an important role of p21 in determining the sensitivity of normal and malignant breast epithelial cells to genistein. Later, we reported genistein-mediated induction of p21 in ER-positive MCF-7 cells as well (Chinni *et al*, 2003). A similar activity of 3, 3′-Diindolylmethane (DIM; obtained from cruciferous vegetables) was also observed, and DIM was found to inhibit the expression of cyclin E2, survivin and Bcl-2, and induce the expression of p27 leading to the induction of cell cycle arrest and apoptosis in multiple breast cancer cell lines (Rahman *et al*, 2006;Wang *et al*, 2008). Effect of DIM on regulators of cell cycle (cyclin E2 and p21) as well as regulators of apoptotic pathways (survivin and Bcl-2) indicated a close connection and a mechanistic link between these pathways that may define the anticancer activity of natural compounds.

Similar to these reports from our laboratory, there are numerous other reports that have documented the anticancer ability of these as well as many other naturally occurring compounds (Sarkar & Li, 2004;Gullett *et al*, 2010). The interest in research on these compounds is largely based on the observation that natural compounds are part of normal diet and, as such, well tolerated. Further, as discussed above, the development of drug resistance often involves cross-talk between multiple pathways. For example, the drug resistance through cyclin D1 is because of its association with so many cancer progression pathways such as transforming growth factor (TGF)-α, EGFR, Ras, phosphoinositide-3-kinase (PI3K)/Akt and NF-κB (Liao *et al*, 2007). Natural agents exhibit their inhibitory effects on carcinogenesis and cancer progression through the regulation of multiple cell signaling pathways. Therefore, regulation of multiple cell signaling pathways for controlling the behavior of cancer cells such as inhibition of cell growth, induction of apoptosis, inhibition of invasion/metastasis as well as re-sensitizing drug-resistant cancer cells requires agents that could target multiple pathways, and it is now believed that many of the natural compounds are perfect examples showing that these natural agents could target multiple pathways.

7. Conclusions and perspectives

The role of cell cycle, and the various regulatory factors during the progression of cancer, is now well appreciated. Therefore, one important parameter to judge the efficacy of anticancer therapeutics is via their modulation of cell cycle regulation. Irregularities in cell cycle regulation are hallmarks of aggressive breast cancers as well as those breast cancers that have turned refractory to drug treatment. A number of anticancer drugs used in the clinic, function through modulation of cell cycle. In addition to direct targeting of cell cycle regulatory factors for anticancer therapy, genes such as FoxM1 that modulate cell cycle machinery (Wang *et al*, 2010a), have also been targeted in breast cancer models leading to the inhibition of proliferation and invasion of aggressive cells (Ahmad *et al*, 2010). Furthermore, the anticancer properties of natural non-toxic compounds are increasingly being realized. Although these compounds are well-tolerated and have low toxicity, still they have not yet made their way to clinic. They suffer from inefficient systemic delivery and bioavailability. To that end, nano-chemoprevention, an application of nanotechnology to enhance the efficacy of natural compounds has shown promise (Siddiqui *et al*, 2009). Another approach is to increase the efficacy as well as bioavailability of natural compounds by synthesizing novel analogs of natural compounds, as demonstrated by our recent work on a synthetic analog of curcumin (Padhye *et al*, 2009).

Another emerging area of cancer research involves the regulation of genes by tiny non-coding RNA molecules, microRNAs (miRNAs). It is interesting to note that natural compounds, that have been shown to induce cell cycle arrest, have also been reported to regulate miRNAs (Li *et al*, 2010). Moreover, it is increasingly being realized that the regulation of miRNAs is a good strategy to overcome the problem of drug resistance (Wang *et al*, 2010b). In breast cancer, the role of miRNAs in tamoxifen resistance, through regulation of cell cycle regulatory proteins, has been suggested. In particular, ectopic expression of miR-221/miR-222 was found to render ER-positive MCF-7 cells resistant to tamoxifen. This was mediated through significant down-regulation of their target p27 (Miller *et al*, 2008). Expression of miR-221 and miR-222 was also found to be significantly increased in Her2-positive primary human breast cancer tissues indicating an interrelationship between miR-221/222 expression and Her2 over-expression in primary breast tumors that are generally resistant to tamoxifen therapy. These preliminary reports are encouraging and a better understanding of the mechanisms, that cause deregulated cell cycle thereby leading to cancer progression, would result in the development of novel anticancer therapeutics.

8. References

Abbas, T. & Dutta, A. (2009). p21 in cancer: intricate networks and multiple activities. *Nat.Rev.Cancer*, Vol. 9, No.6, pp. 400-414.

Abukhdeir, A.M. & Park, B.H. (2008). P21 and p27: roles in carcinogenesis and drug resistance. *Expert.Rev.Mol.Med*, Vol. 10e19.

Abukhdeir, A.M., Vitolo, M.I., Argani, P., De Marzo, A.M., Karakas, B., Konishi, H., Gustin, J.P., Lauring,J., Garay, J.P., Pendleton, C., Konishi, Y., Blair, B.G., Brenner, K., Garrett-Mayer, E., Carraway, H., Bachman, K.E., & Park, B.H. (2008). Tamoxifen-stimulated growth of breast cancer due to p21 loss. *Proc.Natl.Acad.Sci.U.S.A*, Vol. 105, No.1, pp. 288-293.

Ahmad, A., Wang, Z., Kong, D., Ali, S., Li, Y., Banerjee, S., Ali, R., & Sarkar, F.H. (2010). FoxM1 down-regulation leads to inhibition of proliferation, migration and invasion of breast cancer cells through the modulation of extra-cellular matrix degrading factors. *Breast Cancer Res Treat.*, Vol. 122, No.2, pp. 337-346.

Ahnstrom, M., Nordenskjold, B., Rutqvist, L.E., Skoog, L., & Stal, O. (2005). Role of cyclin D1 in ErbB2-positive breast cancer and tamoxifen resistance. *Breast Cancer Res Treat.*, Vol. 91, No.2, pp. 145-151.

Benz, C.C., Scott, G.K., Sarup, J.C., Johnson, R.M., Tripathy, D., Coronado, E., Shepard, H.M., & Osborne, C.K. (1992). Estrogen-dependent, tamoxifen-resistant tumorigenic growth of MCF-7 cells transfected with HER2/neu. *Breast Cancer Res Treat.*, Vol. 24, No.2, pp. 85-95.

Besson, A., Hwang, H.C., Cicero, S., Donovan, S.L., Gurian-West, M., Johnson, D., Clurman, B.E., Dyer, M.A., & Roberts, J.M. (2007). Discovery of an oncogenic activity in p27Kip1 that causes stem cell expansion and a multiple tumor phenotype. *Genes Dev.*, Vol. 21, No.14, pp. 1731-1746.

Blagosklonny, M.V. (2002). Are p27 and p21 cytoplasmic oncoproteins? *Cell Cycle*, Vol. 1, No.6, pp. 391-393.

Cao, W., Chi, W.H., Wang, J., Tang, J.J., & Lu, Y.J. (2005). TNF-[alpha] promotes Doxorubicin-induced cell apoptosis and anti-cancer effect through downregulation of p21 in p53-deficient tumor cells. *Biochemical and Biophysical Research Communications*, Vol. 330, No.4, pp. 1034-1040.

Cao, W., Ma, S.L., Tang, J., Shi, J., & Lu, Y. (2006). A combined treatment TNF-alpha/doxorubicin alleviates the resistance of MCF-7/Adr cells to cytotoxic treatment. *Biochim.Biophys.Acta*, Vol. 1763, No.2, pp. 182-187.

Cardoso, F., Durbecq, V., Laes, J.F., Badran, B., Lagneaux, L., Bex, F., Desmedt, C., Willard-Gallo, K., Ross, J.S., Burny, A., Piccart, M., & Sotiriou, C. (2006). Bortezomib (PS-341, Velcade) increases the efficacy of trastuzumab (Herceptin) in HER-2-positive breast cancer cells in a synergistic manner. *Mol.Cancer Ther.*, Vol. 5, No.12, pp. 3042-3051.

Cariou, S., Donovan, J.C.H., Flanagan, W.M., Milic, A., Bhattacharya, N., & Slingerland, J.M. (2000). Down-regulation of p21WAF1/CIP1 or p27Kip1 abrogates antiestrogen-mediated cell cycle arrest in human breast cancer cells. *Proceedings of the National Academy of Sciences*, Vol. 97, No.16, pp. 9042-9046.

Chinni, S.R., Alhasan, S.A., Multani, A.S., Pathak, S., & Sarkar, F.H. (2003). Pleotropic effects of genistein on MCF-7 breast cancer cells. *Int.J Mol.Med*, Vol. 12, No.1, pp. 29-34.

Chu, I., Blackwell, K., Chen, S., & Slingerland, J. (2005). The dual ErbB1/ErbB2 inhibitor, lapatinib (GW572016), cooperates with tamoxifen to inhibit both cell proliferation- and estrogen-dependent gene expression in antiestrogen-resistant breast cancer. *Cancer Res*, Vol. 65, No.1, pp. 18-25.

Chu, I., Sun, J., Arnaout, A., Kahn, H., Hanna, W., Narod, S., Sun, P., Tan, C.K., Hengst, L., & Slingerland, J. (2007). p27 phosphorylation by Src regulates inhibition of cyclin E-Cdk2. *Cell*, Vol. 128, No.2, pp. 281-294.

Davidovich, S., Ben-Izhak, O., Shapira, M., Futerman, B., & Hershko, D.D. (2008). Over-expression of Skp2 is associated with resistance to preoperative doxorubicin-based chemotherapy in primary breast cancer. *Breast Cancer Res*, Vol. 10, No.4, pp. R63.

De Placido, S., Carlomagno, C., De Laurentiis, M., & Bianco, A.R. (1998). c-erbB2 expression predicts tamoxifen efficacy in breast cancer patients. *Breast Cancer Res Treat.*, Vol. 52, No.1-3, pp. 55-64.

el-Deiry, W.S., Tokino, T., Velculescu, V.E., Levy, D.B., Parsons, R., Trent, J.M., Lin, D., Mercer, W.E., Kinzler, K.W., & Vogelstein,B. (1993). WAF1, a potential mediator of p53 tumor suppression. *Cell*, Vol. 75, No.4, pp. 817-825.

Finn, R.S., Dering, J., Conklin, D., Kalous, O., Cohen, D.J., Desai, A.J., Ginther, C., Atefi, M., Chen, I., Fowst, C., Los, G., & Slamon, D.J. (2009). PD 0332991, a selective cyclin D kinase 4/6 inhibitor, preferentially inhibits proliferation of luminal estrogen receptor-positive human breast cancer cell lines in vitro. *Breast Cancer Res*, Vol. 11, No.5, pp. R77.

Fox, E.M., Bernaciak, T.M., Wen, J., Weaver, A.M., Shupnik, M.A., & Silva, C.M. (2008). Signal transducer and activator of transcription 5b, c-Src, and epidermal growth factor receptor signaling play integral roles in estrogen-stimulated proliferation of estrogen receptor-positive breast cancer cells. *Mol.Endocrinol.*, Vol. 22, No.8, pp. 1781-1796.

Guan, X., Wang, Y., Xie, R., Chen, L., Bai, J., Lu, J., & Kuo, M.T. (2010). p27(Kip1) as a prognostic factor in breast cancer: a systematic review and meta-analysis. *J Cell Mol.Med*, Vol. 14, No.4, pp. 944-953.

Gullett, N.P., Ruhul Amin, A.R., Bayraktar, S., Pezzuto, J.M., Shin, D.M., Khuri, F.R., Aggarwal, B.B., Surh, Y.J., & Kucuk, O. (2010). Cancer prevention with natural compounds. *Semin.Oncol.*, Vol. 37, No.3, pp. 258-281.

Hail, N., Jr. & Lotan, R. (2009). Cancer chemoprevention and mitochondria: targeting apoptosis in transformed cells via the disruption of mitochondrial bioenergetics/redox state. *Mol.Nutr.Food Res.*, Vol. 53, No.1, pp. 49-67.

Harper,J.W., Adami,G.R., Wei,N., Keyomarsi,K., & Elledge,S.J. (1993). The p21 Cdk-interacting protein Cip1 is a potent inhibitor of G1 cyclin-dependent kinases. *Cell*, Vol. 75, No.4, pp. 805-816.

Huang, X., Gao, L., Wang, S., McManaman, J.L., Thor, A.D., Yang, X., Esteva, F.J., & Liu, B. (2010). Heterotrimerization of the growth factor receptors erbB2, erbB3, and insulin-like growth factor-i receptor in breast cancer cells resistant to herceptin. *Cancer Res*, Vol. 70, No.3, pp. 1204-1214.

Ishii, Y., Waxman, S., & Germain, D. (2008). Tamoxifen stimulates the growth of cyclin D1-overexpressing breast cancer cells by promoting the activation of signal transducer and activator of transcription 3. *Cancer Res*, Vol. 68, No.3, pp. 852-860.

Ishii, Y., Pirkmaier, A., Alvarez, J.V., Frank, D.A., Keselman, I., Logothetis, D., Mandeli, J., O'Connell, M.J., Waxman, S., & Germain, D. (2006). Cyclin D1 Overexpression and Response to Bortezomib Treatment in a Breast Cancer Model. *Journal of the National Cancer Institute*, Vol. 98, No.17, pp. 1238-1247.

Ishizawar, R. & Parsons, S.J. (2004). c-Src and cooperating partners in human cancer. *Cancer Cell*, Vol. 6, No.3, pp. 209-214.

Jirstrom, K., Ringberg, A., Ferno, M., Anagnostaki, L., & Landberg, G. (2003). Tissue microarray analyses of G1/S-regulatory proteins in ductal carcinoma in situ of the breast indicate that low cyclin D1 is associated with local recurrence. *Br J Cancer*, Vol. 89, No.10, pp. 1920-1926.

Johnson, N., Bentley, J., Wang, L.Z., Newell, D.R., Robson, C.N., Shapiro, G.I., & Curtin, N.J. (2010). Pre-clinical evaluation of cyclin-dependent kinase 2 and 1 inhibition in anti-estrogen-sensitive and resistant breast cancer cells. *Br J Cancer*, Vol. 102, No.2, pp. 342-350.

Kilker, R.L., Hartl, M.W., Rutherford, T.M., & Planas-Silva, M.D. (2004). Cyclin D1 expression is dependent on estrogen receptor function in tamoxifen-resistant breast cancer cells. *J Steroid Biochem.Mol.Biol.*, Vol. 92, No.1-2, pp. 63-71.

Kilker, R.L. & Planas-Silva, M.D. (2006). Cyclin D1 is necessary for tamoxifen-induced cell cycle progression in human breast cancer cells. *Cancer Res*, Vol. 66, No.23, pp. 11478-11484.

Lee, J. & Kim, S.S. (2009). The function of p27 KIP1 during tumor development. *Exp.Mol.Med*, Vol. 41, No.11, pp. 765-771.

Li, Q.Q., Xu, J.D., Wang, W.J., Cao, X.X., Chen, Q., Tang, F., Chen, Z.Q., Liu, X.P., & Xu, Z.D. (2009). Twist1-mediated adriamycin-induced epithelial-mesenchymal transition relates to multidrug resistance and invasive potential in breast cancer cells. *Clin.Cancer Res*, Vol. 15, No.8, pp. 2657-2665.

Li, Y., Kong, D., Wang, Z., & Sarkar, F.H. (2010). Regulation of microRNAs by natural agents: an emerging field in chemoprevention and chemotherapy research. *Pharm.Res.*, Vol. 27, No.6, pp. 1027-1041.

Liao, D.J., Thakur, A., Wu, J., Biliran, H., & Sarkar, F.H. (2007). Perspectives on c-Myc, Cyclin D1, and their interaction in cancer formation, progression, and response to chemotherapy. *Crit Rev.Oncog.*, Vol. 13, No.2, pp. 93-158.

Louie, M.C., McClellan, A., Siewit, C., & Kawabata, L. (2010). Estrogen receptor regulates E2F1 expression to mediate tamoxifen resistance. *Mol.Cancer Res*, Vol. 8, No.3, pp. 343-352.

Lu, Y., Zi, X., & Pollak, M. (2004). Molecular mechanisms underlying IGF-I-induced attenuation of the growth-inhibitory activity of trastuzumab (Herceptin) on SKBR3 breast cancer cells. *Int.J Cancer*, Vol. 108, No.3, pp. 334-341.

Lukyanova,N.Y., Rusetskya,N.V., Tregubova,N.A., & Chekhun,V.F. (2009). Molecular profile and cell cycle in MCF-7 cells resistant to cisplatin and doxorubicin. *Exp.Oncol.*, Vol. 31, No.2, pp. 87-91.

Maya-Mendoza, A., Tang, C.W., Pombo, A., & Jackson, D.A. (2009). Mechanisms regulating S phase progression in mammalian cells. *Front Biosci.*, Vol. 144199-4213.

Miller, T.E., Ghoshal, K., Ramaswamy, B., Roy, S., Datta, J., Shapiro, C.L., Jacob, S., & Majumder, S. (2008). MicroRNA-221/222 confers tamoxifen resistance in breast cancer by targeting p27Kip1. *J Biol.Chem.*, Vol. 283, No.44, pp. 29897-29903.

Moldovan, G.L., Pfander, B., & Jentsch, S. (2007). PCNA, the maestro of the replication fork. *Cell*, Vol. 129, No.4, pp. 665-679.

Nahta, R., Takahashi, T., Ueno, N.T., Hung, M.C., & Esteva ,F.J. (2004). P27(kip1) down-regulation is associated with trastuzumab resistance in breast cancer cells. *Cancer Res*, Vol. 64, No.11, pp. 3981-3986.

Nahta, R., Yu, D., Hung, M.C., Hortobagyi, G.N., & Esteva, F.J. (2006). Mechanisms of disease: understanding resistance to HER2-targeted therapy in human breast cancer. *Nat.Clin.Pract.Oncol.*, Vol. 3, No.5, pp. 269-280.

Nicholson, S., Wright, C., Richard ,C.S., Halcrow, P., Kelly, P., Angus, B., FarnVon, J.R., & Harris, A.L. (1990). Epidermal growth factor receptor (EGFr) as a marker for poor prognosis in node-negative breast cancer patients: Neu and tamoxifen failure. *The Journal of Steroid Biochemistry and Molecular Biology*, Vol. 37, No.6, pp. 811-814.

Padhye, S., Banerjee, S., Chavan, D., Pandye, S., Swamy, K.V., Ali, S., Li, J., Dou, Q.P., & Sarkar, F.H. (2009). Fluorocurcumins as cyclooxygenase-2 inhibitor: molecular docking, pharmacokinetics and tissue distribution in mice. *Pharm.Res*, Vol. 26, No.11, pp. 2438-2445.

Polyak, K., Lee, M.H., Erdjument-Bromage, H., Koff, A., Roberts, J.M., Tempst, P., & Massague, J. (1994). Cloning of p27Kip1, a cyclin-dependent kinase inhibitor and a potential mediator of extracellular antimitogenic signals. *Cell*, Vol. 78, No.1, pp. 59-66.

Rahman, K.W., Li, Y., Wang, Z., Sarkar, S.H., & Sarkar, F.H. (2006). Gene expression profiling revealed survivin as a target of 3,3'-diindolylmethane-induced cell growth inhibition and apoptosis in breast cancer cells. *Cancer Res*, Vol. 66, No.9, pp. 4952-4960.

Roninson, I.B. (2002). Oncogenic functions of tumour suppressor p21(Waf1/Cip1/Sdi1): association with cell senescence and tumour-promoting activities of stromal fibroblasts. *Cancer Lett.*, Vol. 179, No.1, pp. 1-14.

Rostagno, P., Moll, J.L., Birtwisle-Peyrottes, I., Ettore, F., & Caldani, C. (1996). Cell cycle expression of estrogen receptors determined by image analysis on human breast cancer cells in vitro and in vivo. *Breast Cancer Res Treat.*, Vol. 39, No.2, pp. 147-154.

Russo, A.A., Jeffrey, P.D., Patten, A.K., Massague, J., & Pavletich, N.P. (1996). Crystal structure of the p27Kip1 cyclin-dependent-kinase inhibitor bound to the cyclin A-Cdk2 complex. *Nature*, Vol. 382, No.6589, pp. 325-331.

Saleh, E.M., El-Awady, R.A., bdel Alim, M.A., & bdel Wahab, A.H. (2009). Altered expression of proliferation-inducing and proliferation-inhibiting genes might contribute to acquired doxorubicin resistance in breast cancer cells. *Cell Biochem.Biophys.*, Vol. 55, No.2, pp. 95-105.

Sarkar, F.H. & Li, Y. (2004). Cell signaling pathways altered by natural chemopreventive agents. *Mutat.Res.*, Vol. 555, No.1-2, pp. 53-64.

Shattuck, D.L., Miller, J.K., Carraway, K.L., III, & Sweeney, C. (2008). Met receptor contributes to trastuzumab resistance of Her2-overexpressing breast cancer cells. *Cancer Res*, Vol. 68, No.5, pp. 1471-1477.

Sherr, C.J. (1994). G1 phase progression: cycling on cue. *Cell*, Vol. 79, No.4, pp. 551-555.

Shu, L., Cheung, K.L., Khor, T.O., Chen, C., & Kong, A.N. (2010). Phytochemicals: cancer chemoprevention and suppression of tumor onset and metastasis. *Cancer Metastasis Rev.*, Vol. 29, No.3, pp. 483-502.

Siddiqui, I.A., Adhami, V.M., Bharali, D.J., Hafeez, B.B., Asim, M., Khwaja, S.I., Ahmad, N., Cui, H., Mousa, S.A., & Mukhtar, H. (2009). Introducing nanochemoprevention as a novel approach for cancer control: proof of principle with green tea polyphenol epigallocatechin-3-gallate. *Cancer Res*, Vol. 69, No.5, pp. 1712-1716.

Skog, S., He, Q., Khoshnoud, R., Fornander, T., & Rutqvist, L.E. (2004). Genes related to growth regulation, DNA repair and apoptosis in an oestrogen receptor-negative (MDA-231) versus an oestrogen receptor-positive (MCF-7) breast tumour cell line. *Tumour.Biol.*, Vol. 25, No.1-2, pp. 41-47.

Staalesen, V., Leirvaag, B., Lillehaug, J.R., & Lonning, P.E. (2004). Genetic and epigenetic changes in p21 and p21B do not correlate with resistance to doxorubicin or mitomycin and 5-fluorouracil in locally advanced breast cancer. *Clin.Cancer Res*, Vol. 10, No.10, pp. 3438-3443.

Stendahl, M., Kronblad, A., Ryden, L., Emdin, S., Bengtsson, N.O., & Landberg, G. (2004). Cyclin D1 overexpression is a negative predictive factor for tamoxifen response in postmenopausal breast cancer patients. *Br J Cancer*, Vol. 90, No.10, pp. 1942-1948.

Stendahl, M., Nilsson, S., Wigerup, C., Jirstrom, K., Jonsson, P.E., Stal, O., & Landberg, G. (2010). p27Kip1 is a predictive factor for tamoxifen treatment response but not a prognostic marker in premenopausal breast cancer patients. *Int.J Cancer*, Vol. 127, No.12, pp. 2851-2858.

Stewart, Z.A., Westfall, M.D., & Pietenpol, J.A. (2003). Cell-cycle dysregulation and anticancer therapy. *Trends in Pharmacological Sciences*, Vol. 24, No.3, pp. 139-145.

Sutherland, R.L. & Musgrove, E.A. (2009). CDK inhibitors as potential breast cancer therapeutics: new evidence for enhanced efficacy in ER+ disease. *Breast Cancer Res*, Vol. 11, No.6, pp. 112.

Toyoshima, H. & Hunter, T. (1994). p27, a novel inhibitor of G1 cyclin-Cdk protein kinase activity, is related to p21. *Cell*, Vol. 78, No.1, pp. 67-74.

Upadhyay, S., Neburi, M., Chinni, S.R., Alhasan, S., Miller, F., & Sarkar, F.H. (2001). Differential sensitivity of normal and malignant breast epithelial cells to genistein is partly mediated by p21(WAF1). *Clin.Cancer Res*, Vol. 7, No.6, pp. 1782-1789.

Wang,Z., Ahmad,A., Li,Y., Banerjee,S., Kong,D., & Sarkar,F.H. (2010a). Forkhead box M1 transcription factor: a novel target for cancer therapy. *Cancer Treat.Rev.*, Vol. 36, No.2, pp. 151-156.

Wang, Z., Li, Y., Ahmad, A., Azmi, A.S., Kong, D., Banerjee, S., & Sarkar, F.H. (2010b). Targeting miRNAs involved in cancer stem cell and EMT regulation: An emerging concept in overcoming drug resistance. *Drug Resist.Updat.*, Vol. 13, No.4-5, pp. 109-118.

Wang, Z., Yu, B.W., Rahman, K.M., Ahmad, F., & Sarkar, F.H. (2008). Induction of growth arrest and apoptosis in human breast cancer cells by 3,3-diindolylmethane is associated with induction and nuclear localization of p27kip. *Mol.Cancer Ther.*, Vol. 7, No.2, pp. 341-349.

Wilcken, N.R., Prall, O.W., Musgrove, E.A., & Sutherland, R.L. (1997). Inducible overexpression of cyclin D1 in breast cancer cells reverses the growth-inhibitory effects of antiestrogens. *Clin.Cancer Res*, Vol. 3, No.6, pp. 849-854.

Wu, Y., Shang, X., Sarkissyan, M., Slamon, D., & Vadgama, J.V. (2010). FOXO1A is a target for HER2-overexpressing breast tumors. *Cancer Res*, Vol. 70, No.13, pp. 5475-5485.

Xia, M., Knezevic, D., & Vassilev, L.T. (2011). p21 does not protect cancer cells from apoptosis induced by nongenotoxic p53 activation. *Oncogene*, Vol. 30, No.3, pp. 346-355.

Yang, Q., Sakurai, T., Yoshimura, G., Takashi, Y., Suzuma, T., Tamaki, T., Umemura, T., Nakamura, Y., Nakamura, M., Utsunomiya, H., Mori, I., & Kakudo, K. (2000). Overexpression of p27 protein in human breast cancer correlates with in vitro resistance to doxorubicin and mitomycin C. *Anticancer Res*, Vol. 20, No.6B, pp. 4319-4322.

9

Multidrug Resistence and Breast Cancer

Gengyin Zhou and Xiaofang Zhang
Shandong University of Medicine,
China

1. Introduction

Millions of new cancer patients are diagnosed each year and over half of these patients die from this disease. As the second leading cause of cancer deaths, breast cancer is estimated to be diagnosed in over one million people worldwide and to cause more than 400,000 deaths each year [1]. Chemotherapy is part of a successful treatment to many cases; however, the development of multidrug resistance (MDR) to it becomes a major obstacle so as to as few as half of the breast cancer patients treated benefit from chemotherapy.

MDR is a term used to describe the phenomenon characterized by the ability of drug resistant tumors to exhibit simultaneous resistance to a number of structurally and functionally unrelated chemotherapeutic agents [2]. The cytotoxic drugs that are most frequently associated with MDR are hydrophobic, amphipathic natural products, such as the taxanes (paclitaxel and docetaxel), vinca alkaloids (vinorelbine, vincristine, and vinblastine), anthracyclines (doxorubicin, daunorubicin, and epirubicin), epipodophyllotoxins (etoposide and teniposide), antimetabolites (methorexate, fluorouracil, cytosar, 5-azacytosine, 6-mercaptopurine, and gemcitabine) topotecan, dactinomycin, mitomycin C and so on[3].

At present, many mechanisms have been found to be responsible for it, including overexpression of the members of the adenosine triphosphate (ATP)-binding cassette (ABC) membrane transporter family, changes of apoptosis-related genes, the alteration of DNA-repair gene, cancer stem cells and so on. And up to date, many methods were adopted to overcome MDR, for example natrual drugs, chemical drugs and genetic therapy.

Herein, we will introduce the mechanisms and therapy of MDR of breast cancer briefly.

2. Mechanisms of MDR

2.1 The adenosine triphosphate (ATP)-binding cassette (ABC) membrane transporter family

Elevated expression of ATP-binding cassette (ABC) transporters is considered to be the main cause of MDR in breast cancer. ATP-binding cassette (ABC) transporters are a family of transporter proteins that contribute to drug resistance via adenosinetriphosphate (ATP)-dependent drug efflux pumps, which can result in an increased efflux of the cytotoxic drugs from the cancer cells, thus lowering their intracellular concentrations [4]. Up to date, more than 100 ABC transporters from prokaryotes to humans and 48 human ABC genes have been identified that share sequence and structural homology [3]. The proteins which are related to the MDR in breast cancer are mainly including p-glycoprotein (p-gp), multidrug resistence- related protein (MRP) and breast cancer resistence protein (BCRP).

In mammals, the functionally active typical ABC proteins consist of at least four core domains, two transmembrane domains (TMDs) and two nucleotide-binding domains (NBDs). The two TMDs of each ABC transporter consist of multiple membrane-spanning α-helices (typically, but not always, six α-helices per domain) and form the pathway through which substrate crosses the membrane. The two NBDs play a role in cleaving ATP (hydrolysis) to derive energy necessary for transporting cell nutrients such as sugars, amino acids, ions and small peptides [5]. Normally, they have important physiological function, such as the excretion of toxins from the liver, kidneys, and gastrointestinal tract [6]. Overexpression of these transporters has been observed in many types of human malignancies and correlated with poor responses to chemotherapeutic agents.

2.1.1 P-glycoprotein

In 1970s, a carbohydrate-containing protein, 170 kDa in molecular weight, was found in multidrug-resistant Chinese hamster ovary cells. The glycoprotein was named P-glycoprotein (P-gp) because the protein can modulate membrane permeability with respect to a number of apparently unrelated drugs including actinomycin D, methotrexate, daunomycin, and colchicine [7]. The MDR mediated by P-gp is also called" classical MDR".

Gene sequence membrane analysis for mammalian P-gp has revealed the presence of two similar halves, each containing 6 putative transmembrane segments, and an ATP-binding consensus motif. The human protein is comprised of 1280 amino acids with 12 transmembrane domains and 43% sequence homology between the two halves. Three glycosylation sites on the first extracytoplasmic domain are present [8]. The gene encoding p-glycoprotein was termed mdr1.The gene with 28 exon and 1.2 kb and is located on chromosome 7q21.12.

There are three known isoforms of P-gp, namely, class I, II and III. Rodent cells have all three P-gp genes, whereas human cells only have class I and III P-gp [9]. Classes I and II P-gp genes confer MDR when transfected into sensitive wild type (WT) cells, whereas the class III P-gp gene is not shown to be associated with drug resistance. All three types of P-gp expressed in several normal tissues. In mammalian tissues, class I P-gp is found in epithelium, intestinal, endothelial cells, bone marrow progenitor peripheral blood lymphocytes, natural killer cells and so on. The class III P-GP is localized in hepatocytes, cardiac and striated muscle [10]. The distribution displays that p-gp plays an important role in normal physiological function. Evident confirmed that P-gp take part in the transepithelial secretion of substrates into bile, urine, or gastrointestinal tract lumen. P-gp may also confer a protective role to mediate xenobiotic efflux in tissues such as the brain, testis, and placenta.

P-gp substrates are widespread. Although their structures are very different, they share many physical properties including high hydrophobicity, an amphiphilic nature and a net positive charge[11]. It is important for us to understanding the modulation of P-gp. Evident shows that p-gp is phosphorylated by protein kinase C (PKC) and PKC blockers can reduce P-gp phosphorylation and increase drug accumulation. However, there is evidence that PKC inhibitors directly interact with P-gp and inhibit drug transport by a mechanism independent of P-gp phosphorylation [12]. Experiments using transient transfection of the MDR1 promoter region (linked to a reporter gene) into the cells as well as stable transfection of some other genes showed that genes p53, ras and raf can influence the activity of introduced MDR1 promoter or the expression of the endogenous cellular MDR1. Genes c-fos and c-jun also were shown to confer the regulation of MDR1 activity [13].

For a long time, P-gp was believed to be the only protein capable of conferring MDR in mammalian tumor cells. Over 50% breast cancer expressed P-gp [14]. Moreover, prior exposure to chemotherapy or hormonal therapy has been shown to increase the proportion of breast cancers expressing P-gp by 1.8-fold [15]. However, pre-chemotherapy P-gp expression showed no association with shorter progression-free survival (PFS) so the clinical relevance of this observation in terms of screening patients and treatment selection remains unclear[16].

2.1.2 Multidrug resistence- related protein 1(MRP)

In 1992, Susan Cole and Roger Deeley observed amplification and increased expression of a novel gene in non-P-gp expressing small cell lung cancer DOX resistant cell lines and this is the MRP1 (ABCC1) (MDR related protein) gene.The following study shows that the protein encoded by this gene is also a member of ABC transporters [17].

The multidrug-resistance-associated protein (MRP or MRP1) is a 190 kDa protein and is constituted by 1531 amino acids. Like other members of ABC transporters, MRP1 has 3 membrane spanning domains, 2 NBDs and extracellular N-terminal. Up to now, several isoforms of MRP1 have been identified. Included among these are five human MRP1-related proteins, designated MRP2, MRP3, MRP4, MRP5 and MRP6. MRP7, MRP8 and MRP9 are recent additions to the family which have not yet been characterised[18].

Physiologiclly, MRP1 also plays a normal role in the ATP-dependent unidirectional membrane transport of glutathione conjugates, such as leukotriene C4, S-(2,4-dinitrophenyl)glutathione and leukotriene receptor antagonists could inhibit this function[19]. Besides multidrug-resistance cancer cells, MRP is also expressed in normal human tissues, such as muscle, lung, spleen, bladder, adrenal gland and gall bladder [2]. MRP2 (or cannalicular multispecific organic anion transporter or cMOAT) was first shown to be expressed in the liver which functions in the excretion of glutathione and glucuronate conjugates across the cannalicular membrane into bile. In addition, MRP2/ cMOAT is also expressed in the human kidney proximal tubule epithelia on the apical side. Therefore, it is implicated that MRP2 may play a role in the renal excretion of endogenous substances and xenobiotics, in normal conditions. MRP3 is expressed in liver and involved in the efflux of organic anions from the liver into the blood in case of biliary obstruction. MRP4 and MRP5 transport nucleosides and confer resistance to antiretroviral nucleoside analogs. MRP6 is a lipophilic anion pump with a wide spectrum of drug resistance. Among the members of MRP family, only MRP1 has been widely accepted to cause clinical drug resistance[3].

Like other members of ABC translporters, MRP1 can pump anti-tumor drugs out of the tumor cells, cause reduced intracellular accumulation of drugs and lead to resistance. Whereas P-gp transports neutral and positively charged molecules in their unmodified form, MRP1 overexpression is associated with an increased ATP-dependent glutathione-S conjugate transport activity. Reduced glutathione (GSH) has been suggested as an important component of MRP mediated MDR and drug transport. MRP1 is able to transport a range of substrates as such or conjugated to GSH, glucuronide, and sulfate [20]. The anticancer drugs that are substrates of MRP1 mainly include anthracyclines such as doxorubicin and daunorubicin, vinca alkaloids and etoposide. Several findings indicate that MRP1 reduces drug accumulation by effluxing drugs by a GSH co-transport mechanism or after their conjugation to GSH [21]. But the mechanism by which GSH facilitates transport of some compounds by MRP1 is still a matter of debate.

2.1.3 Breast cancer resistance protein (BCRP)

Breast cancer resistance protein (BCRP) is the latest ABC transporter involved in MDR and it was cloned by Ross and Doyle in 1998 from a mitoxantrone-resistant subline of the breast cancer cell line MCF-7/Adr/Vp which does not express other known multidrug efflux transporters such as P-glycoprotein (P-gp) or the multidrug resistance protein 1 (MRP1) [22]. Two almost identical proteins as BCRP with only a few amino acid differences were later discovered independently by other laboratories from mitoxantrone-resistant human cancer cell lines (so named as MXR) and humanplacenta (so named as ABCP)[23].

The BCRP gene is located on chromosome 4q22. The full length of BCRP gene is 66kb and the length of mRNA is about 2.4kb [23].The product of the gene is a 72KD protein with 655 amino acid that contains an ATP-binding domain and six transmembrane domains, and it is a half transporter member of the ABCG subfamily [24]. As a half transporter, BCRP functions as a homodimeric/oligomeric efflux pump [25], and in a manner that is similar to other ABC transporters. Besides that, BCRP can also transport hydrophilic conjugated organic anions, particularly the sulfated conjugates with high affinity, for example BCRP can detoxify irinotecan and SN-38 by glucuronidation via the activity of UDP-glucuronyltransferase [26]. BCRP substrates include not only chemotherapeutic agents such as mitoxantrone, methotrexate, topotecan, irinotecan and its active analog SN-38, and tyrosine kinase inhibitors imatinib and gefitinib, but non-chemotherapy drugs such as prazosin, glyburide, nitrofurantoin, dipyridamole, statins, and cimetidine as well as nontherapeutic compounds such as the dietary flavonoids, porphyrins, estrone 3-sulfate (E1S), and the carcinogen PhIP [27].

Similar to P-gp and MRP1, BCRP is widely expressed in normal cells and tissues including the capillary endothelial cells, the hematopoietic stem cells [28], the maternal - fetal barrier of the placenta and the blood-brain barrier [29]. In these tissues, BCRP play a protective role against xenobiotics and their metabolites. Whereas, the apical localization of BCRP in the intestinal epithelium and in the bile canalicular membrane also suggests the intestinal absorption and hepatobiliary excretion of BCRP substrates [30].

Unexpectedly, many mutant forms of BCRP proteins were found in drug-selected cells such as those of the S1-M1-80 and MCF7/AdVp3000 cell lines and up to now, more than 50 mutations have been identified including natural variants and non-natrual mutations [27]. The most important natural variant is Q141K, which occurs in Japanese and Chinese populations at high allele frequencies (30 –60%) and in Caucasians and African-American populations at relatively low allele frequencies (5 – 10%) [27]. Several studies consistently revealed that Q141K had a lower protein expression level than wild-type BCRP in both transfected cells and human tissues. A recent study has revealed that Q141K undergoes increased lysosomal and proteasomal degradations than wild-type BCRP, possibly explaining the lower level of protein expression of the variant [31]. The R482T and R482G variants of BCRP detected from MCF7/ AdVp3000 and S1-M1-80 cells belong to non-natural mutants. The non-natural mutants have different effects on BCRP expression, distribution and functions. Some mutations do not affect plasma membrane expression, but alter substrate specificity and/or overall transport activity. For example, the R482T and R482G lose their methotrexate-transporting activity but at the same time confer increased mitoxantrone resistance, so they are highly resistant to both mitoxantrone and doxorubicin[32]. Wild-type BCRP does not transport Rhodamine 123 and Lyso-Tracker Green; however, the mutants R482T and R482G do [33]. These findings confirmed that the transmembrane region of BCRP plays important roles in its activity. Some mutations affect biogenesis with decreased stability, lower expression and/or altered subcellular distribution of BCRP. A typical example is mutations of Arg383 which results in a significant decrease in the protein level, partial retention in the endoplasm reticulum, and altered glycosylation and the treatment with mitoxantrone assisted in protein maturation [34]. Some mutations influence the chemical modifications of BCRP such as N-linked glycosylation or disulfide bond formation in BCRP such as the mutation Asn596. Otherwise, there are also many mutations which do not have major effects on both plasma membrane expression and function of BCRP, including K473A and H630X. The research on the mutations of BCRP could help us to further understand the structures and functions of ABC transportes.

Up to date, BCRP was detected in many resistance tumor cells such as human colon cancer cell line S1-M1-80, prostate cancer cell lines and breast cancer cell line MCF7/AdVp3000 [35]. Many clinical sample were also found BCRP expression, including acute myelogenous leukemia (AML), acute lymphocytic leukemia (ALL), non-small cell lung cancer and so on[36-38]. And it has been suggested that the expression of BCRP is associated with a poor response to cancer chemotherapy and may be responsible for clinical drug resistance. However, the studies on the expression characters of BCRP in breast cancer clinical samples are still very few.

2.2 Apoptosis and MDR

2.2.1 P53

As a tumor suppressor, p53 plays a pivotal role in inducing apoptosis in response to cellular damage, including DNA damage. However, mutant P53 plays an opposite role in the regulation of apoptosis, that is mutant p53 is an anti-apoptosis factor. In a study from the National Cancer Institute (NCI), the majority of breast cancer cell lines were mutant for p53 [39]. About 50% of all tumours have an approximately 25% occurrence of deletions and point mutations in sporadic breast cancers[40]. Many anti-tumor drugs can lead cellular death by inducing cellular apoptosis. When p53 mutations or deletions occur, the cellular apoptosis can be inhibited and the cells exhibit MDR phenotype. Mutations in p53 have been verified to be related with resistance to doxorubicin in breast cancer patients[41].

Many data show the correlation of P53 and ABC transporters. The first experiments implied that a mutant p53 (mtP53)specifically stimulated the MDR1 promoter and wild-type p53(wtP53) exerted specific repression[42]. In the follow-up study, a p53 consensus binding sequence was also found in the promoter of the rat ABCB1 gene. Both promoter function and endogenous mdr1b expression were shown to be up-regulated by wtp53[43]. More studies displayed that the mutations of p53 can dramatically activate the ABCB1 promoter in multiple cell lines including Saos-2, Caco-2, MCF-7 and so on[44]. Linn et al. assessed the status of p53 and ABCB1 in both primary operable and advanced-staged tumors and their results revealed that nuclear p53 accumulation and coexpression of ABCB1 were more prevalent in locally advanced breast cancers and that these markers provided a strong prognostic indication of shorter survival[45,46]. Similar results were also found in other studies.

Recently, Wang et al investigated the effects of wild-type and mutant p53, and nuclear factor kappa-B (NF-kappaB) (p50) on BCRP promoter activity in MCF-7 cells, and the results show that wild-type p53 induced transcriptional suppression of breast cancer resistance protein (BCRP) through the NF-kappaB pathway in MCF-7 cells[47].

2.2.2 Other apoptosis related genes and MDR

Mitochondrial (intrinsic pathway) and cell surface receptor (Fas) mediated (extrinsic pathway) apoptosis are the two main routes leading to programmed cell death. MCF-7 cells can undergo apoptosis by the sequential activation of caspases-9 (associated with mitochondrial mediated apoptosis), -7, and -6. Recently, a splice variant form of caspase-3 has been shown to be overexpressed in chemoresistant, locally advanced breast cancers, and is particularly associated with response to cyclophosphamide[48].

Bcl-2 is a member of a large family of genes coding both anti-apoptotic proteins (for example, Bcl-2, Bcl-XL) and pro-apoptotic proteins (Bax, Bad Bic, etc.). Bcl-2 protein is able to inhibit the apoptosis induced by p53 in response to genotoxic stress. There are data showing that Bcl-2 overexpression results in the resistance of cells to different drugs, including DOX, taxol, etoposide, camptothecin, mitoxantrone and cisplatin[49] . When Bcl-2 is over expressed and contributes as a resistance mechanism, it has been shown that the anticancer drugs promote cell cycle arrest; however, their effects are cytostatic rather than cytotoxic[2]. The phosphorylation state of the Bcl-2 oncoproteins has been shown to modulate response to taxanes[50].

Survivin is another apoptosis-related gene which has been confirmed to confer MDR in tumors. It is a structurally unique inhibitor of apoptosis (IAP), substances which block apoptosis induced by a variety of nonrelated apoptosis triggers. Survivin is known to directly or indirectly bind and inhibit the terminal effector cell death protease cascades, caspase 3 and 7, as well as inhibit the activation of caspase 9[51]. Furthermore, it has been reported that the expression of survivin was significantly higher after treatment with anti-cancer drugs in many cancer cells and may be involved in radio- and chemo-resistance[52]. Liu et al. documented that survivin might modulate the turnover of P-gp or transport by P-gp in the cell, which then resulted in anti-apoptosis and drug resistance in breast cancer cells[51]. However, the role of survivin in MDR breast cancer in the presence of P-gp is still not clear.

In addition, some other apoptosis-related genes were found to take part in the regulation of MDR, such as CD95, TRAIL and so on.

2.3 MDR-related enzyme

2.3.1 Glutathione S-transferase (GST)

GST is a member of phase II detoxification enzymes that catalyses the conjugation of glutathione (GSH) to a wide variety of endogenous and exogenous electrophilic compounds. Because of their capacity to react with electrophiles, radicals and reactive oxygen species, GSTs, together with GSH, have a major role in the protection against oxidative stress [53].

GSTs are divided into two super-family members: the membrane microsomal and cytosolic GSTs(c-GSTs). Microsomal GSTs (m-GSTs) are structurally distinct from the cytosolic in that they homo- and heterotrimerize rather than dimerize to form a single active site and the microsomal GSTs are mainly involved in the metabolism of endogenous compounds, like leukotrienes and prostaglandins. The cytosolic GSTs also conjugate exogenous compounds and the cytosolic GSTs are subject to significant genetic polymorphisms in human populations. Up to date, the cytosolic GSTs are divided into seven classes, Alpha (A), Mu (M), Omega (O), Pi (P), Sigma (S), Teta (T) and Zeta (Z) which have a promiscuous substrate specificity and are localized in different tissues with organ specific expression patterns [54]. The GST-Pi have been confirmed to be closely related with MDR.

Many data show that GST confers the development and expression of MDR. Increased expression of GSTpi—detected as strong immunoreactivity—has been documented to contribute to drug resistance of ovarian carcinomas, head and neck cancer, lung squamous-cell carcinoma, breast cancers and so on[55]. Cells with GST isozyme transfections yield mild increases in resistance (mostly in the 2-5 fold range) to a number of different anticancer drugs [54]. While inhibition of GST expression by antisense cDNA increased the sensitivity to several anticancer drugs [56]. Besides, exposure of cells to a specific inhibitor of c-GCS, buthionine sulfoximine (BSO), decreases multidrug resistance to doxorubicin and vincristine[57]. The substrates of GST reported include chlorambucil, melphalan, nitrogen mustard, phosphoramide mustard, acrolein, carmustine, hydroxyalkenals, ethacrynic acid and steroids. And the MDR mediated by GST is related to mitomycin C, adriamycin, cisplatin and carboplatin.

How GSTs affect MDR in tumor cells? There are mainly two mechanisms found now. First, GST-Pi plays a key role in regulating the MAP kinase pathway via protein: protein interactions. GST-Pi was shown to be an endogenous inhibitor of c-Jun N-terminal kinase 1 (JNK1), a key member of MAP pathway which involved in stress response, apoptosis, and cellular proliferation [58]. In nonstressed cells, low JNK activity is observed due to the sequestration of the protein in a GST- Pi : JNK complex. Direct protein : protein interactions between the C-terminal of JNK and GST-pi were reported with a binding constant of approximately 200 nm. The second, there is a coordinate action of phase II enzymes and MRP in MDR[59]. The already mentioned connection between a MRP drug resistance profile and an increased GST-pi expression, shown in many cell lines, is indeed indicative for a shared regulatory mechanism of MRP and GSTs expression [60]. Studies demonstrated that Nrf2 may be play a key role between MRP and GSTs. A study on Nrf2 knockout mice displayed that: disruption of the Nrf2 gene decreased both the constitutive as well as the inducible expression of class Alpha, class Mu and class Pi glutathione transferases[61]. Meanwhile, Nrf2 was also shown to be necessary for the constitutive and inducible expression of MRP1 in mouse embryo fibroblast[62].

GSTpi immunoreactivity was reported not to correlate with response to chemotherapy in cervical carcinoma, but many data show that in primary breast cancers, expression of GST-Pi was associated with poor prognosis. Fengxi Su et al analyzed the relationship between GST-Pi and the FAM (5-fluorouracil, adriamycin, mitomycin) protocol and the result showed that the presence of GSTpi in breast cancer tissue was a bad prognostic indicator, and these tumors were largely resistant to chemotherapy[55]. In cultured breast cancer cells, GST-pi is exclusively expressed in estrogen receptor-negative (ER−) cells but not in receptor-positive (ER+) cells [63]. In 1997, Mona S. Jhaveri verified that that methylation status of the promoter contributes significantly to the levels of GSTP1 expressed in ER− and ER+ breast cancer cell lines [64].

2.3.2 DNA topoisomerase II (topo II)

DNA topoisomerase II (topo II) is a nuclear phosphoprotein involved in DNA replication and chromosome dynamics. These enzymes catalyse the ATP-dependent passage of one DNA duplex (the transport or T-segment) through a transient, double-stranded break in another (the gate or G-segment), navigating DNA through the protein using a set of dissociable internal interfaces, or 'gates' [65,66]. The family of DNA topoisomerase II includes two related but genetically distinct isoforms isforms TOPIIα and IIβ in mammalian cells.

The human topoisomerase II α gene (TOP2 α) is localized on chromosome 17q21-22 [67] whereas TOPIIβ maps to chromosome 3p24 [68]. The cDNAs for the human α and β isoforms encode p170 and p180 proteins of 1531- and 1621-amino-acid [68], respectively. TOP2α lies close to the epidermal growth factor-like receptor gene ERBB2 (HER2) and the retinoic acid receptor locus RARK in a region of chromosomal 17 which is amplified in some human breast cancer [69]. The two enzymes are closely similar in structure each comprising three functional domains de¢ned by sites of cleavage by trypsin or staphylococcal V8 proteases: an N-terminal ATPase domain (approximately residues 1-400); a DNA breakage-reunion region (400-1220); and the C-terminal domain which carries a multitude of phosphorylation sites[70].

In addition to its role in cell division, TOP2α is also found to be related to the MDR in tumor.It is the major molecular target for a large group of clinically relevant, structurally different cytotoxic agents known as TOP2α inhibitors including the anthracycline class of antitumor cytotoxic agents [71]. These drugs all act by forming covalent bonds with TOP2α, creating a complex that introduces permanent double-strand breaks in DNA leading to apoptosis. Reduced topoisomerase II expression or function can contribute to resistance to agents such as anthracyclines and epipodophyllotoxins [72]. In vitro studies of breast tumor cell lines have shown that amplification of the TOP2α gene leads to protein overexpression and sensitivity to anthracyclines [73,74]. Similarly, deletion of TOP2α genomic alterations in breast cancer leads to a marked decrease in TOP2α protein expression, which results in chemoresistance to TOP2α inhibitor anticancer drugs in cell culture.

The HER-2 gene is another gene on chromosome 17 and it encodes for a ligandless, transmembrane glycoprotein receptor with intrinsic tyrosine–kinase activity. HER-2 gene amplification or protein overexpression occurs in about 20% of patients with breast cancer and is a recognized poor prognostic marker, often associated with endocrine resistant, high grade disease[75]. Recently research reported that the expression of TOP2α is closely related to the expression of HER2 gene and co-expression of them may be a useful tool in predicting benefit from chemotherapy. Top IIα is reported to be either amplified or deleted in nearly 90% of HER-2 amplified primary breast cancers[76]. Recent review of the Canadian-MA.5 trial assessed TOP2α alterations and HER-2 amplification by FISH on tissue microarrays in 438 patients [77]. Top IIα alterations occurred in 18% patients (12% amplification, 6% deletions) and were more common in large tumors and in HER-2 positive tumors. In patients with Top IIα alterations, relative benefits of therapy were seen with CEF having statistical superiority over CMF in terms of RFS (adjusted HR 0.35, 95% CI 0.17 - 0.73, p = 0.005) and OS (adjusted HR 0.33, 95% CI 0.15 - 0.75, p = 0.008). However, there are also diffusing evidents. An analysis displayed topo IIa mRNA overexpression in 19% of HER-2 negative patients [78]. In conclusion, the relationship between TOP II, HER2 and chemosensitivity needs further investigation.

2.3.3 Glucosylceramide synthase

Sphingolipids, which include ceramides and sphingosine, were first isolated and characterized in the late 1800s. Recent years, many studies have shown that they are not only structural and insert components of cell membranes but also associated with myriad process of cells including the proliferation, survival and death of cells. As an important member of sphingolipid metabolism, ceramide have been proven to be a second messager of apoptosis [79, 80]. Cellular stress is known to increase ceramide levels in cells. So it is easily

to understand that increased ceramide has been oberserved in response to many anti-cancer drugs, such as doxorubicin, vincristine, paclitaxel, etoposide, PSC 833 and fenretinide.
Many enzymes have been confirmed to be responsible for the regulation of ceramide levels, such as ceramide synthase and sphingomyelinase which are responsible for the ceramide generation, and sphingomyelin synthase and ceramidase which take part in the ceramide metabolization[81]. Glucosylceramide synthase (GCS) is one of them. As an enzyme which catalyzes the first step in glycosphingolipid synthesis, GCS transfers UDP–glucose to ceramide to form glucosylceramide, which have been found to involve in many cellular processes such as cell proliferation, oncogenic transformation, differentiation, and tumor metastasis[82].In additon, many studies show that GC was related with MDR in many tumor cells. In 1996, Lavie Y et al first reported that chemotherapy resistant MCF-7-AdrR breast cancer cells accumulate GC in comparison to wild-type MCF-7 cells[83].After that, GC was found to confer to MDR in many other cancers [84-86].So some people guessed that elevated GCS activity may be a novel form of multidrug resistance.
Then, Liu etc found that increased competence to glycosylate ceramide conferred adriamycin resistance in MCF-7 breast cancer cells by transfection with GCS cDNA[8], while using GCS inhibitor 1-phenyl-2-palmitoylamino-3- morpholino-propanol (PPMP) or transfection of doxorubicin-resistant MCF-7-AdrR cells with GCS antisense both restored cell sensitivity to doxorubicin or vinblastine and paclitaxeland[86,87]. Ladisch found that blocking GCS with D, L-threo-phenyl-2-hexadecanoylamino-3-pyrrolidino-1- propanol (PPPP), was able to elevate ceramide levels and enhance vincristine cytotoxicity via programmed cell death[88]. All the following works demonstrated that GCS was potentially one MDR-related drug resistance mechanism.
Recently, Yong-Yu Liu et al reported that glucosylceramide synthase upregulates MDR1 expression in the regulation of cancer drug resistance through cSrc and β-catenin signaling in the ovarian cell line NCI/ADR-RES which was ever named MCF-7/AdrR [89]. This study revealed the importance of GCS in the mechanism of cancer drug resistance.
Further studies demonstrated that a GC-rich/Sp1 promoter binding region was of importance in the regulation of GCS expression and doxorubicin could induce activation of Sp1 and up-regulation of GCS and apoptosis in Leukimia drug-resistance cell line HL-60/ADR and ovarian cell line NCI/ADR-RES [81,90].
In 2009, Eugen Ruckhäberle et al analyzed microarray data of GCS expression in 1,681 breast tumors and found that expression of GCS was associated with a positive estrogen receptor (ER) status, lower histological grading, low Ki67 levels and ErbB2 negativity ($P < 0.001$ for all) [91]. This study revealed the expression profile of GCS in breast cancer.But, the study also found that GCS has no clearly correlation with mdr1.So the relationship between GCS and mdr1 in breast cancer is still a puzzle.

2.4 Cancer stem cells and MDR

Stem cells are defined as cells with both self-renewal capacity and the ability to produce multiple distinct differentiated cell types to form all the cell types that are found in the mature tissue[92]. Thus, these two characteristics of stem cells confer the unique property of asymmetric division. Stem cells are quiescent or slowly cycling cells maintained in an undifferentiated state until normal functioning of the organism needs their participation. Stem cells are classified into two principal types: embryonic and adult stem cells[93].

Recent studies have revealed that they play important role in cancer biology. Cancer stem cells (CSC) have been detected in many tumors, such as retinoblastoma and melanoma [94,95]. In breast cancer, a CD44+/CD24-or low/Lin- cell population was first identified as CSC [96].Later, aldehyde dehydrogenase (ALDH) 1 activity was reported to be associated with stem/progenitor properties in breast cancer [97].

Although the origin of cancer stem cells has not yet been elucidated, researchers proposed that the malignant transformation of a normal stem cell, or a progenitor cell that has acquired self-renewal ability may be the reason. Up to now, Three major pathways have been identified to be related with the regulation and maintenance of stem cells in adult life: Wnt, Hedgehog, and Notch[92].

It is well known that cancer chemotherapy targets dividing cells. Because stem cells are quiescent or slowly cycling cells under normal situation, it is easy to understand that cancer stem cells could escape from the killing of anti-tumor drugs.

Besides, the side-population (SP) cells may be another reasons why stem cells become multi-drug resistant. The isolation of SP cells is based on the technique described by Goodell et al. in 1996 [98]. While experimenting with staining of murine bone marrow cells with the vital dye, Hoechst 33342, they discovered that the display of Hoechst fluorescence simultaneously at two emission wavelengths (red 675 nm and blue 450 nm) localizes a distinct, small, nonstained cell population (0.1% of all cells) that express stem cells markers (Sca1+linneg/low), which were named SP cells. At first, they thought the exclusion of Hoechst 33342 by SP cells is an active process involving multidrug resistance transporter 1 (MDR1). But the following study show that MDR1 can not be taken as a single marker to identify and isolate SP cells. Zhou et al. have demonstrated the breast cancer resistance protein (BCRP) may also attend the SP phenotype[28]. The SPs from breast cancer contain primitive stem cell-like cells that can differentiate into epithelial tumors in vitro and in vivo and express stemness genes [28,99]. The characterization of cells within SP demonstrates that they are immature, poorly differentiated, and highly tumorigenic. Gene expression profiles of SP show that these cells are less differentiated than non-SP cells [100].

The ABC transporters may play three functions in CSCs. First, the ABC transporters can protect the CSCS against exogenous products able to penetrate the cell membrane barrier by active exclusion.Second, there is mounting speculation that ABC transporters repress the maturation and differentiation of stem cells. For example, the overexpression of ABCG2 inhibits hematopoietic development.The last, protection from hypoxia appears to be another function of ABC transporters in CSCS[101].

In conclusion, although the mechanisms of cancer stem cell are still unclear, the cancer stem cells must become target of chemotherapy.

2.5 Sex hormones and MDR

2.5.1 ER

Estrogens play key roles in development and maintenance of normal sexual and reproductive function. The most potent estrogen produced in the body is 17β-estradiol(E2). Two metabolites of E2, estrone and estriol, although they are high-affinity ligands are much weaker agonists on estrogen receptors (ERs)[102]. Up to now, two type of ERs have been found which named ERα(NR3A1) and ERβ(NR3A2). At the regulation of some genes, particularly those involved in proliferation, ERα and ERβ can have opposite actions [103], a finding which suggests that the overall proliferative response to E2 is the result of a balance between ERα and ERβ signaling.

The expression of ERα is closely associated with breast cancer biology, especially the development of tumors; estrogen hormones induce expression of c-myc and c-fos protooncogenes sufficient for cell division and breast cancer progression[104].Many studies demonstrated that breast carcinomas which lack ERα expression often reveal more aggressive phenotypes. Furthermore, ERα expression in tumor tissues is a favorable predictor of prognosis in endocrine treatment[105]. ERα typically functions as a transcription factor to regulate specific gene expression which binds to estrogen response elements (ERE)upstream of the target genes. The study of Lisa D. Coles et al. demonstrated that E2 could up-regulate the expression of p-gp in P-gp Overexpressing Cells (NCI-ADR-RES) [106].

Anti-estrogens, designed to block ERα, are widely and effectively used clinically in the treatment of breast cancer.The most common drugs including tamoxifen and toremifene.Some researches show that antiestrogens such as tamoxifen, metabolites of tamoxifen (4-hydroxytamoxifen and N-desmethyltamoxifen), droloxifen, and toremifene stimulated the p-gp ATPase activity and are substrates of p-gp. These results suggest that the antiestrogens may be potent drugs that reverse the multidrug-resistant phenotype mediated by P-gp[107]. However, another study displayed that tamoxifen activates CYP3A4 and MDR-1 genes through steroid and xenobiotic receptor (SXR) in breast cancer cells [108].But, some other anti-estrogens seem to be more effective on reversing MDR. A study shows that the pure anti-oestrogen ICI 164 could enhance doxorubicin and VBL toxicity to MCF-7/Adr cells 25- and 35-fold, respectively and the pure anti-oestrogens iodotamoxifens completely reversed VBL resistance in the mdr1 transfected lung cancer cell line [109].

Besides affection on p-gp, there are many data showing the relationship between anti-estrogens and BCRP. Imai et al. demonstrated that BCRP mRNA expression was induced by 17b-estradiol in T47D:A18 cells [110].Our research indicated that BCRP expression is upregulated by 17 β -estradiol via a novel pretranscriptional mechanism which might be involved in 17β-estradiol-ER complexes binding to the ERE of BCRP promoter via the classical pathway to activate transcription of the BCRP gene[111]. Besides, we also found that tamoxifen and toremifene could reverse MDR mediated by BCRP in breast cancer cells[104].

2.5.2 Progesterone receptor (PR)

Like estrogens, the physiological effects of progesterone are mediated by interaction of the hormone with the progesterone receptor. Up to now, two types of PRs were detected, named as PRA and PRB, respectively. The two PRs are expressed from a single gene as a result of transcription from two alternative promoters[112]. In general, PRB acts as a stronger transcriptional activator, whereas PRA functions as a transcriptional inhibitor of PRB and ER[113]. PR expression in breast cancer is also an important indicator of likely responsiveness to endocrine agents. It has been shown that PRA and PRB are expressed in similar amounts in most breast tumors[114]. Some data indicated that progesterone via PRs may be related to the regulation of MDR in breast cancer.

In 1994, Rao US et al found that at 50 microM, progesterone stimulated the P-gp ATPase activity as effectively as verapamil and is a potent drugs inducing p-gp mediated MDR[115]. Recently study displays that transcriptional regulation by E2 and progesterone (P4) likely contributes to the modulation of P-gp levels[116].

Besides that, the relationship between PR and BCRP has also been focus on. Wang et al found there were progesterone response elements on the upstream of BCRP promoter[114] and they note that the identified PRE is exactly the same as the estrogen response element published by Ee et al[117]. They found that PRB is a strong activator of transcription of the BCRP promoter, and PRA represses the PRB activity in the human placental choriocarcinoma BeWo cells. But the real situation in breast cancer may be complex. Because 17β-estradiol can induce PRB expression and down-regulate BCRP expression through posttranscriptional modification[118]; On the other hand, PRA can repress the estrogen receptor activity[113]. So the relationship between progesterone receptor and BCRP needs further data.

2.6 EMT and MDR

Tumor invasiveness, and metastasis, as well as MDR are still great puzzle in the development and treatment of tumors. The interconversion between epithelial and mesenchymal cells (designated as epithelialmesenchymal or mesenchymal-epithelial transition, EMT or MET, respectively) has received special attention and emerging evidence suggests that epithelial-mesenchymal transitions (EMTs) may take part in the above processes. An epithelial-mesenchymal transition (EMT) is a biologic process that allows a polarized epithelial cell, which normally interacts with basement membrane via its basal surface, to undergo multiple biochemical changes that enable it to assume a mesenchymal cell phenotype, which includes enhanced migratory capacity, invasiveness, elevated resistance to apoptosis, and greatly increased production of ECM components[119].

Kalluri R and Weinberg RA divided EMT into three types[119]. Type 1 EMTs can generate mesenchymal cells (primary mesenchyme) that have the potential to subsequently undergo a MET to generate secondary epithelia during implantation, embryogenesis, and organ development. Type 2 EMTs, the program begins as part of a repair-associated event that normally generates fibroblasts and other related cells in order to reconstruct tissues following trauma and inflammatory injury.

Type 3 EMTs occur in neoplastic cells that have previously undergone genetic and epigenetic changes, specifically in genes that favor clonal outgrowth and the development of localized tumors. Envidents show that EMT is critically linked with up-regulated invasion, metastasis, and angiogenesis. Figure 1 displays the relationship between EMT and progression of tumors. During the acquisition of EMT characteristics, cells loose epithelial cell–cell junctions, undergo actin cytoskeleton reorganization and decrease in the expression of proteins that promote cell–cell contact such as E-cadherin and β-catenin, and gain in the expression of mesenchymal markers such as vimentin, fibronectin,γ-smooth muscle actin (SMA), N-cadherin as well as increased activity of matrix metalloproteinases (MMPs) like MMP-2, MMP-3 and MMP-9, associated with an invasive phenotype[120].

The modulation of EMT is complicated. Many genes or signal transduction pathways are confirmed to take part in the regulation, such as hepatocyte growth factor (HGF)[121], transforming growth factor beta (TGF-β)[122], epidermal growth factor (EGF)[123], MMP-3[124] and so on. In addition, some transcriptional factors including snail and twist also play important role in EMT[125,126].

Recent studies have shown an intimate relationship between the EMT phenotype and MDR. Kajiyama et al. found that paclitaxel-resistant ovarian cancer cells showed phenotypic changes consistent with EMT[127]. These results were confirmed in other types of tumors like gemcitabine-resistant pancreatic cancer cells, oxaliplatin-resistant colorectal cancer cells, lapatinib-resistant breast cancer[120]. In addition, tamoxifen-resistant breast cancer cells undergone EMT with altered β-catenin phosphorylation[128]. It has been indicated that mesenchymal-like cancers might be more sensitive to DNA damaging agents such as doxorubicin, whereas epithelial-like cancers are more sensitive to targeted therapies, such as EGFR and HER2 antagonists [129].That may be the reason why mesenchymal-like, basal breast cancers are initially more sensitive to chemotherapy than epithelial-like luminal breast cancers[130]. However, it was discussed that basal, mesenchymal-like breast cancers possibly would be more prone to develop drug resistance. So more works need to do to investigate the links of EMT and MDR.

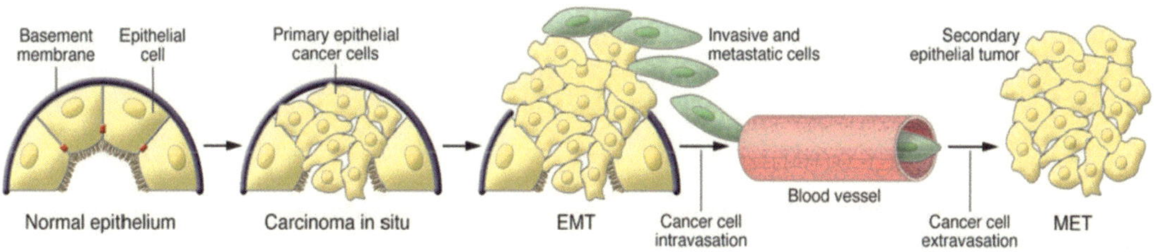

Fig. 1. The relationship between EMT and progression of tumors. Nomal epithelial cells transform to tumor cells. After EMT,tumor cells invade into surrounding normal tissues and distant organs. Then, MET reverse the cells into epithelial cells in the metastasis.

2.7 Methylation and MDR

Cancer is known as a genetic disease. Gain, loss, and mutation of genetic information have long been known to contribute to cancer development and progression. It is being increasingly recognized that epigenetic alterations in cancer often serve as potent surrogates for genetic mutations. Methylation of CpG dinucleotides is an important pattern of epigenetics.

Methylation can directly interfere with the binding of transcription factors to inhibit replication and/or methyl-CpG binding proteins that can bind to methylated DNA, as well as regulatory proteins to inhibit transcription[131]. The patterns of CpG methylation are specie and tissue specific. The biological machinery of this system comprises a variety of regulatory proteins including DNA methyltransferases, putative demethylases, methyl-CpG binding proteins, histones modifying enzymes and chromatin remodeling complexes. Alterations in DNA methylation participate in the development of some human diseases, including tumor [132].

Then whether DNA methylation takes part in the modulation of MDR? The answer is yes. El-Osta et al. used inhibitors of DNA methyltransferase (5-azacytidine [5aC]) and histone deacetylase (trichostatin A [TSA]) to examine gene transcription, promoter methylation status, and the chromatin determinants associated with the MDR1 promoter and their result displayed that 5aC and TSA induced DNA demethylation, leading to reactivation of methylated MDR1[133] . Nakayama et al. demonstrated the hypomethylation status of the MDR1 promoter region might be a necessary condition for MDR1 gene overexpression and establishment of P-glycoprotein-mediated multidrug resistance in AML patients[134]. Detailed mapping of MDR1 promoter showed that its promoter is always hypermethylated in drug-sensitive cells, while the drugresistant cells have hypomethylated MDR1 promoter[135]. Gayatri Sharma et al used methylation-specific PCR to investigate the promoter methylation status of MDR1 in tumor and serum of 100 patients with invasive ductal carcinomas of breast (IDCs) and MDR1 was hypomethylated in 47% tumors and 44% paired serum of IDC patients [136].

The methylation of BCRP has also been focus on. To et al. have shown an active CpG island within the proximal ABCG2 promoter region contributing to inactivation of ABCG2[137]. A follow-up research by Turner et al. demonstrated that ABCG2 expression in multiple myeloma patients and in cell lines is regulated in part by promoter methylation[138].

DNA methylation has been found to anticipate the regulation of other MDR-related genes. Chekhun VF et al. found that the promoter regions of MDR1, GST-pi, genes were highly methylated in MCF-7 cell line but not in its MCF-7/R drug resistant variant. The results suggests that acquirement of doxorubicin resistance of MCF-7 cells is associated with DNA hypomethylation of the promoter regions of the MDR1, GST-pi[139].

3. Strategies to reverse MDR

Since MDR phenomena have been recognised, the war fighting against it has been continuing. Many strategies have been devised to overcome it and mainly divided into three types: modulators, immunotherapy and genetic therapy.

3.1 Modulators of MDR

Because P-gp is the best characterized gene conferring MDR and its wide effects, most modulators target for it. So herein, we divide the modulators into two types: modulators targeting P-gp and targeting other genes.

3.1.1 Modulators of P-gp

Up to now, numerous compounds have been shown to inhibit the drug efflux function of P-gp and therefore, reverse cellular resistance. Since P-gp was first detected in 1976, three generation of modulators are found or synthesis. The process of chemosensitization involves the co-administration of a MDR modulator with an anticancer drug in order to cause enhanced intracellular accumulation via impairing the P-gp function[2].

3.1.1.1 First generation modulators

The first compounds documented to reverse MDR was verapamil (VRP), one of the calcium channel blocker[140]. Studies displayed that VRP enhanced intracellular accumulation of many anticancer drugs, including DOX in numerous cell lines. Subsequent studies revealed that this MDR reversing character is shared by many other calcium channel blockers, clinically available calcium antagonists, and calmodulin antagonists, such as felodipine and trifluorperazine[141]. Indole alkaloids, the anti-malarial quinine and the anti-arrhythmic quinidine, have also been shown to reverse MDR in vitro in experimental cell lines [142].Cyclosporin A, a commonly used immunosuppressant for organ transplantation, remains one of the most effective first generation of MDR modulators[2].

A number of these first generation MDR modulators, such as VRP and CsA, displayed excellent MDR reversal activities both preclinically and clinically. However, a unique property shared by most first generation modulators is that they are therapeutic agents and typically reverse MDR at concentrations much higher than those required for their individual therapeutic activity and at these elevated doses, both compounds exhibited severe and sometimes life-threatening toxicities[2].

3.1.1.2 Second generation modulators

In order to solve the high toxicity of the first generation modulators, many newer analogs of the first generation are researched which were more potent and considerably less toxic.
Analogs of VRP, including dexverapamil (less cardiotoxic R-enantiomer of VRP), emopamil, gallopamil, and Ro11-2933 (a tiapamil analog) which reversed MDR in vitro to a degree equivalent to VRP, but with marginal toxicity in animal models were documented[2]. The non-immunosuppressive analog of CsA, PSC 833, has demonstrated superior MDR reversal efficacy in conjunction with daunorubicin, DOX, vincristine, vinblastine, taxol, or mitoxantrone in many cell lines in vitro at concentrations of 0.5–2 mM[143].
Although these agents circumvented many of the problems experienced with first generation MDR modulators, when these agents were co-administered with anticancer agents for modulating P-gp-based MDR, they influenced the pharmacokinetics and biodistribution properties of the anticancer drugs, which resulted in increased toxicity to normal organs such as liver and kidney[144].

3.1.1.3 Third generation modulators

The third generation modulators of p-gp have recently been developed using structure-activity relationships and combinatorial chemistry approaches. These agents required low doses (in the nanomolar range (20–100 nM)) to achieve effective reversing concentrations in vivo.
The cyclopropyldibenzosuberane LY 335979 is the representative and is currently under investigation in phase II clinical trials. This substance is highly effective on P-gp-mediated MDR at the concentration of 0.1–0.2μM and shows a very strong affinity for P-gp[145]. Compared to CsA, LY 335979 is characterized by a 10-fold increased potency, latent modulating activity and a blockade specific for P-gp. Another drug the acridonecarboxamide GF 120918 exihibits similar characteristics to LY 335979, but seems to be more effective than LY 335979[146]. The effective concentration of it is 20–100 nM and is one of the most potent and selective MDR modulators disclosed thus far. Both of them are specific for P-gp-mediated MDR since it does not modulate MRP-mediated resistance. In addition, some bispecific chemosensitizers that block both P-gp and MRP were found, such as VX-710 and VX-853[2].
In summary, all the modulators of p-gp can be divided into 10 classifications. Table 1 selected list the modulators of p-gp of each classification reported.

3.1.2 Modulators of other genes

Besides agents targeting P-gp, drugs that inhibit other genes have also been developing. Table 2 displays the selected list of modulators that inhibit other MDR-related genes. Although these agents appear to be well tolerated in combination with anticancer drugs such as DOX, the lack selectivity for the tumor tissue P-GP is still their deficiency which is the cause of adversely affect therapy.

3.2 Immunotherapy of MDR

Another method of MDR reversal is the use of monoclonal antibodies, several of which can inhibit P-gp-mediated drug efflux in vitro. The monoclonal antibody (mAb) MRK16 is the

Immunosuppressant	Anti-arrhythmic agent
Cyclosporin A	Quinidine
Valspodar (PSC833)	Antifungal agent
HIV protease inhibitors	Ketoconazole
Ritonavir	Sedative
Saquinavir	Midazolam
Nelfi navir	Acridone carboxamide
Calcium channel blocker	LY 335979(zosoquidar)
Verapamil	GG918 (GF120918)
Bepridil	Peptide chemosensitiser
Diltiazem	Reversin 121
Flunarizine	Reversin 205
Progesterone antagonist	Anti-oestrogen
Mifepristone (RU486)	Tamoxifen

Table 1. Selected list of P-gp modulators[149]

Name	inhibitors
MRP1[3]	MS-209
	XR-9576 (tariquidar)
	VX-710 (biricodar)
	Isothiocyanates
	tRA 98006
	Agosterol A
	Rifampicin
	NSAIDs
BCRP(ABCG2)[3]	GF-120918 (elacridar)
	tRA 98006
	Flavonoids
	Phytoestrogens
	Imatinib mesylate
	Fumitremorgin C
	TAG- 139
GST-pi[150]	Clofibrate
	Ethacrynic acid
	GSH analogs
	Gossypol
	Indomethacin
	Misonidazole
	Piriprost
	Quinones
	Quercetin
	Sulfasalazine
GCS[91]	PDMP
	PPMP
	Miglustat

Table 2. Selected list of modulator targeting other MDR-related genes

first antibody used for reversing MDR by Hamada and Tsuruo[147]. The results found that MRK16 increased intracellular accumulation and cytotoxicity of vincristine and actinomycin D in some MDR cell lines, but had no effect on doxorubicin cytotoxicity. An increase in the accumulation ofvincristine and actinomycin D was also observed with two other anti-Pgp mAbs, HYB-241 and HYB-612[148].

3.3 Genetic therapy of MDR

The genetic therapy of MDR mainly includes two methods.The first method was established by Gottesman et al.They produced multidrug resistant bone marrow cells by transfecting them with vectors carrying the MDR1 cDNA and this process allowed bone marrow cells to apply a chemotherapeutic regimen at otherwise unacceptable doses, and thus overcoming MDR[149].

The other method is inhibiting MDR proteins including transcriptional/translational inhibition through the introduction of antisense oligonucleotides or ribozymes or RNA interference.Recently, researchers has done many work targeting different genes, such as mdr1, MRP1, BCRP, GCS and so on. These techniques were proved to have considerable effects on overcoming MDR in vitro and in animal models. However, as many of these methods require gene targeting and transfer, they are unlikely to produce any really significant in vivo applications anytime soon[149].

In summary, although many approaches have been adopted to battle with MDR, it will be for a long time to ovecome it completely.

4. References

[1] Germano S, O'Driscoll L. Breast cancer: understanding sensitivity and resistance to chemotherapy and targeted therapies to aid in personalised medicine. Curr Cancer Drug Targets. 2009; 9(3):398-418.

[2] Rajesh Krishna, Lawrence D. Mayer. Multidrug resistance (MDR) in cancer Mechanisms, reversal using modulators of MDR and the role of MDR modulators in influencing the pharmacokinetics of anticancer drugs. European Journal of Pharmaceutical Sciences.2000; 11(4): 265–283.

[3] Tomris Ozben. Mechanisms and strategies to overcome multiple drug resistance in cancer. FEBS Letters.2006; 580 (12): 2903–2909

[4] Gottesman MM, Fojo T and Bates SE. Multidrug resistance in cancer: role of ATP-dependent transporters. Nat Rev Cancer. 2002; 2(1), 48–58

[5] Higgins CF, Hiles ID, Salmond GPC, Gill DR, Downie JA, Evans IJ, Holland IB, Gray L, Buckel SD, Bell AW, Hermodson MA. A family of related ATP-binding subunits coupled to many distinct biological processes in bacteria. Nature.1986; 323(6087): 448–450.

[6] Sarkadi B, Ozvegy-Laczka C, Német K, Váradi A. ABCG2--a transporter for all seasons. FEBS Lett. 2004; 567(1):116-20.

[7] Juliano, R L, Ling, V. A surface glycoprotein modulating drug permeability in mutants Chinese hamster ovary cells. Biochim Biophys Acta.1976; 455(1): 152–162.

[8] Chen CJ, Chin JE, Ueda K, Clark DP, Pastan I, Gottesman MM, Roninson IB. Internal duplication and homology with bacterial transport proteins in the mdr1 (P-glycoprotein) gene from multidrug resistant human cells. Cell. 1986; 47(3):381-389.

[9] Lee CH, Bradley G, Zhang JT, Ling V.Differential expression of P-glycoprotein genes in primary rat hepatocyte culture. J Cell Physiol. 1993; 157(2):392-402.

[10] Krishna R, Mayer LD.Multidrug resistance (MDR) in cancer. Mechanisms, reversal using modulators of MDR and the role of MDR modulators in influencing the pharmacokinetics of anticancer drugs. Eur J Pharm Sci. 2000; 11(4):265-283.
[11] Frézard F, Pereira-Maia E, Quidu P, Priebe W, Garnier-Suillerot A. Garnier Suillerot. P-glycoprotein preferentially effluxes compounds containing free basic versus charged amine. Eur. J. Biochem.2001; 268 (6): 1561–1567.
[12] Conseil G, Perez-Victoria JM, Jault JM, Gamarro F, Goffeau A, Hofmann J, Di Pietro A.Protein kinase C effectors bind to multidrug ABC transporters and inhibit their activity. Biochemistry. 2001; 40(8):2564-2571.
[13] Stavrovskaya AA. Cellular mechanisms of multidrug resistance of tumor cells. Biochemistry (Mosc). 2000; 65(1): 95-106
[14] Klappe K, Hinrichs JW, Kroesen BJ, Sietsma H, Kok JW. MRP1 and glucosylceramide are coordinately over expressed and enriched in rafts during multidrug resistance acquisition in colon cancer cells. Int J Cancer. 2004;110(4):511-522.
[15] Rudas M, Filipits M, Taucher S, Stranzl T, Steger GG, Jakesz R, Pirker R, Pohl G. Expression of MRP1, LRP and Pgp in breast carcinoma patients treated with preoperative chemotherapy. Breast Cancer Res Treat 2003;81(2):149−157.
[16] Clarke R, Leonessa F, Trock B. Multidrug resistance/P-glycoprotein and breast cancer: review and metaanalysis.Semin Oncol. 2005; 32(6 Suppl 7):S9−15.
[17] Leonard GD, Fojo T, Bates SE.The role of ABC transporters in clinical practice. Oncologist. 2003; 8(5):411-24.
[18] Teodori E, Dei S, Scapecchi S, Gualtieri F. The medicinal chemistry of multidrug resistance (MDR) reversing drugs. Farmaco. 2002; 57(5):385-415.
[19] Jedlitschky G, Leier I, Buchholz U, Center M, Keppler D. ATP-dependent transport of glutathione S-conjugates by the multidrug resistance-associated protein.Cancer Res. 1994; 54(18):4833-4836.
[20] Manciu L, Chang XB, Riordan JR, Ruysschaert JM. Multidrug resistance protein MRP1 reconstituted into lipid vesicles: secondary structure and nucleotide-induced tertiary structure changes. Biochemistry. 2000; 39(42):13026-13033.
[21] Keppler D, Leier I, Jedlitschky G, König J.ATP-dependent transport of glutathione S-conjugates by the multidrug resistance protein MRP1 and its apical isoform MRP2. Chem Biol Interact. 1998; 111-112:153-161.
[22] Doyle LA, Yang W, Abruzzo LV, Krogmann T, Gao Y, Rishi AK, Ross DD.A multidrug resistance transporter from human MCF-7 breast cancer cells. Proc. Natl. Acad. Sci. USA. 1998; 95(26): 15665–15670.
[23] Bailey-Dell KJ, Hassel B, Doyle LA, Ross DD.Promoter characterization and genomic organization of the human breast cancer resistance protein (ATP-binding cassette transporter G2 gene. Biochim Biophys Acta. 2001; 1520(3):234-241
[24] J.D. Allen, A.H. Schinkel. Multidrug resistance and pharmacological protection mediated by the breast cancer resistance protein (BCRP/ABCG2), Mol. Cancer Ther.2002; 1 (6): 427-434.
[25] Bhatia A, Schäfer HJ, Hrycyna CAOligomerization of the human ABC transporter ABCG2: evaluation of the native protein and chimeric dimers. Biochemistry. 2005; 44(32):10893-10904.
[26] Nakatomi K, Yoshikawa M, Oka M, Ikegami Y, Hayasaka S, Sano K, Shiozawa K, Kawabata S, Soda H, Ishikawa T, Tanabe S, Kohno S. Transport of 7ethyl-10-hydroxycamptothecin (SN-38) by breast cancer resistance protein ABCG2 in human lung cancer cells, Biochem. Biophys Res Commun. 2001; 288 (4): 827–832.

[27] Ni Z, Bikadi Z, Rosenberg MF, Mao Q.Structure and function of the human breast cancer resistance protein (BCRP/ABCG2). Drug Metab. 2010; 11(7):603-617.
[28] Zhou S, Schuetz JD, Bunting KD, Colapietro AM, Sampath J, Morris JJ, Lagutina I, Grosveld GC, Osawa M, Nakauchi H, Sorrentino BP.The ABC transporter Bcrp1/ABCG2 is expressed in a wide variety of stem cells and is a molecular determinant of the side-population phenotype. Nat Med. 2001; 7(9):1028-1034.
[29] Maliepaard M, Scheffer GL, Faneyte IF, van Gastelen MA, Pijnenborg AC, Schinkel AH, van De Vijver MJ, Scheper RJ, Schellens JH.Subcellular localization and distribution of the breast cancer resistance protein transporter in normal human tissues. Cancer Res. 2001; 61(8): 3458-3564.
[30] Hirano M, Maeda K, Matsushima S, Nozaki Y, Kusuhara H, Sugiyama Y.Involvement of BCRP (ABCG2) in the biliary excretion of pitavastatin. Mol Pharmacol. 2005; 68(3):800-807.
[31] Furukawa T, Wakabayashi K, Tamura A, Nakagawa H, Morishima Y, Osawa Y, Ishikawa T. Major SNP (Q141K) variant of human ABC transporter ABCG2 undergoes lysosomal and proteasomal degradations. Pharm Res. 2009; 26(2): 469-479.
[32] Noguchi K, Katayama K, Mitsuhashi J, Sugimoto Y.Functions of the breast cancer resistance protein (BCRP/ABCG2) in chemotherapy. Adv Drug Deliv Rev. 2009; 61(1):26-33.
[33] Honjo Y, Hrycyna CA, Yan QW, Medina-Perez WY, Robey RW, van de Laar A, Litman T, Dean M, Bates SE. Acquired mutations in the MXR/BCRP/ABCP gene alter substrate specificity in MXR/BCRP/ABCP-overexpressing cells. Cancer Res. 2001; 61(18):6635-6639.
[34] Polgar O, Ediriwickrema LS, Robey RW, Sharma A, Hegde RS, Li Y, Xia D, Ward Y, Dean M,Ozvegy-Laczka C, Sarkadi B, Bates SE. Arginine 383 is a crucial residue in ABCG2 biogenesis.Biochim Biophys Acta 2009; 1788(7):1434–1443.
[35] Honjo Y, Hrycyna CA, Yan QW, Medina-Pérez WY, Robey RW, van de Laar A, Litman T, Dean M, Bates SEAcquired mutations in the MXR/BCRP/ABCP gene alter substrate specificity in MXR/BCRP/ABCP-overexpressing cells. Cancer Res. 2001; 61(18):6635-6639.
[36] Ross DD, Karp JE, Chen TT, Doyle LA.Expression of breast cancer resistance protein in blast cells from patients with acute leukemia. Blood. 2000; 96(1):365-368.
[37] Benderra Z, Faussat AM, Sayada L, Perrot JY, Chaoui D, Marie JP, Legrand O.Breast cancer resistance protein and P-glycoprotein in 149 adult acute myeloid leukemias. Clin Cancer Res. 2004 Dec 1;10(23):7896-902.
[38] Usuda J, Ohira T, Suga Y, Oikawa T, Ichinose S, Inoue T, Ohtani K, Maehara S, Imai K, Kubota M, Tsunoda Y, Tsutsui H, Furukawa K, Okunaka T, Sugimoto Y, Kato H.Breast cancer resistance protein (BCRP) affected acquired resistance to gefitinib in a "never-smoked" female patient with advanced non-small cell lung cancer. Lung Cancer. 2007;58(2):296-299.
[39] O'Connor PM, Jackman J, Bae I, Myers TG, Fan S, Mutoh M, Scudiero DA, Monks A, Sausville EA, Weinstein JN, Friend S, Fornace AJ Jr, Kohn KW.Characterization of the p53 tumor suppressor pathway in cell lines of the National Cancer Institute anticancer drug screen and correlations with the growth-inhibitory potency of 123 anticancer agents. Cancer Res. 1997; 57(19):4285-4300.
[40] Gasco M, Yulug IG, Crook T. TP53 mutations in familial breast cancer: functional aspects. Hum Mutat. 2003; 21(3): 301-306.

[41] Aas T, Børresen AL, Geisler S, Smith-Sørensen B, Johnsen H, Varhaug JE, Akslen LA, Lønning PE. Specific P53 mutations are associated with de novo resistance to doxorubicin in breast cancer patients. Nat Med. 1996; 2(7):811-814.

[42] Chin KV, Ueda K, Pastan I, Gottesman MM. Modulation of activity of the promoter of the human MDR1 gene by Ras and p53. Science. 1992; 255(5043): 459-462.

[43] Zhou G, Kuo MT. Wild-type p53-mediated induction of rat mdr1b expression by the anticancer drug daunorubicin. J Biol Chem. 1998; 273(25): 15387-15394.

[44] Bush JA, Li G. Cancer chemoresistance: the relationship between p53 and multidrug transporters. Int J Cancer. 2002; 98: 323-330.

[45] Linn SC, Honkoop AH, Hoekman K, van der Valk P, Pinedo HM, Giaccone G. p53 and P-glycoprotein are often co-expressed and are associated with poor prognosis in breast cancer. Br J Cancer. 1996; 74: 63-68.

[46] Linn SC, Pinedo HM, van Ark-Otte J, van der Valk P, Hoekman K, Honkoop AH, Vermorken JB, Giaccone G.. Expression of drug resistance proteins in breast cancer, in relation to chemotherapy. Int J Cancer. 1997; 71(5): 787-795.

[47] Wang X, Wu X, Wang C, Zhang W, Ouyang Y, Yu Y, He Z.. Transcriptional suppression of breast cancer resistance protein (BCRP) by wild-type p53 through the NF-kappaB pathway in MCF-7 cells. FEBS Lett. 584(15): 3392-3397.

[48] Coley HM. Mechanisms and strategies to overcome chemotherapy resistance in metastatic breast cancer. Cancer Treat Rev. 2008; 34(4): 378-390.

[49] Stavrovskaya AA. Cellular mechanisms of multidrug resistance of tumor cells. Biochemistry (Mosc). 2000; 65(1): 95-106.

[50] Shitashige M, Toi M, Yano T, Shibata M, Matsuo Y, Shibasaki F. Dissociation of Bax from a Bcl-2/Bax heterodimer triggered by phosphorylation of serine 70 of Bcl-2. J Biochem. 2001; 130(6): 741-748.

[51] Liu F, Xie ZH, Cai GP, Jiang YY. The effect of survivin on multidrug resistance mediated by P-glycoprotein in MCF-7 and its adriamycin resistant cells. Biol Pharm Bull. 2007; 30(12): 2279-2283.

[52] Zhang M, Latham DE, Delaney MA, Chakravarti A. Survivin mediates resistance to antiandrogen therapy in prostate cancer. Oncogene. 2005; 24(15): 2474-2482.

[53] Devling TW, Lindsay CD, McLellan LI, McMahon M, Hayes JD.Utility of siRNA against Keap1 as a strategy to stimulate a cancer chemopreventive phenotype. Proc Natl Acad Sci USA. 2005; 102:7280-5A.

[54] Meijerman I, Beijnen JH, Schellens JH.Combined action and regulation of phase II enzymes and multidrug resistance proteins in multidrug resistance in cancer. Cancer Treat Rev. 2008; 34(6):505-520.

[55] Su F, Hu X, Jia W, Gong C, Song E, Hamar P.Glutathion S transferase pi indicates chemotherapy resistance in breast cancer. J Surg Res. 2003 ;113(1):102-108.

[56] Ban N, Takahashi Y, Takayama T, Kura T, Katahira T, Sakamaki S, et al. Transfection of glutathione S-transferase (GST)-pi antisense complementary DNA increases the sensitivity of a colon cancer cell line to adriamycin, cisplatin, melphalan, and etoposide. Cancer Res 1996; 56: 3577–3582.

[57] Akan I, Akan S, Akca H, Savas B, Ozben T. Multidrug resistance-associated protein 1 (MRP1) mediated vincristine resistance: effects of N-acetylcysteine and buthionine sulfoximine. Cancer Cell Int 2005;5:22.

[58] Adler V, Yin Z, Fuchs SY, Benezra M, Rosario L, Tew KD, Pincus MR, Sardana M, Henderson CJ, Wolf CR, Davis RJ, Ronai Z.Regulation of JNK signaling by GSTp. EMBO J. 1999; 18(5):1321-1334.

[59] Benet LZ, Cummins CL, Wu CY. Unmasking the dynamic interplay between efflux transporters and metabolic enzymes.Int J Pharm. 2004; 277:3–9.
[60] Tew KD, Monks A, Barone L, Rosser D, Akerman G, Montali JA. Glutathione-associated enzymes in the human cell lines of the National Cancer Institute Drug Screening Program. Mol Pharmacol. 1996; 50:149–159.
[61] Chanas SA, Jiang Q, McMahon M, McWalter GK, McLellan LI, Elcombe CR, et al. Loss of the Nrf2 transcription factor causes a marked reduction in constitutive and inducible expression of the glutathione S-transferase Gsta1, Gsta2, Gstm1, Gstm2, Gstm3 and Gstm4 genes in the livers of male and female mice. Biochem J. 2002;365:405–416.
[62] Hayashi A, Suzuki H, Itoh K, Yamamoto M, Sugiyama Y.Transcription factor Nrf2 is required for the constitutive and inducible expression of multidrug resistance-associated protein 1 in mouse embryo fibroblasts. Biochem Biophys Res Commun. 2003;310:824–829.
[63] Moscow JA, Townsend AJ, Goldsmith ME, Whang-Peng J, Vickers PJ, Poisson R, Legault-Poisson S, Myers CE, Cowan KH.Isolation of the human anionic glutathione S-transferase cDNA and the relation of its gene expression to estrogen-receptor content in primary breast cancer. Proc Natl Acad Sci U S A. 1988;85(17):6518-6522.
[64] Jhaveri MS, Morrow CS.Methylation-mediated regulation of the glutathione S-transferase P1 gene in human breast cancer cells. Gene. 1998; 210(1):1-7.
[65] Berger JM, Gamblin SJ, Harrison SC, Wang JC. Structure and mechanism of DNA topoisomerase II. Nature. 1996; 379(6562):225-232
[66] Schmidt BH, Burgin AB, Deweese JE, Osheroff N, Berger JM, A novel and unified two-metal mechanism for DNA cleavage by type II and IA topoisomerases. Nature. 2010 Jun 3;465(7298):641-644.
[67] Tsai-Pflugfelder M, Liu LF, Liu AA, Tewey KM, Whang-Peng J, Knutsen T, Huebner K, Croce CM, Wang JC. Cloning and sequencing of cDNA encoding human DNA topoisomerase II and localization of the gene to chromosome region 17q21-22. Proc Natl Acad Sci U S A. 1988 Oct;85(19):7177-7781.
[68] Jenkins JR, Ayton P, Jones T, Davies SL, Simmons DL, Harris AL, Sheer D, Hickson ID.Isolation of cDNA clones encoding the L isozyme of human DNA topoisomerase II and localization of the gene to chromosome 3p24, Nucleic Acids Res. 1992; 20(21):5587-5592.
[69] Keith WN, Douglas F, Wishart GC, McCallum HM, George WD, Kaye SB, Brown R. Co-ampli¢cation or erbB2, topoisomerase IIαand the retinoic acid receptor α genes in breast cancer and allelic loss at topoisomerase I on chromosome 20. Eur J Cancer 1993(29A): 1469-1473.
[70] Sng JH, Heaton VJ, Bell M, Maini P, Austin CA, Fisher LM. Molecular cloning and characterization of the human topoisomerase IIalpha and IIbeta genes: evidence for isoform evolution through gene duplication. Biochim Biophys Acta. 1999; 1444(3): 395-406.
[71] Jarvinen TA, Liu ET. HER-2/neu and topoisomerase Iialphasimultaneous drug targets in cancer. Comb Chem High Throughput Screen. 2003;6:455 -470.
[72] Valkov NI, Sullivan DM. Drug resistance to DNA topoisomerase I and II inhibitors in human leukemia, lymphoma, and multiple myeloma. Semin Hematol. 1997; 34:48-62.

[73] Järvinen TA, Tanner M, Rantanen V, Bärlund M, Borg A, Grénman S, Isola J.. Amplification and deletion of topoisomerase IIalpha associate with ErbB-2 amplification and affect sensitivity to topoisomerase II inhibitor doxorubicin in breast cancer. Am J Pathol 2000;156(3):839- 847.
[74] Withoff S, Keith WN, Knol AJ, Coutts JC, Hoare SF, Mulder NH, de Vries EG.. Selection of a subpopulation with fewer DNA topoisomerase II alpha gene copies in a doxorubicinresistant cell line panel. Br J Cancer 1996;74(4):502- 507.
[75] Oakman C, Moretti E, Galardi F, Santarpia L, Di Leo A. The role of topoisomerase IIa and HER-2 in predicting sensitivity to anthracyclines in breast cancer patients. Cancer Treat Rev. 2009 Dec;35(8):662-7.
[76] Jarvinen TA, Liu ET. HER-2/neu and topoisomerase II alpha in breast cancer. Breast Cancer Res Treat 2003;78(3): 299-311.
[77] O'Malley FP, Chia S, Tu D, Shepherd LE, Levine MN, Bramwell VH, Andrulis IL, Pritchard KI.. Topoisomerase II alpha and responsiveness of breast cancer to adjuvant chemotherapy. J Natl Cancer Inst 2009;101(9): 644–650.
[78] Gennari A, Sormani M, Pfeffer U. TOP mRNA expression in HER2 negative breast cancer. San Antonio Breast Cancer Sympos. 2008:6036.
[79] Hannun YA, Luberto C, Argraves KM. Enzymes of sphingolipid metabolism: from modular to integrative signaling. Biochemistry. 2001;40(16):4893-4903.
[80] Kolesnick R. The therapeutic potential of modulating the ceramide/sphingomyelin pathway. J Clin Invest. 2002; 110(1):3-8.
[81] Uchida Y, Itoh M, Taguchi Y, Yamaoka S, Umehara H, Ichikawa S, Hirabayashi Y, Holleran WM, Okazaki T. Ceramide reduction and transcriptional up-regulation of glucosylceramide synthase through doxorubicin-activated Sp1 in drug-resistant HL-60/ADR cells. Cancer Res. 2004; 64(17):6271-6279.
[82] Shukla A, Shukla GS, Radin NS. Control of kidney size by sex hormones: possible involvement of glucosylceramide. Am J Physiol. 1992; 262(1 pt 2):F24-29.
[83] Lavie Y, Cao H, Bursten SL, Giuliano AE, Cabot MC. Accumulation of glucosylceramides in multidrug-resistant cancer cells. J Biol Chem 1996;271(32):19530-19536.
[84] Lucci A, Cho WI, Han TY, Giuliano AE, Morton DL, Cabot MC.Glucosylceramide: a marker for multiple-drug resistant cancers. Anticancer Res. 1998;18(1B):475-480.
[85] Yamashita T, Wada R, Sasaki T, Deng C, Bierfreund U, Sandhoff K, Proia RL. A vital role for glycosphingolipid synthesis during development and differentiation. Proc Natl Acad Sci U S A. 1999; 96(16):9142-9147.
[86] Liu YY, Han TY, Giuliano AE, Cabot MC. Expression of glucosylceramide synthase, converting ceramide to glucosylceramide, confers adriamycin resistance in human breast cancer cells. J Biol Chem 1999;274(2):1140-1146.
[87] Liu YY, Han TY, Giuliano AE, Hansen N, Cabot MC. Uncoupling ceramide glycosylation by transfection of glucosylceramide synthase antisense reverses adriamycin resistance. J Biol Chem. 2000;275(10):7138-7143.
[88] Olshefski RS, Ladisch S. Glucosylceramide synthase inhibition enhances vincristine-induced cytotoxicity. Int J Cancer. 2001; 93(1):131-138.
[89] Liu YY, Gupta V, Patwardhan GA, Bhinge K, Zhao Y, Bao J, Mehendale H, Cabot MC, Li YT, Jazwinski SM. Glucosylceramide synthase upregulates MDR1 expression in the regulation of cancer drug resistance through cSrc and beta-catenin signaling. Mol Cancer.2010;9:145.

[90] Liu YY, Yu JY, Yin D, Patwardhan GA, Gupta V, Hirabayashi Y, Holleran WM, Giuliano AE, Jazwinski SM, Gouaze-Andersson V, Consoli DP, Cabot MC...A role for ceramide in driving cancer cell resistance to doxorubicin. FASEB J. 2008;22(7):2541-2551.
[91] Ruckhäberle E, Karn T, Hanker L, Gätje R, Metzler D, Holtrich U, Kaufmann M, Rody A. Prognostic relevance of glucosylceramide synthase (GCS) expression in breast cancer. J Cancer Res Clin Oncol. 2009;135(1):81-90.
[92] Nguyen NP, Almeida FS, Chi A, Nguyen LM, Cohen D, Karlsson U, Vinh-Hung V Molecular biology of breast cancer stem cells: potential clinical applications.Cancer Treat Rev. 2010; 36(6):485-91. Review.
[93] Fuchs E, Segre JA. Stem cells: a new lease on life, Cell. 2000; 100(1):143-55. Review.
[94] Seigel GM, Campbell LM, Narayan M, Gonzalez-Fernandez F. Gonzalez-Fernandez. Cancer stem cell characteristics in retinoblastoma, Mol Vis. 2005 Sep 12;11:729-37.
[95] Grichnik JM, Burch JA, Schulteis RD, Shan S, Liu J, Darrow TL, Vervaert CE, Seigler HF. Melanoma, a tumor based on a mutant stem cell? J. Invest. Dermatol.2006; 126 (1) 142–153.
[96] Al-Hajj M, Wicha MS, Benito-Hernandez A, Morrison SJ, Clarke MF. Prospective identification of tumorigenic breast cancer cells. Proc Natl Acad Sci USA. 2003; 100(7): 3983–3988
[97] Ginestier C, Hee Hur M, Charafe-Jauffret E, Monville F, Dutcher J, Brown M, Jacquemier J, Viens P, Kleer CG, Liu S, Schott A, Hayes D, Birnbaum D, Wicha MS, Dontu G. ALDH1 is a marker of normal and malignant human mammary stem cells and a predictor of poor clinical outcome. Cell Stem Cell.2007; 1(5): 555–567
[98] Goodell MA, Brose K, Paradis G,et al. Isolation and functional properties of murine hematopoietic stem cells that are replicating in vivo. J Exp Med, 1996; 183(4):1797-806.
[99] Patrawala L, Calhoun T, Schneider-Broussard R, Zhou J, Claypool K, Tang DG. Side population is enriched in tumorigenic, stem-like cancer cells, whereas ABCG2+ and ABCG2- cancer cells are similarly tumorigenic. Cancer Res, 2005; 65(14):6207-6219.
[100] Decraene C, Benchaouir R, Dillies MA, Israeli D, Bortoli S, Rochon C, Rameau P, Pitaval A, Tronik-Le Roux D, Danos O, Gidrol X, Garcia L, Piétu G. Global transcriptional characterization of SP and MP cells from the myogenic C2C12 cell line: effect of FGF6, Physiol. Physiol Genomics. 2005 Oct 17;23(2):132-149.
[101] Hadnagy A, Gaboury L, Beaulieu R, Balicki D.SP analysis may be used to identify cancer stem cell populations. Exp Cell Res. 2006; 312(19):3701-3710.
[102] Heldring N, Pike A, Andersson S, Matthews J, Cheng G, Hartman J, Tujague M, Ström A, Treuter E, Warner M, Gustafsson JA. Estrogen Receptors: How Do They Signal and What Are Their Targets. Physiol Rev. 2007; 87(3):905-31. Review
[103] Liu MM, Albanese C, Anderson CM, Hilty K, Webb P, Uht RM, Price RH Jr, Pestell RG, Kushner PJ. Opposing action of estrogen receptors alpha and beta on cyclin D1 gene expression. J Biol Chem. 2002; 277: 24353–24360,.
[104] Zhang Y, Wang H, Wei L, Li G, Yu J, Gao Y, Gao P, Zhang X, Wei F, Yin D, Zhou G. Transcriptional modulation of BCRP gene to reverse multidrug resistance by toremifene in breast adenocarcinoma cells. Breast Cancer Res Treat. 2010;123(3):679-689.
[105] Hayashi SI, Eguchi H, Tanimoto K, Yoshida T, Omoto Y, Inoue A, Yoshida N, Yamaguchi Y. The expression and function of estrogen receptor alpha and beta in

human breast cancer and its clinical application. Endocr Relat Cancer. 2003; 10(2):193-202.

[106] Coles LD, Lee IJ, Voulalas PJ, Eddington ND. Estradiol and progesterone-mediated regulation of P-gp in P-gp overexpressing cells (NCI-ADR-RES) and placental cells (JAR). Mol Pharm. 2009; 6(6):1816-1825.

[107] Rao US, Fine RL. Scarborough GA.Antiestrogens and steroid hormones: substrates of the human P-glycoprotein. Biochem Pharmacol. 1994; 48(2):287-292.

[108] Nagaoka R, Iwasaki T, Rokutanda N, Takeshita A, Koibuchi Y, Horiguchi J, Shimokawa N, Iino Y, Morishita Y, Koibuchi N.Tamoxifen activates CYP3A4 and MDR1 genes through steroid and xenobiotic receptor in breast cancer cells. Endocrine. 2006; 30(3):261-268.

[109] Kirk J, Syed SK, Harris AL, Jarman M, Roufogalis BD, Stratford IJ, Carmichael. . Reversal of P-glycoprotein-mediated multidrug resistance by pure anti-oestrogens and novel tamoxifen derivatives. J Biochem Pharmacol. 1994;48(2):277-85.

[110] Imai Y, Ishikawa E, Asada S, Sugimoto Y. Estrogenmediated post transcriptional down-regulation of breast cancer resistance protein/ABCG2. Cancer Res.2005; 65:596–604.

[111] Zhang Y, Zhou G, Wang H, Zhang X, Wei F, Cai Y, Yin D. Transcriptional upregulation of breast cancer resistance protein by 17beta-estradiol in ERalpha-positive MCF-7 breast cancer cells. Oncology. 2006; 71(5-6):446-455.

[112] Kastner P, Krust A, Turcotte B, Stropp U, Tora L, Gronemeyer H, Chambon P. Two distinct estrogen-regulated promoters generate transcripts encoding the two functionally different human progesterone receptor forms A and B. EMBO J. 1990; 9(5): 1603-1614.

[113] Giangrande PH, McDonnell DP. The A and B isoforms of the human progesterone receptor: two functionally different transcription factors encoded by a single gene. Recent Prog Horm Res. 1999; 54: 291-313.

[114] Wang H, Lee EW, Zhou L, Leung PC, Ross DD, Unadkat JD, Mao Q.. Progesterone receptor (PR) isoforms PRA and PRB differentially regulate expression of the breast cancer resistance protein in human placental choriocarcinoma BeWo cells. Mol Pharmacol. 2008; 73: 845-854.

[115] Rao US, Fine RL, Scarborough GA. Antiestrogens and steroid hormones: substrates of the human P-glycoprotein. Biochem Pharmacol. 1994; 48: 287-292.

[116] Coles LD, Lee IJ, Voulalas PJ, Eddington ND. Estradiol and progesterone-mediated regulation of P-gp in P-gp overexpressing cells (NCI-ADR-RES) and placental cells (JAR). Mol Pharm. 2009; 6: 1816-1825.

[117] Ee PL, Kamalakaran S, Tonetti D, He X, Ross DD, Beck WT. Identification of a novel estrogen response element in the breast cancer resistance protein (ABCG2) gene. Cancer Res. 2004; 64: 1247-1251.

[118] Wang H, Zhou L, Gupta A, Vethanayagam RR, Zhang Y, Unadkat JD, Mao Q. Regulation of BCRP/ABCG2 expression by progesterone and 17beta-estradiol in human placental BeWo cells. Am J Physiol Endocrinol Metab. 2006; 290: E798-807.

[119] Kalluri R, Weinberg RA. The basics of epithelial-mesenchymal transition. J Clin Invest. 2009; 119: 1420-1428.

[120] Wang Z, Li Y, Ahmad A, Azmi AS, Kong D, Banerjee S, Sarkar FH. Targeting miRNAs involved in cancer stem cell and EMT regulation: An emerging concept in overcoming drug resistance. Drug Resist Updat.2010; 13()4-5: 109-118.

[121] Balkovetz DF, Pollack AL, Mostov KE. Hepatocyte growth factor alters the polarity of Madin-Darby canine kidney cell monolayers. J Biol Chem. 1997; 272: 3471-3477.

[122] Janda E, Lehmann K, Killisch I, Jechlinger M, Herzig M, Downward J, Beug H, Grünert S. Janda E, Lehmann K, Killisch I, et al. Ras and TGF[beta] cooperatively regulate epithelial cell plasticity and metastasis: dissection of Ras signaling pathways. The Journal of cell biology. 2002; 156(2): 299-313.

[123] Lu Z, Ghosh S, Wang Z, Hunter T. Downregulation of caveolin-1 function by EGF leads to the loss of E-cadherin, increased transcriptional activity of beta-catenin, and enhanced tumor cell invasion. Cancer Cell. 2003; 4: 499-515.

[124] Radisky DC, Levy DD, Littlepage LE, Liu H, Nelson CM, Fata JE, Leake D, Godden EL, Albertson DG, Nieto MA, Werb Z, Bissell MJ.. Rac1b and reactive oxygen species mediate MMP-3-induced EMT and genomic instability. Nature. 2005; 436(7047): 123-127.

[125] Li QQ, Xu JD, Wang WJ, Cao XX, Chen Q, Tang F, Chen ZQ, Liu XP, Xu ZD. Twist1-mediated adriamycin-induced epithelial-mesenchymal transition relates to multidrug resistance and invasive potential in breast cancer cells. Clin Cancer Res. 2009; 15(8): 2657-2665.

[126] de Herreros AG, Peiro S, Nassour M, Savagner P. Snail family regulation and epithelial mesenchymal transitions in breast cancer progression. J Mammary Gland Biol Neoplasia. 15: 135-147.

[127] Kajiyama H, Shibata K, Terauchi M, Yamashita M, Ino K, Nawa A, Kikkawa F.Chemoresistance to paclitaxel induces epithelial-mesenchymal transition and enhances metastatic potential for epithelial ovarian carcinoma cells. Int J Oncol. 2007 ;31(2):277-283

[128] Kim MR, Choi HK, Cho KB, Kim HS, Kang KW.Involvement of Pin1 induction in epithelial-mesenchymal transition of tamoxifen-resistant breast cancer cells. Cancer Sci. 2009 Oct;100(10):1834-1841.

[129] Singh, A., Settleman, J., 2010. EMT, cancer stem cells and drug resistance: an emerging axis of evil in the war on cancer. Oncogene, doi:10.1038/onc.2010.215.

[130] Carey, L.A., Dees, E.C., Sawyer, L., Gatti, L., Moore, D.T., Collichio, F., Ollila, D.W., Sartor, C.I., Graham, M.L., Perou, C.M., 2007. The triple negative paradox: primary tumor chemosensitivity of breast cancer subtypes. Clin. Cancer Res. 13, 2329–2334.

[131] Segura-Pacheco B, Perez-Cardenas E, Taja-Chayeb L, Chavez-Blanco A, Revilla-Vazquez A, Benitez-Bribiesca L, Duenas-González A. Global DNA hypermethylation-associated cancer chemotherapy resistance and its reversion with the demethylating agent hydralazine. J Transl Med. 2006; 4: 32.

[132] Rodriguez-Dorantes M, Tellez-Ascencio N, Cerbon MA, Lopez M, Cervantes A. DNA methylation: an epigenetic process of medical importance. Rev Invest Clin. 2004; 56: 56-71.

[133] El-Osta A, Kantharidis P, Zalcberg JR, Wolffe AP. Precipitous release of methyl-CpG binding protein 2 and histone deacetylase 1 from the methylated human multidrug resistance gene (MDR1) on activation. Mol Cell Biol. 2002; 22: 1844-1857.

[134] Nakayama M, Wada M, Harada T, Nagayama J, Kusaba H, Ohshima K, Kozuru M, Komatsu H, Ueda R, Kuwano M.. Hypomethylation status of CpG sites at the promoter region and overexpression of the human MDR1 gene in acute myeloid leukemias. Blood. 1998; 92(11): 4296-4307.

[135] Sharma D, Vertino PM. Epigenetic regulation of MDR1 gene in breast cancer: CpG methylation status dominates the stable maintenance of a silent gene. Cancer Biol Ther. 2004; 3: 549-550.

[136] Sharma G, Mirza S, Parshad R, Srivastava A, Datta Gupta S, Pandya P, Ralhan R. CpG hypomethylation of MDR1 gene in tumor and serum of invasive ductal breast carcinoma patients. Clin Biochem. 43: 373-379.

[137] To KK, Zhan Z, Bates SE. Aberrant promoter methylation of the ABCG2 gene in renal carcinoma. Mol Cell Biol. 2006; 26: 8572-8585.

[138] Turner JG, Gump JL, Zhang C, Cook JM, Marchion D, Hazlehurst L, Munster P, Schell MJ, Dalton WS, Sullivan DM.. ABCG2 expression, function, and promoter methylation in human multiple myeloma. Blood. 2006; 108(12): 3881-3889.

[139] Chekhun VF, Kulik GI, Yurchenko OV, Tryndyak VP, Todor IN, Luniv LS, Tregubova NA, Pryzimirska TV, Montgomery B, Rusetskaya NV, Pogribny IP. Role of DNA hypomethylation in the development of the resistance to doxorubicin in human MCF-7 breast adenocarcinoma cells. Cancer Lett. 2006; 231(1): 87-93.

[140] Tsuruo T, Iida H, Tsukagoshi S, Sakurai Y. Overcoming of vincristine resistance in P388 leukemia in vivo and in vitro through enhanced cytotoxicity of vincristine and vinblastine by verapamil. Cancer Res. 1981; 41: 1967-1972.

[141] Hollt V, Kouba M, Dietel M, Vogt G. Stereoisomers of calcium antagonists which differ markedly in their potencies as calcium blockers are equally effective in modulating drug transport by P-glycoprotein. Biochem Pharmacol. 1992; 43: 2601-8.

[142] Sehested M, Jensen PB, Skovsgaard T, Bindslev N, Demant EJ, Friche E, Vindeløv L. Inhibition of vincristine binding to plasma membrane vesicles from daunorubicin-resistant Ehrlich ascites cells by multidrug resistance modulators. Br J Cancer. 1989; 60(6): 809-814.

[143] Watanabe T, Naito M, Oh-hara T, Itoh Y, Cohen D, Tsuruo T. Modulation of multidrug resistance by SDZ PSC 833 in leukemic and solid-tumor-bearing mouse models. Jpn J Cancer Res. 1996; 87: 184-193.

[144] Lum BL, Gosland MP. MDR expression in normal tissues. Pharmacologic implications for the clinical use of P-glycoprotein inhibitors. Hematol Oncol Clin North Am. 1995; 9: 319-336.

[145] Dantzig AH, Law KL, Cao J, Starling JJ. Reversal of multidrug resistance by the P-glycoprotein modulator, LY335979, from the bench to the clinic. Curr Med Chem. 2001; 8: 39-50.

[146] Wallstab A, Koester M, Bohme M, Keppler D. Selective inhibition of MDR1 P-glycoprotein-mediated transport by the acridone carboxamide derivative GG918. Br J Cancer. 1999; 79: 1053-1060.

[147] Hamada H, Tsuruo T. Functional role for the 170- to 180-kDa glycoprotein specific to drug-resistant tumor cells as revealed by monoclonal antibodies. Proc Natl Acad Sci U S A. 1986 Oct;83(20):7785-7789.

[148] Mechetner EB, Roninson IB.Efficient inhibition of P-glycoprotein-mediated multidrug resistance with a monoclonal antibody. Proc Natl Acad Sci U S A. 1992 Jul 1;89(13):5824-8.

[149] Luqmani YA. Mechanisms of drug resistance in cancer chemotherapy. Med Princ Pract. 2005;14 Suppl 1:35-48.

[150] Tew KD, Dutta S, Schultz M. Inhibitors of glutathione S-transferases as therapeutic agents. Adv Drug Deliv Rev. 1997; 26: 91-104.

10

Multiple Molecular Targets of *Antrodia camphorata*: A Suitable Candidate for Breast Cancer Chemoprevention

Hsin-Ling Yang[1], K.J. Senthil Kumar[2] and You-Cheng Hseu[2]
[1]*Institute of Nutrition,*
[2]*Department of Cosmaceutics, College of Pharmacy,*
China Medical University, Taichung,
Taiwan

1. Introduction

Data from cancer registries reported that cancer incidence is increasing every year and cancer claimed the second leading causes of death worldwide, surpassed only by cardiovascular disease. National Cancer Research Institute classified that the breast cancer ranks second as a cause of cancer death in women, followed by lung cancer. Globally, more than 1.1 million women are diagnosed with breast cancer every year at the same time nearly 410, 000 women are queued for die due to the breast cancer (Cancer factors and Figures, 2010, American Cancer Society). The incidence of breast cancer varies greatly around the world. Lowest breast cancer incidence was observed in less developed countries, whereas highest in the more developed countries. In United States alone, annually more than 240, 000 women are diagnosed breast cancer and nearly 180, 000 women are diagnosed with the most deadly invasive breast cancer. It is also notable that about 1 in 8 women in the United States (12%) will develop invasive breast cancer of her life time. In 2010, an estimated 207, 090 new cases of invasive breast cancer were expected to be diagnosed in women in the U.S., along with 54, 000 new cases of non-invasive (*in situ*) breast cancer. In addition, approximately 2000 men are expected to be diagnosed with invasive breast cancer in 2010. The survival rate for women diagnosed with localized breast cancer (cancer that has not spread to lymph nodes or other location in outside the breast) is 98%. If the invasive cancer that has spread to nearby or distant lymph nodes or organs, the five years survival is 84% or 23%, respectively. However, the surprising result is the five year relative survival for female breast cancer patients has improved from 63% in the early 1960's to 90% today.
Women is primary risk factor for developing breast cancer, because, women's naturally have more breast cells than men. The main reason for develop more breast cells in women due to the constant exposure of growth-promoting effects of the female hormones especially, estrogen and progesterone. Aside from being female, age is the most important risk factor for breast cancer. Potentially modifiable risk factors include weight gain after age 18. About 1 out of 8 invasive breast cancer are found in women younger than 45, while 2 out of 3 invasive breast cancer are common in women age 55 or older. Many studies have shown that being over weight adversely affects survival for postmenopausal women with breast

cancer risk and those women who are more physically active and less to die from the disease than women who are in active. The actual fact that only 20-30% of women are diagnosed with breast cancer has significant family history of breast cancer. However, a women's risk of breast cancer approximately doubles if she has a first-degree relative (mother, sister, and daughter) who has been diagnosed with breast cancer. Apart from the family history of breast cancer, personal breast cancer history also a major risk factor for further onset. For an example, A women with cancer in one breast has a 3 to 4-fold increased risk of developing a new cancer in the other breast or other part of the same breast. This is unlike from first breast cancer recurrence.

Mammography and ultrasonography are still the most effective for women with non-dense and dense breast tissues, respectively. Additionally, MRI, lymphatic mapping, the nipple-sparing mastectomy, partial breast irradiation, neoadjuvant systemic therapy, and adjuvant treatment are promising for subgroups of breast-cancer patients. Although, there few drugs are commercially available, the well known tamoxifen can be offered for endocrine-responsive disease, aromatase inhibitors are increasingly used. Assessment of potential molecular targets is now important in primary diagnosis. Tyrosine kinase inhibitors and other drugs with anti-angiogenesis and cancer cell metastasis inhibitors are currently undergoing preclinical investigations. Recent study show the experimental drug iniparib ultimately shrank tumors and increased the time they took to progress, in addition iniparib prolonging survival in women with what's known as triple-negative breast cancers. This type of breast cancer lacks receptors for estrogen and progesterone and doesn't have large quantities of HER-2/neu protein, which the most successful cancer therapies target. This means that may currently available drugs simply won't affect it. Therefore, new class of chemotherapeutic drug that can potentially inhibit the growth of estrogen-nonresponsible breast cancer are highly warranted.

The indigenous Taiwanese medicinal mushroom *A. camphorata (Syn, Antrodia cinnamomea; Taiwanofungus camphoratus)*, locally known as "Niu Chang Chih" is a parasitic fungus grown in the inner cavity on the aromatic tree *Cinnamomum kaneirai* Hay (Lauraceae). This species is endemic to Taiwan and has been widely used as a Chinese folk medicine and functional food. In Taiwanese culture, it is believed that *Niu Chang Chih* is a valuable gift from the haven. Thereby, it claimed "National treasure of Taiwan". This species was first published by Zang & Su (1990). Dr. Su, a residential chemist, knew Niu Cheng Chih" very well from his chemical studies of various medicinal fungus (Wu et al., 1997) *A. camphorata* is starting to attract interest due to their abundant bioactive phytocompounds including, triterpenoids, flavonoids, polysaccharides, maleic/succinic acid, benzenoids and benzoquinone derivatives. The current scientific world's particular interest in *A. camphorata* and its curative properties originated from the realm of traditional practice. Till the dates there are more then three hundred scientific reports were published regarding the therapeutic potential of *A. camphorata* or it's derived pure compounds. Both the fruiting bodies and mycelium of *A. camphorata* has been shown to exhibit a wide range of health promoting benefits for the hepatic, neurological and cardiovascular systems. It also shown to inhibit variety of inflammation, viral infection, oxidative stress, atheroslerosis and the growth of a variety of cancer cells (Ao et al., 2009; Geethangili & Tzeng, 2009).

1.1 Clinical studies on *A. camphorata* as an adjuvant therapy for cancer

The anticancer potential of *A. camphorata* was recognized as early as 2002, when it was shown to inhibit proliferation and enhanced apoptosis in cultured human premyelocytic leukemia HL-60 cells (Hseu et al., 2002; 2004). Thereafter extensive studies have verified the cancer-preventing or anti-cancer properties of *A. camphorata* and their derived pure compounds in various murine models of human cancer cell lines. Both the fruiting bodies and mycelium of *A. camphorata* have potent anti-proliferative activity against various cancers *in vitro* and *in vivo* (Table. 1). Its chemopreventive action against various cancer cells *via* modulating multiple signaling pathways at various cellular levels, the ultimate outcomes of which are apoptosis, call cycle arrest, growth inhibition, anti-angiogenesis and inhibition of metastasis. Figure 1, illustrating the molecular targets modulated by *A. camphorata*.

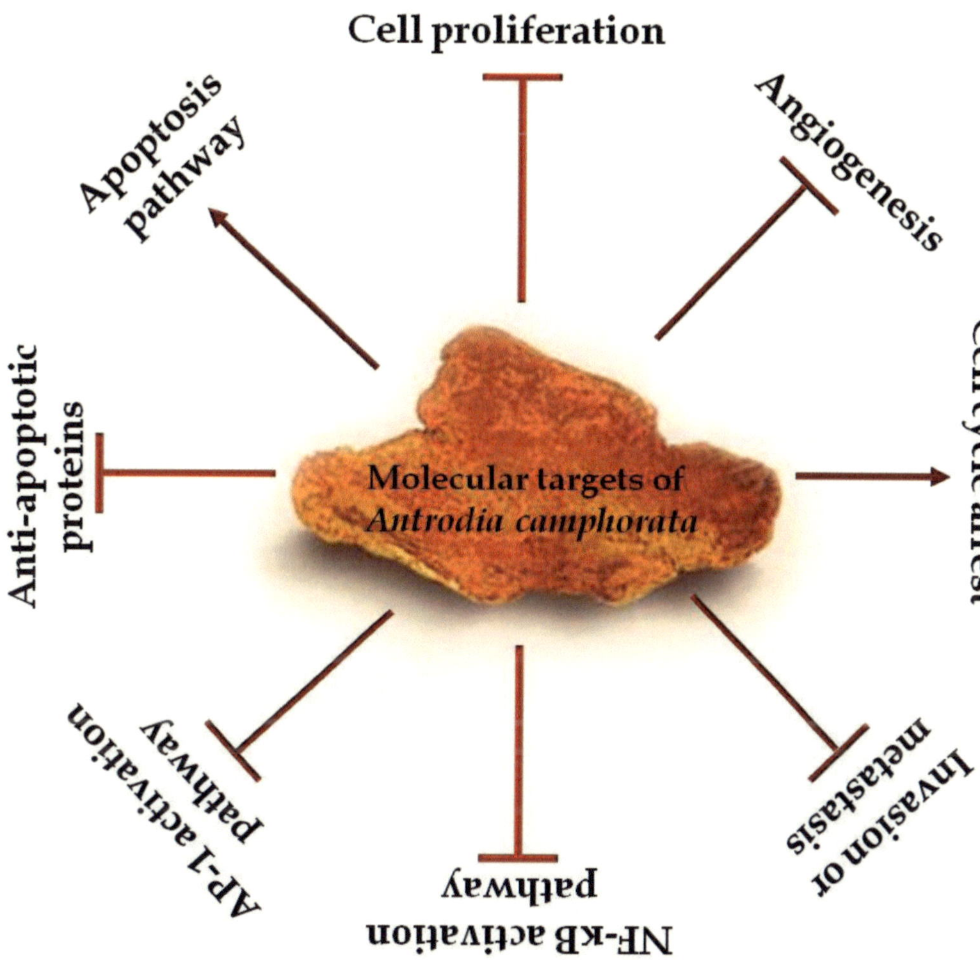

Fig. 1. Molecular targets of *A. camphorata* on various cancers

Agent	Mechanism	Target	Model	Cell lines or animal
A. camphorata	Cell cycle arrest	Cell cycle regulatory proteins	*In vitro*	PC3 & LNCap human prostate cancer cells
A. camphorata	Inhibits tumorigenesis	COX-2 and MDR-1 activity	*In vitro*	HepG2 human liver cancer cell
A. camphorata	Inhibits tumorigenesis	COX-2 and MDR-1 activity	*In vitro*	HepG2 human liver cancer cell
A. camphorata	Immunomodulation	HER-2/neu activity	*In vivo*	Inbreed female C3H/HeN mice
A. camphorata	Induce apoptosis	Caspase activity	*In vitro*	MDA-MB-231 breast cancer cell*
A. camphorata	Induce apoptosis	Caspase activity	*In vitro*	HepG2 human liver cancer cell
A. camphorata	Induce apoptosis	Caspase activity	*In vitro*	HL-60 human premyelotic leukemia
A. camphorata	Cell cycle arrest	Cell cycle regulatory proteins	*In vitro*	T24 bladder cancer cell
A. camphorata	Induce apoptosis	Caspase activity	*In vitro*	MCF-7 human breast cancer cell*
A. camphorata	Inhibits proliferation	Cytokines activity	*In vitro*	HepG2, MCF & colon-205 cancer cells*
A. camphorata	Induce apoptosis	Ca^{2+} activity	*In vitro*	PC3 human prostate cancer cell
A. camphorata	Induce apoptosis	Ca^{2+} and MAPK activity	*In vitro*	OC2 human oral cancer cell
A. camphorata	Induce apoptosis	Caspase activity	*In vitro*	HepG2 and PLC/PRF/5 human cancer cells
A. camphorata	Induce apoptosis	Ca2+/calpain activity	*In vitro*	HepG2 human liver cancer cell
A. camphorata	Induce apoptosis	Caspase activity	*In vitro*	A549 & NSCLC human lung cancer cells
A. camphorata	Inhibits metastasis	KF-	*In vitro*	PLC/PRF/5 human liver cancer cell
A. camphorata	Induce senescence	Cell cycle regulatory proteins	*In vitro*	RT4, TSGH-8301 and T_24 carcinomas
A. camphorata	Inhibits metastasis	NF-	*In vitro*	MDA-MB-231 human breast cancer cell*
A. camphorata	Cell cycle arrest	Cell cycle regulatory proteins	*In vitro*	MDA-MB-231, athymic nude mice (BALB/c-nu)*
A. camphorata	Induce apoptosis	Fas activity	*In vitro*	HepG2 human liver cancer cell
Triterpinoids	Induce apoptosis	Caspase activity	*In vitro*	A549 & NSCLC human lung cancer cell
Polysaccharides	Inhibits angiogenesis	VEGF expression	*In vitro*	Bovine aortic endothelial cells
Polysaccharides	Inhibits angiogenesis	VEGF expression	*In vivo*	HL-60 & HUVECs
Polysaccharides	Inhibits tumorigenesis	Cytokines activity	*In vitro*	U937 human leukemia & ICR mice
Polysaccharides	Inhibits angiogenesis	VEGF activity	*In vitro*	Bovine aortic endothelial cells
MMHO-1	Induce apoptosis	Mitotic-catastrophe	*In vitro*	U937 & BxPC3 pancreatic cancer cell
Antroquinonol	Cell cycle arrest	AMPK and mTOR activity		HCCs, HepG2, HepG2.2.15, Mahlavu, PLC/PRF/5, SK-Hept & Hep3B cancer calls
Antroquinonol	Induce cytotoxicity	Unknown	*In vitro*	MCF-7, MDA-MB-231, HepG2, Hep3B, Du-145 & LNCaP*
Antroquinonol	Cell cycle arrest	mTOR activity	*In vitro*	NSCLC human non-small lung cancer cell line
Antroquinonol	Inhibits proliferation	COX-2 and MDR1 activity	*In vitro*	HepG2 human liver cancer cell
Anticinate	Inhibits metastasis	Akt/mTOR activity	*In vitro*	MDA-MB-231 human breast cancer cell*
Methyl anticinate-A	Induce apoptosis	Caspase activity	*In vitro*	HepG2 and Hep3B human liver cancer cells
Methyl anticinate-A	Induce apoptosis	Caspase activity	*In vitro*	OEC-M1 and OC-2 human oral cancer cells

Table 1. Anti-cancer activity of *A. camphorata* and it's components against various cancer models

2. *A. camphorata* regulates cell cycle progression

In mammalian cells, cell cycle progression is tightly coordinated by the cyclin-dependent protein kinases (Cdk1, Cdk2, Cdk4 and Cdk6), regulatory cyclin subunits (cyclin-A, cyclin-B, cyclin-Ds and cyclin-E) and their inhibitors including $p21^{WAF1}$ and $p27^{KIP1}$ (Athar et al., 2009). Cyclin-E/Cdk1 (Cdc2) complex is the key components of the cell cycle check point pathway that delays mitotic entry in response to stalled replication or DNA damage. In addition to Cdk1, cyclin-Ds/Cdk4/6, and cyclin-A/Cdk2 are also required for G1/S transition and progression through S phase, while cyclin-A,B/Cdk1 complex activates are required for entry into mitosis (Fig. 1). Although, cyclin-B/Cdk1 complex are maintained inactive during interphase through the phosphorylation of Cdk1 at Thr 14 and Tyr 15 residues, which are catalysed by Wee1 and Myt1 (Thomas et al., 2005). Cyclin-D1 is a rate limiting activator for the G1/S transition, another cell cycle check point. The G1/S transition requires the activation of the cyclinD/Cdk4/Cdk6 and cyclin-E/Cdk2 complexs, which in turn phosphorylates the retinoblastoma protein (Rb). The subsequent dissociation of E2Fs from Rb activates a serious of target genes that are required for cell entering S phase (Athar et al., 2009). Rb was the first tumor suppressor gene, which is essentially hypophosphorylated when cells are in G0 and become progressively phosphorylated by G1 phase cyclin/Cdk complexes as cells enter G1, becoming hypophosphorylated on a larger number of serine and thrionine residues as cells advance through the R point., Rb remaines hypophosphorylated through the reminder of the cell cycle. The phosphorylate groups on Rb are removed by the protein phosphatase (PPI) as cells exit mitosis. Therefore, Rb plays a critical role in cell cycle progression as the molecular governor of the R-point transition (Mathhews & Gerritsen, 2010). Besides, Cdk2 activation, entry into mitosis requires nuclear translocation of active Cdc2/cyclin-B1 complexes. Normally, most Cdc2/cyclin-B1 complexes accumulate in the nucleus during prophase while Cdc25C phosphatase activates them by dephosphorylating Cdc2 on both Thr14 and Tyr15 (Thomas et al., 2005).

Cell cycle kinases are frequently upregulated in human cancer due to the over expression of their cyclin partners or inactivation of the Cdks inhibitors. Indeed, deregulation of cyclin-D1-Rb axis is very common in human cancers as cyclin-D1 accumulation is found in various types of human malignancies including breast, skin, lung, liver etc., and affect cell cycle modulation perhaps its most extensively studied target (Athar et al., 2009). Number of researchers has been reported on the cancer preventive and therapeutic effects of *A. camphorata* in different *in vitro* and *in vivo* test models. As summarized in Table. 1, various parts including mycelium and fruiting body, extracts (ethanol, methanol and ethyl acetate extracts) and chemical ingredients such as polysaccharides, triterpinoids, sesquiterpine, steroids, phenol compounds, adenosine, cordycepin, ergosterol etc., possessed potent anticancer activity. Besides, breast cancer cells are highly resistant to chemotheraphy, and there is still no effective cure for patients with advanced stages of the disease, specifically in cases of hormone-independent cancer (Rao et al., 2011). In addition, the cost of this therapy is significant, and therefore

The inhibition of breast cancer cell proliferation by *A. camphorata* was strongly associated with cell cycle arrest and/or induction of apoptosis. Exposure of human breast cancer cells (MCF-7) against *A. camphorata* caused significant arrest of cell progression (Fig. 2) in G1 phase (Yang et al., 2006). It was further confirmed by estrogen non-responsive human breast cancer cell line (MDA-MB-231) showed that approximately 70% of *A. camphorata* treated MDA-MB-231 cells were arrested in sub-G1 (Fig. 2) phase (Hseu et al., 2008). It has been documented that *A. camphorata* also arrest androgen-responsive-LNCaP and androgen-independent PC-3 human prostate cancer cells in a similar G1/S (Fig. 2) phase arrest (Chen et al., 2007), but caused G0/G1 arrest in human hepatoma HepG2 cells (Song et al., 2005), whereas, human urinary bladder cancer (T24) cells were arrested in G2/M (Fig. 2) phase (Peng et al., 2007). The reasons as to why *A. camphorata* causes G1 arrest in breast cancer cells, but G2/M phase arrest in other cells are still unknown. Therefore, *A. camphorata* has been shown to modulate the major cell cycle mediators at lower microgram concentrations, arresting breast cancer cells at the G1/S phase of the cell cycle. The anti-proliferative activity of *A. camphorata* involves the induction of p21^{WAFI} and p27KIP1 and down-regulation of cyclin-A/D1/E, cdc2, and CDK4 (Hseu et al., 2008).

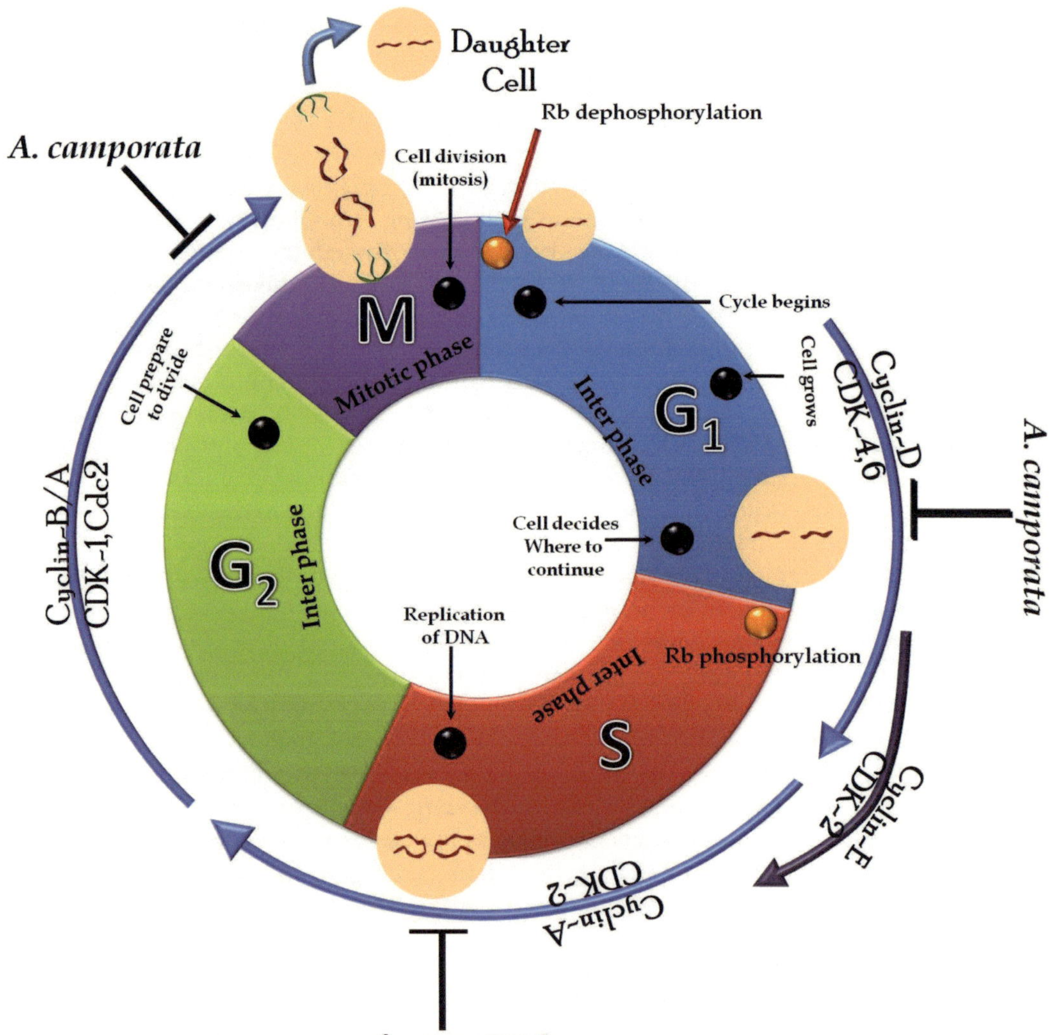

Fig. 2. Schematic diagram of *A. camphorata*-induced cell cycle arrest in various cancer cells

3. *A. camphorata* regulates apoptosis and cell survival

The major strategies of the underlying case of cancer was attributed to accelerated or dysregulated proliferation leading to cellular expansion and accumulation of tissue mass. It is well understood that key regulators of the cell cycle are frequently altered in many tumor types, with a consequent impact on elements of proliferative control such as cell cycle checkpoints and the response to DNA damage. Therefore, modern chemotherapeutic approaches are designed to exploit such aberration to induce cytotoxicity and tumor regression or cytostasis to control tumor progression. Uncontrolled cell proliferation, however, is only part of the picture. Recent cancer research progress has broadened our understanding underlying etiology to encompass aberrant cellular survival, as a consequence of failing to appropriately induce apoptosis or cell death, which are major contributor to the transformed state. Apoptosis, also known as programmed cell death, is a well-regulated and ordered process that occurs both in development and in response to stress to help maintain tissue homeostasis. Environmental and physico-chemicals stimulates accumulation of mutations or carcinogens that critically alter cell proliferation, cell cycle regulation, cell-cell or cell-extra cellular matrix (ECM) interactions, which eventually leads malignancy. However, apoptosis induction helps to prevent malignancies via eliminating damaged cells (Leibowitz & Yu, 2010). Apoptosis occurred *via* multiple pathways, and the extrinsic death receptor-mediated and the intrinsic mitochondrial-mediated cell death pathway (Fig. 3) are the ones better characterized in molecular terms (Fulda & Debatin, 2006).

The role of mitochondria as principal crossroad of the apoptotic process and emerged since 1990's, when it was shown that mitochondria of apoptosing cell death (Ghibelli & Diederich, 2010). The intrinsic pathway is characterized by the rapid release of cytochrome *c* from the mitochondrial inner membrane space into the cytosol. This critical event is absolutely required for caspase-dependent cell death (Kasibhatla & Tseng, 2003). The term mitochondrial outer membrane permeabilization (MOMP) was coined (Green & Kroemer, 2004), which indicates release of inter-membrane proteins rather than ion passage. However, the topological features and size concerns questioned about cytochrome *c* release *via* phospholipids transfer protein (PTP). A channel linking the inter-membrane mitochondrial space to the cytosol was sought to explain release of cytochrome *c*. The release of cytochrome c also depended activation of pro-apoptotic proteins such as Bax/Bid, which was stimulated by physico-chemical-induced cell stress. During the stimulation, cytochrome c nucleates the assembly of a multi-protein complex, known as apoptosomes, functionally analog to the DISC, further recruits and activates the other upstream caspases, including caspase-9 and caspase-8. Caspase-8 and caspase-9 converge into proteolytic activation of caspase-3, results cells undergo execution phase of apoptosis and/or cell dismantling (Ghibelli & Diederich, 2010).

Number of investigations critically characterized the anticancer potential of *A. camphorata*, regarding to the potential cytotoxic effect of various cancer cells derived from different human origins including lung, liver, breast, prostate, colon and oral cells (Table. 1). The viability of these cancer cells was significantly decreased by *A. camphorata* treatment in a dose-dependent manner. However, different cancer cells responded to *A. camphorata* with different sensitivities. A crude aqueous extract obtained from the fermented culture broth of *A. camphorata* exerted a potent effect in reducing the viability of different human breast cancer cell lines, including estrogen-responsive MCF-7 and estrogen-nonresponsive MDA-

MB-231 cells with an IC_{50} value of 57 and 136 μg/mL, respectively (Yang et al., 2006; Hseu et al., 2008; Yang et al., 2011). Meanwhile, the highest dose of *A. camphorata* (>100 μg/mL) was used to treat normal human endothelial cells for 24 hours, there was no cytotoxic effects were found. Furthermore, the chloroform extracts of fruiting bodies of *A. camphorata* significantly inhibited the growth of human breast cancer (MCF-7) cells with an IC_{50} value of 65 μM (Rao et al., 2007). This indicated the differential cytotoxic effects of *A. camphorata* crude extract on different kinds of breast cancer cells, with no harmful effects on normal cells at higher concentrations (Hseu et al., 2002).

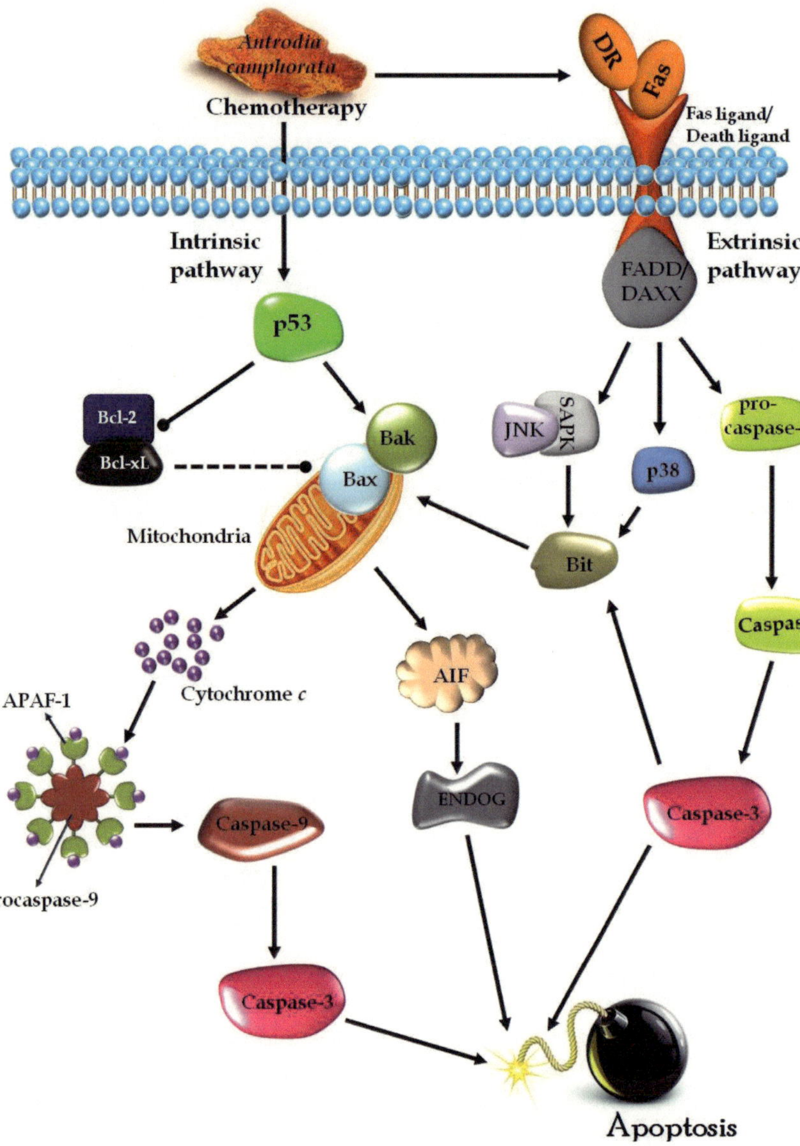

Fig. 3. Schematic representation of *A. camphorata*-induced apoptosis in *via* intrinsic and extrinsic pathways

In recent years much interest has been focused investigation onto the cancer preventive compositions of *A. camphorata* rather crude extract. There are two review articles available, thus, extensively summarized potent bioactive components, which are present in *A. camphorata* (Ao et al., 2009; Geethangili & Tzeng, 2009). It is believed that the anti-cancer and anti-metastasis properties of this mushroom are derived from its diversified chemical constituents, although it is comprised primarily of two types of compounds: polysaccharides and triterpenes (Shao et al., 2008). Yeh et al. demonstrated that five lanostanes (dehydroeburicoic acid, 15α-acetyl dehydrosulphurenic acid, 24-triene-21-oic acid, dehydrosulphurenic acid and sulphurenic acid) and three ergostane-type triterpenes (zhankuic acid, zhankuic acid-A and zhankuic acid-C) isolated from fruiting bodies of *A. camphorata* exhibits in vitro cytotoxic effect to various cancer cell lines, including MDA-MB-231. Zhankuic acid and suphurenic acid showed significant cytotoxic effect to the human breast cancer cells MDA-MB-231 and MCF-7 with an IC_{50} value of 25.1 and 89.2; and 57.8 and 357.0 μM, respectively. Indeed, sulphurenic acid is selectively cytotoxic to estrogen-nonresponsive MDA-MB-231 cells, and the only one compound that does not contain the diene structure with in the rings at position 7 and 9 and instead possesses a single double bond in the rings at the position 8 (Yeh et al., 2009). This result also provides another hallmark that cytotoxic effect of bioactive compounds also depends on structural activity relationship. Antroquinonol, an ubiquinone derivatives, was isolated from the solid state fermented mycelium of *A. camphorata* exhibits cytotoxic effect against MDA-MB-231 and MCF-7 human breast cancer cells with an IC_{50} value of 2.64 and 2.1 μM, respectively (Lee et al., 2007). A very similar result were obtained from an another pure compound antrocin, isolated from the fruiting bodies of A. camphorata showed the most anti-proliferative effect against MDA-MB-231 and MCF-7 cells (Rao et al., 2011). Notably, non-tumorigenic breast epithelial MCF-10A cells were not affected by antrocin treatment.

The morphological changes of human breast cancer (MCF-7) cells after *A. camphorata* treatment were further investigated to elucidate the underlying process of reduced viability treatment. The typical morphological characteristics for cell apoptosis, such as cell condensation, plasma membrane blabbing and formation of apoptotic bodies, were confirmed under phase contrast microscopy (Yang et al., 2006). The hallmark of cell apoptosis, DNA fragmentation was also demonstrated in *A. camphorata* treated human breast cancer cells including MCF-7 and MDA-MB-231. Caspase-3 activity in *A. camphorata*-treated MCF-7 breast cancer cells was shown to be increased, which further confirmed that *A. camphorata* could induce apoptosis in human breast cancer cells (Yang et al., 2006). An addition to *A. camphorata* crude extract, antrocin, a pure compound isolated from the fruiting bodies of *A. camphorata* significantly induced apoptosis in MDA-MB-231 breast cancer cells through the activation of caspase-3 (Rao et al., 2011). *In vivo* study, we showed that the tumor formation in BALB/c-*nu* mice with the implantation of MDA-MB-231 cells could be inhibited by the administration of the aqueous fermented culture broth of *A. camphorata*. The initial tumor development was dose-dependently inhibited by *A. camphorata*. The significant suppression of tumor development was directly demonstrating the *in vivo* anti-tumor effect of *A. camphorata* (Hseu et al., 2008). Comparably there was no cytotoxic effect was observed in control mice that received *A. camphorata* alone.

The mechanism of apoptosis induced by *A. camphorata* with various cancer cell lines were extensively studied (Table. 1) and demonstrated the relevant pathways of apoptosis (Fig. 3). There is an increase of the Bax/Bcl-2 ratio associated with the apoptosis induced by *A. camphorata* treatment in MCF-7 and MDA-MB-231 cells (Fig. 3). MCF-7 cells exposed to *A.*

camphorata significantly enhanced Bax protein expression, whereas, Bcl-2 the anti-apototic protein was not affected (Yang et al., 2006). Rao et al. studied that antrocin, a pure compound isolated from the fruting bodies of *A. camphorata* markedly augmented Bax:Bcl-2/Bcl-xL ratio in MDA-MB-231 cells (Rao et al., 2011). In an *in vivo* model, Bcl-2-positive cells were observed in MDA-MB-231 cells implanted cells mice tumor tissue. Furthermore, TUNEL assay showed that *A. camphorata*-induced Bcl-2 inhibition was directly proportional to apoptotic cells in mice tumor tissue (Hseu et al., 2008). This study also confirmed that *A. camphorata*-induced tumor suppression was mediated by cell-cycle arrest, as evidenced by reduction of cyclin-D and PCNA protein levels in mice tumor tissues. The down-regulation of Bcl-2 expression is known to be involved in the release of cytochrome *c* from mitochondria from the intrinsic pathway (Fig. 2). Further we investigated the *A. camphorata*-induced mitochondria membrame permeability and cytochrome *c* release in MCF-7 cells. Cells treated with *A. camphorata* significantly increased cytochrome *c* accumulation in cytoplasm, which supports *A. camphorata*-induced mitochondrial membrane potential. This data also provided another possible mechanism that *A. camphorata*-induced apoptosis was mediated by mitochondrial membrane potential followed by cytochrome *c* release in human breast cancer cells (Yang et al., 2006).

Another important mediator of apoptosis in immune cells is the Fas receptor/ligand signaling system. The critical elements of the Fas pathway that link receptor-ligand interaction and down-stream activation of caspases, including caspase-3, have been identified (Hung et al., 2010). Recent studies also indicate that widely used chemotherapeutic agents induce apoptosis in susceptible cells. Thereby, the chemotherapeutic agents required an alternative mediator. Recent studies revealed that Fas/Fas ligand (FasL) or death ligand/death receptor (DR) can activate the downstream extrinsic apoptotic pathway (Fig. 2). Gene expressions of both Fas/FasL were induced in human hepatoma HepG2 cells by treatment with methanolic extract of mycelium of *A. camphorata*. However, *A. camphorata* treatment dose-dependently inhibits death receptors (DR-4 and DR-5) and TNF-α receptors (TNFR-I and TNFR-II) in HepG2 cells.

Indeed, these results well demonstrate that *A. camphorata* induced apoptosis possibly by involving up-regulation of Fas expression, which promotes the ligation of Fas and FasL and then passes the death message to cytosolic messengers. As a result, procaspase-8 is activated to caspase-8, which triggers the caspase activation cascade. In addition, this study also demonstrates that *A. camphorata*-induced apoptosis was mediated by mitochondrial-independent pathway (Song, 2005).

4. *A. camphorata* up-regulates tumour-suppressor genes

The p53 tumor suppressor gene encodes a multifunctional protein involved in the comphrehensive control of cellular responses to genotoxic stress. p53 mediated tumor suppressor effects are mediated by a variety of mechanisms including cell cycle arrest, apoptosis and cellular senescence that prevent cells with damaged DNA to pass on their genome to progeny. Recently much attention has been focused towards p53, because it is once of the main effectors of cell cycle check point. However, the precise molecular mechanisms of its action are still controversial. Several reports indicate that p53 directly arrest cells in G1 phase in response to DNA damage, thus preventing DNA synthesis from damaged templates (Wahl et al., 1997). Apart from this p53 is involved in regulating the cell cycle at transition of G1/S and G2/M and with in S phase (Talos & Moll, 2010). Evidence for a possible role of p53 in M phase came from observations that p53 contributes to the control of centrosome duplication and to the prevention of DNA replication is impaired by spindle inhibitors (Talos and Moll, 2010).

In recent reports indicate that both estrogen receptor positive (MCF-7) and triple negative (MDA-MB-231) breast cancer cells were exposed to synthetic or natural derived anti-cancer drugs remarkable arrest cell cycle via accumulation in G2/M phase through the inhibition of Akt activity and p53-independent or p53-dependent activation of p53 inducible proteins such as p21/p53R2 /CDKN1A and GADD45A (De Santi et al., 2011; Hahm et al., 2011; Hsieh et al., 2011). It is noteworthy that *A. camphorata* significantly up-regulates p53 tumor suppressor gene in human colorectal carcinoma cells (Lien et al., 2009), and human prostate cancer cell lines (Chen et al., 2007). However, the potential up-regulation of p53 tumor suppressor gene product by *A. camphorata* was yet to be illustrated in human breast cancer cell lines. Our current work is fascinating *A. camphorata* induced up-regulation of p53 in triple negative MDA-MB-231 cells. We believe coming future this result may give vital evidence that anti-tumor activity of *A. camphorata* through the up-regulation of p53 tumor suppressor gene.

5. *A. camphorata* down-regulates invasion and metastasis

Metastasis is characterized that the multistep processes by which cancer spreads from the place at which it first arose as a primary tumor to distant location and establish itself in a new site in the body through blood stream or lymphatic system. Metastasis depends on the cancer cells acquiring two separate abilities increased motility and invasiveness cells that metastasize are basically identical to the original tumor. For example if cancer arises in the breast and metastasizes to the lung, the cancer cells in lung are similar breast cancer cells. Normally our body has many safeguards to prevent cells from adverse cancerous effects. However, many cancer cells itself have the ability to overcome these safeguards. In recent years much research has been focused on to understanding how cancer cells are mutated to circumvent the body's defenses and freely travel to another location. In normal tissue, cells adhere both to one another and a mesh of proteins are filled the space between them, this outer membrane proteins are known as extracellular matrix. The connection between cells and extracellular matrix is particularly characterized that from skin, mouth, lung, stomach and other organs. During invasion, cells spreads, it must break away not only from the cells around it, but also from the extracellular matrix. Cells are tightly bonded with cell-to-cell adhesion molecules. These adhesion molecules also allow interactions between numerous proteins on the cells surface. In cancerous cells, the adhesion molecules seem to be missing or compromised.

Cadherins, a family of Ca^{2+}-dependent intracellular adhesion protein molecules, which playing vital role for connecting two individual cells. Cadherins also regulates cells morphology, motility and hence tumor invasiveness. The cadherin molecules have three major regions. There is an extracellular region that mediates specific adherins, a transmembrane domain that spans the cell membrane, and a cytoplasmic domain that extends into the cell. The normal pattern of E-cadherin, α-, β-, γ- and p20-catenin are strong membraneous staining with localization at the intracellular border of luminal cells. Abnormal (absent, reduced or localized to cell compartments other than cell membrane) expression of E-cadherin and catenin has been reported in various human cancers and has been associated with tumor progression. The degradation of β-catenin involves its phosphorylation through complex formation with tumor suppressor gene products such as adenomatous polyposis coli (APC), glycogen synthase kinase-3β (GSK3β) and axin (Davidson et al., 2000). In tumor cells, E-caherin is either partly or entirely missing. This allows tumor cells to detach from each other, and from the matrix which holds everything in place. Recent clinical studies reveled that E-cadherin is important to regulate metastasis. E-cadherin-mediated cell-cell adhesion is associated with the progression of many carcinomas, including breast, bladder and squamous head and neck carcinomas (Davidson et al., 2000).

Abnormal expression of E-cadherin and catenin is very common in lobular than ductal carcinomas. However, its expression appears not to be involved into the early stage of neoplasia but to correlate with high grade invasive ductal carcinoma (Nakopoulou et al., 2002). Reduced expression of E-cadherin is seen in about 50% of ductal carcinomas of the breast and is associated with high histological grade, nodal metastases and poor prognosis. Addition to cadherins, a number of proteolytic enzymes contribute to the degradation of environmental barriers, such as the extracellular matrix and the basement membrane. Thus, degradation of the extracellular matrix and components of the basement membrane, mediated by the concerted action of proteinases, such as matrix metalloproteinases (MMPs) and urokinase plasminogen activator (uPA), play a critical role in tumor invasion and metastasis (Westermarck & Kahari, 1999).

Increasing expression of MMP-2, MMP-9 and angiogenic cytokine vascular endothelial growth factor (VEGF) in human breast cancer cell lines including estrogen receptor positive (MCF-7), triple negative (MDA-MB-231) and ductal epithelial tumor (T47D) cells has been suggested to be associated with the highly metastatic potential of breast cancer (Shibata et al., 2002; H.S. Lee et al., 2008). The promoter region of MMP-2 contains various cis-acting elements, including potential binding sites for the transcription factors nuclear factor-kappa B (NF-κB), activator protein-1 (AP-1), and stimulatory protein-1 (SP-1) (Lin et al., 2010). NF-kB is critically involved in tumor progression through transcriptional regulation of invasion related factors, such as MMP-2/MM-9, uPA and VEGF (Shibata et al., 2002; Yang et al., 2011). In addition, the involvement of mitogen-activated protein kinase (MAPK) pathways in NF-kB activation has been demonstrated to play an important role in tumor metastasis (Yang et al., 2011). Therefore, the inhibition of MMPs- and/or uPA-mediated migration or invasion could be a potential treatment for preventing or inhibiting cancer metastasis.

Once breast cancer has spread beyond the breast and under arm lymph nodes, it is considered a "systemic" disease, meaning that it is necessary to treat the whole body rather than just one particular spot. If breast cancer cells has traveled through the blood stream or lymphatic system, there are likely to be breast cancer cells in many different parts of the body, even scans only shows few spots. Therefore, the treatment that reaches all parts of the body. Chemotheraphy or hormonal therapy, are more suggestible treatment are used to treat metastic breast cancer instead of treatments that just treat one part of the body, just as surgery. In general, a women might be treated with a hormonal theraphy if she has a hormone responsive (estrogen or progesterone receptor positive) tumor, whereas, tumor that are not responsive to hormonal therapy, further choice is chemotherapy. There are many different types of chemotherapy that are used for breast cancer. In recent years, there has been much interest in developing new types of medicines that kill breast cancer cells in new and different way. Some of these drugs are only work against a specific type of breast cancer. To overcome this problem, current drug discovery system more fascinating a target protein or signaling cascades rather than specific type of breast cancer cells.

It was well demonstrated that metastasis is responsible for the majority of failures in cancer treatment, and is the major case of death from cancer. Therefore, chemotherapy is suggested to prevent local recurrence of the primary tumor and the spread of tumor cells (Weng & Yen, 2010). However, commercially available synthetic chemotherapeutic agents have severe side effects. Recent studies demonstrated that phytochemicals derived from plant source potentially prevents cancer metastasis (Sliva, 2008). As I mentioned that *A. camphorata* has been used in traditional Chinese medicine for various ills, including cancer. The mechanisms of action of *A. camphorata* against cancer cells includes inhibition of cell proliferation, induction of apoptosis and suppression of the motility of highly invasive breast cancer cells were intensively studied (Yang et al., 2006; Hseu et al., 2008). Although there are different compounds with various pharmacological activities were extracted from mycelia, fruiting bodies, spores and fermented culture broth of *A. camphorata*. The anticancer and anti-metastatic activities of this medicinal mushroom were primarily relied on its polysaccharide, benzenoids, lignans, diterpenes, triterpinod and steroid components (Ao et al., 2009; Geethangili & Tzeng, 2011).

Our recent study was clearly demonstrated that the anti-invasive and anti-metastatic effects of *A. camphorata* against highly metastatic human breast cancer cells (MDA-MB-231) is due to the inhibition of invasion and metastasis regulatory proteins such as MMP-2, MMP-9, uPA, uPA receptor and VEGF through the down-regulation of MAPK/NF-κB signaling pathway (Yang et al., 2011). *A. camphorata* inhibits invasion and metastasis of breast cancer cells not only through the suppression of MMPs/uPA, it also enhance endogenous MMPs/uPA inhibitors, TIMP-1, TIMP-2 and PAI respectively. It is also well understood that *A. camphorata* potentially modulates MAPKs cascades (Geethangili & Tzeng, 2009). Our investigation also revealed that the inhibition of MMPs/uPA due to the down-regulation of MAPK cascades such as ERK1/2, JNK and p38. Further we observed the major MMP's transcription factor NF-κB also significantly inhibited by *A. camphorata* treatment in MDA-MB-231 human breast cancer cell (Yang et al., 2011).

Moreover, there is substantial evidence on the inhibition of MMP-9/MMP-2 and suppression of invasiveness and metastases of cancer cells using various chemopreventive or chemotherapeutic agents (Ho et al., 2002; Abiru et al., 2002). Based on the observation, *A. camphorata* eventually decreased the activity or protein levels of tumor metastasis-related proteins, including MMP-9, MMP-2, uPA, and uPAR, and increase the expression of their endogenous inhibitors, TIMP-1, TIMP-2, and PAI-1, in MDA-MB-231 cells. Therefore, *A. camphorata* could be a potential agent for the prevention of breast cancer metastasis.

6. *A. camphorata* down-regulates tumour angiogenesis

Angiogenesis is the development of a new blood supply from an existing vasculature. Normal cells can stimulate new blood vessels to grow. This happens to repair damaged tissue when wounds are healing. Therefore, normal cells have genes that can produce proteins known as angiogenic factors, which switch blood vessels growth on. However, cells also have genes that produce certain molecules called anti-angiogenic factors, which slow down blood vessel growth (Papetti & Herman, 2002).

Accumulating evidences indicate that progressive tumor growth is dependent on angiogenesis. It also plays an important role in the growth and spread of cancer. New blood vessels "feed" the cancer cells with oxygen and nutrients, allowing these cells to grow, invade nearby tissue, spread to other parts of the body, and form new colonies of cancer cells (Maliwal et al., 2009). Every cancer begins its existence as a tiny cluster of abnormal tumor cells growing in an organ. Without its own blood supply to bring in oxygen and nutrients, the tumor cannot grow larger than 1-2 millimeters in diameter (about the size of a small pea). While this early stage of tumor growth can last for month or even years, eventually a few cancer cells gain the ability to produce angiogenic growth factors. These growth factors are released by the tumor into nearby tissues, and stimulate new blood vessels to sprout vigorously from existing healthy blood vessels toward and into the tumor. In addition, increased angiogenesis has also been observed in preneoplastic conditions (Sharma et al., 2001), indicating that it plays a key role in the early processes of carcinogenesis.

Various angiogenic regulators have been identified since the introduction of angiogenesis in the scientific community. As we mentioned above that the stability of vasculature is highly regulated by the homeostasis between angiogenic stimulators and inhibitors. The best characterized angiogenic stimulators including, angiopoietin, vascular endothelial growth factor (VEGF), platelet-derived growth factor (PDGF), fibroblast growth factor (FGF), endothelial growth factor (EGE) and hepatocyte growth factor (HGF) (Liekens et al., 2001; Takeya et al., 2008). Number of research is going on onto anti-angiogenic therapy. The research has found that the amounts of these angiogenic factors are expressed very high at the outer edge of tumor. Anti-angiogenic drugs may stop a cancer from growing into surrounding tissue or spreading. They will probably not be able to get rid of a cancer, but may be able to halt new blood vessel growth and starve a tumor by cutting off its blood supply. There ate more than three hundred angiogenesis inhibitor molecules have been discovered so far: Some angiogenesis inhibitors are naturally present in the human body (endogenous angiogenic inhibitors) results healthy tissues appear to resist cancer growth by containing these antiangiogenic compounds. The endogenous angiogenic inhibitors are classified into five major groups; 1) endothelial cell specific inhibitors, 2) avascular tissue-derived inhibitors, 3) anti-angiogenic cytokines, 4) angiogenic factor antagonists and 5) other inhibitors (Cao, 2001; Grant & Kullar, 2005). Other angiogenesis inhibitors occur naturally in substances found in green tea, soy beans, fungi, mushrooms, tree bark, shark tissues, snake venom and many other plants and animals. Still other angiogenesis inhibitors have been manufactured synthetically in the laboratory.

Conventional chemotherapy preferentially targets rapidly dividing cancer cells. However, certain normally dividing cells (hair cells, intestinal cells, mucous membranes, bone marrow cells) are also destroyed, which causes the well-known severe chemotherapy side effects of hair loss, diarrhea, mouth ulcer, infection, and low blood counts. Some chemotherapy regimens work very well at treating cancers that are diagnosed early. Most of the anti-angiogenic therapies targets only growing new blood vessel (endothelial) cells. Since blood vessels do not grow in normal, healthy tissues, the side effects of anti-angiogenic therapy are concentrated primarily at the cancer site. Most anti-angiogenic drugs do not kill cancer cells directly and are therefore better tolerated compared to chemotherapy, with fewer and less severe side effects. To keep cancers from re-growing, it is possible that some patients may need to take anti-angiogenic drugs as a chronic therapy, although this hypothesis is still being tested in clinical studies. In response to targeted affects anti-angiogenic agents are classified into three major class; they are 1) agent that block new bllod vessel from sprouting (true angiogenic inhibitors), 2) assault a tumor's established blood supply (vascular targeting agents) and 3) attack both the cancer cells as well as blood vessel cells (the double-barreled approach). Recent clinical studies in different cancer types have shown that anti-angiogenic therapy generally works best when used in combination with cytotoxic chemotherapy or radiation. Most experts believe that such combinations will ultimately provide cancer patients with the greatest benefit.

A recent study has shown that ethyl acetate extracts of fruiting bodies of *A. camphorata* not only suppressed tumor growth in human liver cancer cell PLC/PRF/5 xenografted male BALB/cA-*nu* nude mice, but also inhibits tumor angiogenesis (Hsu et al., 2007). It is now known that a decrease in tumor size is often associated with inhibited microvessel formation in the tumor. This study also confirmed that PLC/PRF/5 cells implanted mice greatly induced angiogenesis and the hemoglobin levels (6.4-fold). The amount of hemoglobin level in tumor tissue is considered as a blood vasculature in tumor tissue. However, mice were pretreated with *A. camphorata* significantly inhibits PLC/PRF/5 cells-induced angiogenesis and hemoglobin level in mice tumor tissue (Hsu et al., 2007).

Subsequently, polysaccharides were isolated from the mycelium or fermented culture broth of *A. camphorata* showed potent anti-tumor activity in several in vitro and in vivo models (Liu et al., 2004). Tumor growth and metastasis is angiogenesis dependent. Several lines of direct evidence have shown that angiogenesis is essential for tumor growth and metastasis (Weng & Yen, 2010). The *ex vivo* check chorioallatonic membrane (CAM) assay is commonly employed to examine the anti-angiogenic activity of samples. Polysaccharides with different molecular weight, isolated from *A. camphorata* were tested for its anti-angiogenic properties using CAM assay. The microvasculature was markedly reduced after treatment with polysaccharides (Yang et al., 2009). In addition to CAM assay, Tube forming assays measure a complex series of events involving changes in endothelial cell morphology and migration, leading to the formation of a complex interconnecting network of capillary tubes with identifiable lumens (branching morphogenesis) (Cavell et al., 2011). Polysaccharides from *A. camphorata* also significantly inhibit matrigel-dependent capillary tube formation in human umbilical vein endothelial (HUVEC) cell and bovine aortic endothelial cells (Yang et al., 2009; Chen et al., 2005; Cheng et al., 2005).

Angiogenesis requires endothelial proliferation, migration, and tube formation. Cancer cells are able to produce large amounts of several angiogenic factors including VEGF, EGF, FGF (Liekens et al., 2001). Therefore, VEGF is considered as an important biomarker of angiogenesis. Over expression of VEGF in tumors increases tumor vascularization and growth, while capturing VEGF or blocking its signaling receptor, VEGFR-2, by VEGF receptor tyrosine kinase inhibition, antisense oligonucleotides, vaccination, or neutralizing antibodies reduces tumor angiogenesis and growth. Besides, VEGF induces cyclin D1 expression, which serves as a cell cycle regulatory switch in actively proliferating cells, through PLCg-PKC-MAP kinase pathways. Further to confirm the anti-angiogenic activity of *A. camphorata* the inhibition of VEGF-R tyrosine kinase phosphorylation was monitored. Similarly, polysaccharides from *A. camphorata* have been shown to suppressed VEGFR-2 tyrosine kinase phosphorylation in Tyr1054/1059 residual position. This study also revealed *A. camphorata* significantly inhibits endothelial cell proliferation as evidenced by the reduction of cyclin-D1 protein expression, which is a marker of cell cycle check point (Cheng et al., 2005). These results indicate that *A. camphorata* might be a potent inhibitor of angiogenesis and subsequent tumor promotion.

7. *A. camphorata* down-regulates NF-κB/AP-1 signalling pathway

7.1 Inhibits NF-κB activation

NF-κB (Nuclear Factor-KappaB) is a heterodimeric protein composed of different combinations of members of the Rel family of transcription factors. NF-κB dimers are sequestered in the cytosol of un-stimulated cells *via* non-covalent interactions with a class of inhibitor proteins, called I-κBs. Signals that induce NF-κB activity cause the phosphorylation of I-κBs, their dissociation and subsequent degradation, thereby allowing activation of the NF-κB complex. The degradation of I-κB proteins that permits NF-κB molecules to move into the nucleus is also carried out by the proteasome but only after prior phosphorylation of I-κB by the IKKs. NF-κB can be activated by exposure of cells to LPS or inflammatory cytokines such as TNF-α or IL-1, growth factors, lymphokines, and by other physiological and non physiological stimuli (Li & Verma, 2002; Verma, 2004).

The Rel/NF-κB family of transcription factors are involved mainly in stress-induced, immune, and inflammatory responses. In addition, these molecules play important roles during the development of certain hemopoietic cells, keratinocytes, and lymphoid organ structures (Matsumori, 2004). Moreover, NF-κB family members have been implicated in neoplastic progression and the formation of neuronal synapses (Matsumori, 2004). NF-κB is also an important regulator in cell fate decisions, such as programmed cell death and proliferation control, and is critical in tumorigenesis (Thu & Richmond, 2010). An another study showed that angiocidin, which shown anti-tumor activity by blocking angiogenesis in various cancer cells through the suppression of NF-κB. However, in MDA-MB-231 cells, angiocidin significantly activate NF-κB and the de novo up-regulation of many down-stream genes transcribed by NF-κB, including cytokines, inflammatory mediators and the cell cycle inhibitor p21(waf1) (Godek et al., 2011).

The molecular identification of its p50 subunit (v-REL) as a member of the reticuloendotheliosis (REL) family of viruses that provided the first evidence that NF-κB is linked to cancer (Prasad et al., 2010). Although the transforming ability of the v-REL oncoprotein was established many years ago, recent evidence suggests other human NF-κB family members may be important in oncogenesis (Dolcet et al., 2005). NF-κB DNA binding activity is constitutively increased in many lymphoid and epithelial tumors. The RAS, BCR-ABL, and HER2 oncogenes and transforming viruses can activate NF-κB. Furthermore, several genes thought to be essential to the cancer phenotype those controlling angiogenesis, invasion, proliferation, and metastasis, contain κB binding sites.

Research over the past decade has revealed that NF-κB is an inducible transcription factor for genes involved in cell survival, cell adhesion, inflammation, differentiation and growth. Many of the target genes that are activated are critical to the establishment of early and late stages of aggressive cancers such as expression of cyclin D1, apoptosis suppressor proteins such as Bcl-2 and Bcl-XL and those required for metastasis and angiogenesis such as MMPs and VEGF (Dorai & Aggarwal, 2004). Higher concentration of serum VEGF has been shown to associate with a poorer prognosis in patients with breast cancer. On the other hand, constitutive expression of a transcription factor, NF-κB was correlated with progression and metastasis in a number of human breast cancers, suggesting a possible regulation of VEGF expression by NF-κB. Shibata et al. analyzed the expression of VEGF and constitutive NF-κB activity in three breast cancer cell lines, MCF-7, T47D, and MDA-MB-231. The basal levels of VEGF mRNA expression correlated with those of nuclear NF-κB activity in these cell lines. The highest NF-κB activity in MDA-MB-231 cells was associated with the highest expression of VEGF mRNA, while the activity and the mRNA levels were moderate in MCF cells and the lowest in T47D cells (Shibata et al., 2002). A similar study showed that the triple negative breast cancers (MDA-MB231 and MDA-MB-468) or MCF-7 and T47D implanted mice expressed higher VEGF and NF-κB activation in their tumor tissues (Chougule et al., 2011; Antoon et al., 2011). Recently, Ambs and Glynn revived that inducible nitric oxide synthase (iNOS) has been observed in many types of human tumors. In breast cancer, increased iNOS is associated with markers of poor outcome and decreased survival. iNOS induction will trigger the release of variable amounts of NO into the tumor microenvironment and can activate oncogenic pathways, including the Akt, epidermal growth factor receptor and c-Myc signaling pathways, and stimulate tumor microvascularization. More recent findings suggest that NO induces stem cell-like tumor characteristics in breast cancer. This review, also pointed that NF-κB is the key transcription factor which playing major role for the production of NO *via* iNOS expression in various breast cancer cell lines (Ambs & Glynn, 2011). The over expression of metallothionein-2A (MT-2A) is frequently observed in invasive human breast tumors and has been linked with more aggressive breast cancers. MT-2A over expression led to the induction of MDA-MB-231 breast cancer cell migratory and invasive abilities. Concomitantly, they observed the expression of matrix metalloproteinase-9 (MMP-9) and the transcriptional activity of AP-1 and NF-κB were upregulated by MT-2A overexpression in MDA-MB-231 cells (Kim et al., 2011).

7.2 Inhibits AP-1 activation

Activated protein-1 (AP-1) is another transcription factor that regulates the expression of several genes that are involved in cell differentiation and proliferation. Functional activation of the AP-1 transcription complex is implicated in tumor promotion as well as malignant transformation. This complex consists of either homo or heterodimers of the members of the JUN and FOS family of proteins (Surh, 2003). This AP-1 mediated transcription of several target genes can also be activated by a complex network of signaling pathways that involves external signals such as growth factors, mitogen activated protein kinases (MAPK), extracellular-signal regulated protein kinases (ERK) and JUN-terminal kinases (JNK). Some of the target genes that are activated by AP-1 transcription complex mirror those activated by NF-κB and include Cyclin D1, bcl-2 , bcl-XL, VEGF, MMP and urokinase plasminogen activator (uPA) (Dorai & Aggarwal, 2004). Expression of genes such as MMP and uPA especially promotes angiogenesis and invasive growth of cancer cells. Most importantly, AP-1 can also promote the transition of tumor cells from an epithelial to mesenchymal morphology which is one of the early steps in tumor metastasis. These oncogenic properties of AP-1 are primarily dictated by the dimer composition of the AP-1 family proteins and their post-transcriptional and translational modifications.

7.3 Inhibits COX-2 activity

Several preclinical studies indicated the importance of regulation of cyclooxygenase-2 (COX-2) expression in the prevention and the treatment of several malignancies. This enzyme is overexpressed in practically every pre-malignant and malignant condition involving the colon, liver, pancreas, breast, lung, bladder, skin, stomach, head and neck and esophagus (Aggarwal et al., 2006). Overexpression of this enzyme is a consequence of deregulation of transcriptional and post-transcriptional control. Depending upon the stimulus and the cell type, different transcription factors including AP-1, NF-IL-6, NF-κB can stimulate COX-2 transcription (Surh, 2003). Wild type p53 protein expression can suppress COX-2 transcription while the mutant p53 protein can not. Consistent with this observation, increased COX-2 levels are seen in several epithelial cancers that express mutant p53. Taken together, these findings suggest that the balance between the activation of the oncogenes and the inactivation of the tumor suppressor genes and expression of several pro-inflammatory cytokines can modulate the expression of COX-2 in tumors. Complicating matters further is the fact that conventional cancer therapies such as radiation and chemotherapy can induce COX-2 and prostaglandin biosynthesis. Thus, inhibition of this enhanced COX-2 activity in tumors clearly has a therapeutic potential.

Accumulating evidence to implicate COX-2 function in breast cancer tumorigenesis. Soslowe et al. examined that 56% of infiltrating mammary carcinomas and intraductal carcinomas expressed significant levels of COX-2, while benign breast tissue at least 1 cm from a malignant lesion did not express COX-2 (Soslow et al., 2000). In a murine model of metastatic breast cancer, PGE_2 levels are positively correlated with increased tumorigenic and metastatic potential (Kundu et al., 2001). Perhaps the most convincing evidence that COX-2 causes breast cancer in animals comes from transgenic mice in which COX-2 was overexpressed in mammary tissue by using the mouse mammary tumor virus (MMTV) long-terminal repeat promoter. More than 85% of these mice developed tumors, indicating that COX-2 overexpression alone is sufficient to cause breast tumors (Liu et al., 2001). Ristimaki et al. analyzed the expression of COX-2 protein by immunohistochemistry in tissue array specimens of 1576 invasive breast cancers. Moderate to strong expression of COX-2 protein was observed in 37.4% of the tumors, and it was associated with unfavorable distant disease-free survival. Elevated COX-2 expression was associated with a large tumor size, a high histological grade, a negative hormone receptor status, a high proliferation rate (identified by Ki-67), high p53 expression, and the presence of HER-2 oncogene amplification, along with axillary node metastases and a ductal type of histology (Ristimaki et al., 2002). These results indicate that elevated COX-2 expression is more common in breast cancers with poor prognostic characteristics and is associated with an unfavorable outcome. Therefore the breast cancer treatment also targeted inhibition of COX-2 activity.

A. camphorata extract and its bioactive compounds, polysaccharides and triterpenoids, have been shown to have anti-proliferative, anti-invasive or anti-metastatic activities were observed in various cell lines or animal models. These investigations also revealed the *A. camphorata* regulation on signaling pathways or transcription factors, especially NF-κB involved in the effects of anti-angiogenesis, anti-adhesion and anti-invasion (Fig. 3). Moreover, the mechanism induced by *A. camphorata* with various cancer cell lines was well understood. We also contributed to understand the mechanism involved in breast cancer cells. Triple negative human breast cancer cells, MDA-MB-231 were treated with fermented culture broth of *A. camphorata* induced apoptosis followed by the regulation of Bax:Bcl-2 ratio. The induction of apoptosis was directly correlated with down-regulation of COX-2 expression in MDA-MB-231 cells (Hseu et al., 2007). This data supports *A. camphorata*-induced apoptosis might be associated with the inhibition of COX-2 activity. Very recently, we also observed that the fermented culture broth extracts of *A. camphorata* inhibit invasive behavior of breast cancer MDA-MB-231 cells through suppressing degradation of ECM, down-regulating the expression of MMPs, including MMP-9 and MMP-2; uPA and uPAR expression. This study also provided positive evidence that the inhibition of MMP-2, MMP-

9, uPA and uPAR in MDA-MB-231 cells by *A. camphorata* is through the down-regulation of MAP kinase cascades, including ERK1/2, JNK1/2 and p38. In addition, we also found that the inhibition of MAPKs further suppressed NF-κB nuclear translocation (Yang et al., 2011). Similar NF-κB, AP-1/MAPK and COX-2 inhibitory activity of *A. camphorata* was observed in various cancers and activated cell lines as summarized in (Geethangili & Tzeng, 2009; Ao et al., 2009). However, still certain molecular mechanisms are yet to be understood, especially the involvement *A. camphorata* in AP-1 transcriptional activation of inhibition in human breast cancer cells.

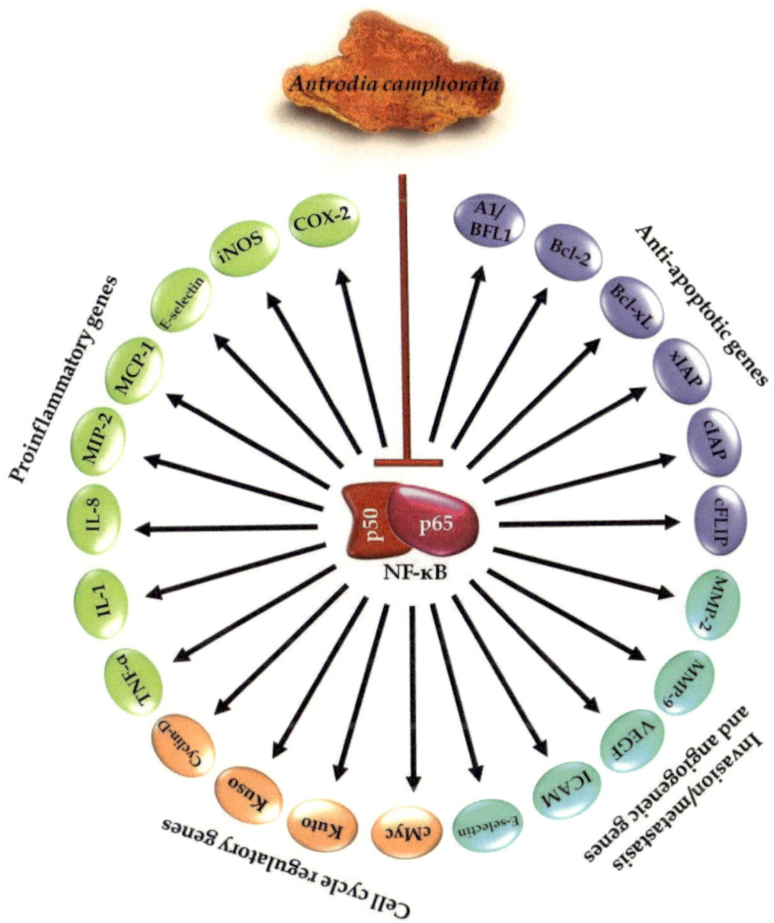

Fig. 4. NF-κB mediated anti-cancer activity of *A. camphorata*

8. Future perspectives

In past two decades *A. camphorata* received pioneering interest for their pharmacological intervention s. It is oblivious that *A. camphorata* exhibits anti-cancer activity against human breast cancer cell lines, including estrogen receptor-positive (MCF) and triple-negative (estrogen, progesterone and Her-2) MDA-MB-231 cell lines *in vitro* and *in vivo*. The pronounced anti-cancer activity was highly connected with its anti-metastasis, anti-angiogenic, and the inhibition of cell cycle progression; and the induction of apoptosis in both intrinsic and extrinsic pathways. Besides, *A. camphorata* possessed various chemical components such as polysaccharides, triterpenes, diterpenes, benzinoids and steroids may be the bioactive compounds responsible for the observed anticancer activity against human breast cancer cells. Still, there are number compounds which presented *A. camphorata* are warranted to extensive study. The presented evidences are confirmed that *A. camphorata* as a potential candidate for breast cancer chemoprevention. However, the chemopreventive agents can be used not just to prevent cancer but also treat cancer. Since, the pharmacological safety, most chemopreventive agents to enhance the effect at lower dose and thus can minimize chemotherapy-induced toxicity to non-cancer cells. It was cleared that *A. camphorata* failed to induce cytotoxic effect against non-cancer cell lines. And the notable point is certain human breast cancer cells are resistance to hormonal therapy or chemotherapy. Thus, agents that can suppress multiple pathways have great potential for the treatment of human breast cancer. *A. camphorata* achieved the target that it can inhibit cancer development in multiple signaling pathways.

9. References

Abiru, S., Nakao, K., Ichikawa, T., Migita, K., Shigeno, M., Sakamoto, M., Ishikawa, H., Hamasaki, K., Nakata, K. & Eguchi, K. (2002) Aspirin and NS-398 inhibit hepatocyte growth factor induced invasiveness of human hepatoma cells, *Hepatology* 35: 1117–24.

Aggarwal, B.B., Ichikawa, H., Garodia, P., Weerasinghe, P., Sethi, G., Bhatt, I.D., Pandey, M.K., Shishodia, S. & Nair, M.G. (2006) From traditional Ayurvedic medicine to modern medicine: identification of therapeutic targets for suppression of inflammation and cancer, *Expert Opin Ther Targets* 10: 87-118.

Ambs, S. & Glynn, S.A. (2011) Candidate pathways linking inducible nitric oxide synthase to a basal-like transcription pattern and tumor progression in human breast cancer, *Cell Cycle* 10: 619-24.

Antoon, J.W., White, M.D., Slaughter, E.M., Driver, J.L., Khalili, H.S., Elliott, S., Smith, C.D., Burow, M.E. & Beckman, B.S. (2011) Targeting NFκB mediated breast cancer chemoresistance through selective inhibition of sphingosine kinase-2, *Cancer biol ther* 11: 678 – 89.

Ao, Z.H., Xu, Z.H., Lu, Z.H., Xu, H.Y., Zhang, X.M. & Dou, W.F. (2009) Niuchangchih (*Antrodia camphorata*) and its potential in treating liver diseases. *J Ethnopharmacol* 121:194-212.

Athar, M., Back, J.H., Kopelovich, L., Bickers, D.R., Kim, A.L. (2009) Multiple molecular targets of resveratrol: Anti-carcinogenic mechanisms, *Arch Biochem Biophys* 486: 95-102.

Cao, Y. (2001) Endogenous angiogenesis inhibitors and their therapeutic implications, *Inter J Biochem Cell Biol* 33: 357-69.

Cavell, B.E., Sharifah, S., Alwi, S., Donlevy, A., Packham, G. (2011) Anti-angiogenic effects of dietary isothiocyanates: Mechanisms of action and implications for human health, *Biochem Pharmacol* 81: 327–36.

Chen, K.C., Peng, C.C., Peng, R.Y., Su, C.H., Chiang, H.S., Yan, J.H., Hsieh-Li, H.M. (2007) Unique formosan mushroom *Antrodia camphorata* differentially inhibits androgen-responsive LNCaP and -independent PC-3 prostate cancer cells, *Nutr Cancer* 57: 111-21.

Chen, S.C., Lu, M.K., Cheng, J.J. & Wang, D.L. (2005) Antiangiogenic activities of polysaccharides isolated from medicinal fungi, *FEMS Microbiol Lett* 249: 247–54.

Chougule, M.B., Patel, A.R., Jackson, T. & Singh, M. (2011) Antitumor Activity of Noscapine in Combination with Doxorubicin in Triple Negative Breast Cancer. *PLoS One* 6: e17733.

Davidson, B., Berner, A., Nesland, J.M., Resberg, B., Berner, H.S., Trope, C.G., Kristensen, G.B., Bryne, M & Florenes, V.A. (2000) E-cadherin and a-, b-, and g-catenin protein expression is up-regulated in ovarian carcinoma cells in serous effusions, *J Pathol* 192: 460-69.

De-Santi, M., Galluzzi, L., Lucarini, S., Paoletti, M.F., Fraternale, A., Duranti, A., De-Marco, C., Fanelli, M., Zaffaroni, N., Brandi, G. & Magnani, M (2011) The indole-3-carbinol cyclic tetrameric derivative CTet inhibits cell proliferation via overexpression of p21/CDKN1A in both estrogen receptor positive and triple negative breast cancer cell lines. *Breast Cancer Res* 13:R33.

Dolcet, X., Llobet, D., Pallares, J., Matias-Guiu, X.(2005) NF-kB in development and progression of human cancer, *Virchows Arch* 446: 475-82.

Dorai, T. & Aggarwal, B.B. (2004) Role of chemopreventive agents in cancer therapy, *Cancer Lett* 215:129-40.

Fulda, S. & Debatin, K.M. (2006) Extrinsic versus intrinsic apoptosis pathways in anticancer chemotherapy, *Oncogene* 25: 4798–811.

Fulda, S. (2010) Resveratrol and derivatives for the prevention and treatment of cancer, *Drug Discov Today* 15: doi:10.1016/j.drudis.2010.07.005.

Geethangili, M. & Tzeng, Y.M. (2009) Review of Pharmacological Effects of *Antrodia camphorata* and Its Bioactive Compounds. *eCAM* 2011, doi:10.1093/ecam/nep108.

Ghibelli, L. & Diederich, M. (2010) Multistep and multitask Bax activation. *Mitochondrion* 10: 604–13.

Godek, J., Sargiannidou, I., Patel, S., Hurd, L., Rothman, V.L., Tuszynski, G.P.(2011) Angiocidin inhibits breast cancer proliferation through activation of epidermal growth factor receptor and nuclear factor kappa (NF-κB), *Exp Mol Pathol* 90: 244-51.

Grant, M.A & Kallur, R. (2005) Structural Basis for the Functions of Endogenous Angiogenesis Inhibitors. *Cold Spring Harb Symp Quant Biol* 70: 399-417.

Green, D.R. & Kroemer, G. (2004) The pathophysiology of mitochondrial cell death, *Science* 305: 626–29.

Hahm, E.R., Lee, J., Huang, Y. & Singh, S.V. (2011) Withaferin A Suppresses Estrogen Receptor-α Expression in Human Breast Cancer Cells, *Mol Carcinogen:* DOI: 10.1002/mc.20760.

Ho, L.L., Chen, W.J., Lin-Shiau, S.Y., Lin, J.K., (2002) Penta-O-galloyl-beta-D-glucose inhibits the invasion of mouse melanoma by suppressing metalloproteinase-9 through down-regulation of activator protein-1, *Eur J Pharmacol* 453: 149–58.

Hseu, Y.C., Chang, W.C., Hseu, Y.T., Lee, C.Y., Yech, J.J, Chen, P.C., Chen, J.Y and Yang, H.L. (2002) Protection of oxidative damage by aqueous extract from Antrodia camphorata mycelia in normal human erythrocytes, *Life Sciences* 14: 469-82.

Hseu, Y.C., Chen, S.C., Chen, H.C., Liao, J.W. & Yang, H.S. (2008) *Antrodia camphorata* inhibits proliferation of human breast cancer cells *in vitro* and *in vivo*, *Food Chem Toxicol* 46: 2680–8.

Hseu, Y.C., Chen, S.C., Tsai, P.C., Chen, C.S., Lu, F.J., Chang, N.W. & Yang, H.S. (2007) Inhibition of cyclooxygenase-2 and induction of apoptosis in estrogen-nonresponsive breast cancer cells by *Antrodia camphorata, Food Chem Toxicol* 45:1107–15.

Hseu, Y.C., Yang, H.L., Lai, Y.C., Lin, J.G., Chen, G.W., Chang, Y.H., (2004) Induction of apoptosis by *Antrodia camphorata* in human premyelocytic leukemia HL-60 cells, *Nutr Cancer* 48: 189–197.

Hsieh, T.C., Wong, C., Bennett, D.J. & Wu, J.M. (2011) Regulation of p53 and cell proliferation by resveratrol and its derivatives in breast cancer cells: an *in silico* and biochemical approach targeting integrin αvβ3, *Inter J Cancer:* DOI: 10.1002/ijc.25930.

Hsu, Y.L., Kuo, P.L., Cho, C.Y., Ni, W.C., Tzeng, T.F., Ng, L.T., Kuo, Y.H. & Lin, C.C. Antrodia cinnamomea fruiting bodies extract suppresses the invasive potential of human liver cancer cell line PLC/PRF/5 through inhibition of nuclear factor κB pathway, *Food Chem Toxicology* 45: 1249–57.

Huang, S.T., Pang, J.H.S. & Yang, R.C. (2010) Anti-cancer Effects of *Phyllanthus urinaria* and Relevant Mechanisms, *Chang Gung Med J* 33: 477-87.

Jing-Jy Cheng, Nai-Kuei Huang, Tun-Tschu Chang, Danny Ling Wang, Mei-Kuang Lu. Study for anti-angiogenic activities of polysaccharides isolated from *Antrodia cinnamomea* in endothelial cells. *Life Sciences* 76 (2005) 3029–3042.

Kasibhatla, S. & Tseng, B. (2003) Why target apoptosis in cancer treatment? *Mol Cancer Ther* 2: 573–80.

Kim, H.G., Kim, J.Y., Han, E.H., Hwang, Y.P., Choi, J.H., Park, B.H., Jeong, H.G. (2011) Metallothionein-2A overexpression increases the expression of matrix metalloproteinase-9 and invasion of breast cancer cells, *FEBS Lett 585*: 421–28.

Kundu, N., Yang, Q., Dorsey, R. & Fulton, A.M. (2001) Increased cyclooxygenase-2 (cox-2) expression and activity in a murine model of metastatic breast cancer, *Int J Cancer* 93: 681-6.

Lee, H.S., Seo, E.Y., Kang, N.E., Kim, W.K. (2008) [6]-Gingerol inhibits metastasis of MDA-MB-231 human breast cancer cells, *J Nutr Biochem* 19: 313–19.

Lee, T.H., Lee, C.K., Tsou, W.L., Liu, S.Y., Kuo, M.T. & Wen, W.C. (2007) A new cytotoxic agent from solid state fermented mycelium of *A. camphorata*. *Planta Medica* 73: 1-3.

Leibowitz, B. & Yu, J. (2010) Mitochondrial signaling in cell death *via* the Bcl-2 family, *Cancer Biol Ther* 9: 417–22.

Li, Q. & Verma, I.M. NF-kappaB regulation in the immune system. *Nat Rev Immunol* 2:725-34.

Liekens, S., Clercq, E.D. & Neyts, J. (2001) Angiogenesis: Regulators and clinical applications. *Biochem Pharmacol* 61: 253-70.

Lien, H.M., Lin, H.W., Wang, Y.J., Chen, L.C., Yang, D.Y., Lai, Y.Y., Ho, Y.S. (2009) Inhibition of Anchorage-Independent Proliferation and G0/G1 Cell-Cycle Regulation in Human Colorectal Carcinoma Cells by 4,7-Dimethoxy-5-methyl-l,3-benzodioxole Isolated from the Fruiting Body of *Antrodia camphorata, eCAM* doi:10.1093/ecam/nep020.

Lin, M.L., Lu, Y.C., Chung, J.G., Wang, S.G., Lin, H.T., Kang, S.E., Tang, C.H., Ko, J.L. & Chen, S.S. (2010) Down-Regulation of MMP-2 Through the p38 MAPK-NF-κB-Dependent Pathway by Aloe-Emodin Leads to Inhibition of Nasopharyngeal Carcinoma Cell Invasion, *Mol Carcinog* 49:783–97.

Liu, C.H., Chang, S.H., Narko, K., Trifan, O.C., Wu, M.T., Smith, E., Haudenschild, C., Lane, T.F. & Hla T. (2001) Overexpression of cyclooxygenase-2 is sufficient to induce tumorigenesis in transgenic mice. *J Biol Chem* 276: 18563-9.

Liu, J.J., Huang, T.S., Hsu, M.L., Chen, C.C., Lin, W.S., Lue, F.J. & Chang, W.H. (2004) Antitumor effects of the partially purified polysaccharides from *Antrodia camphorata* and the mechanism of its action. *Toxicol Appl Pharmacol* 201: 186–93.

Maliwal, D., Patidar, V., Talesara, A., Dave, K. & Jain, N. (2009) Anti-angiogenic natural products in cancer therapy. *J Her Med Toxicol* 3: 157-9.

Matsumori, A. (2004) The role of NF-kappaB in the pathogenesis of heart failure and endotoxemia. *Drugs Future* 29: 733.

Matthews, D.J. & Gerritsen, M.E. (2010) *Targeting Protein Kinases for Cancer Therapy*, John Wiley & Sons Inc. New Jersey.

Nakopoulou, L., Gakiopoulou-Givalou, H., Karayiannakis, A.J., Giannopoulou, I., Keramopoulos, A., Davaris, P. & Pignatelli, M. (2002) Abnormal alpha-catenin expression in invasive breast cancer correlates with poor patient survival, *Histopathology* 40:536-46.

Papetti, M. & Herman, I.M. (2002) Mechanisms of normal and tumor derived angiogenesis, *Am J Physiol Cell Physiol* 282: C947-70.

Peng, C.C., Chen, K.C., Peng, R.Y., Chyau, C.C., Su, C.H., Hsieh-Li, H.M. (2007) *Antrodia camphorata* extract induces replicative senescence in superficial TCC, and inhibits the absolute migration capability in invasive bladder carcinoma cells, *J Ethnopharmacol* 109: 93–103.

Prasad, S., Ravindran, J. & Aggarwal, B.B. (2010) NF-kappaB and cancer: how intimate is this relationship, *Mol Cell Biochem* 336:25-37.

Rao, Y.K., Fang, S.H. & Tzeng, W.M. (2007) Evaluation of the anti-inflammatory and anti-proliferation tumoral cells activities of *Antrodia camphorata*, *Cordyceps sinensis*, and *Cinnamomum osmophloeum* bark extracts, *J Ethnopharmacol* 114: 78–85.

Rao, Y.K., Wu, A.T.H., Geethangili, M., Huang, M.T., Chao, W.J., Wu, C.H., Deng, W.P., Yeh, C.T. & Tzeng, W.M. (2011) Identification of Antrocin from *Antrodia camphorata* as a Selective and Novel Class of Small Molecule Inhibitor of Akt/mTOR Signaling in Metastatic Breast Cancer MDA-MB-231 Cells, *Chem Res Toxicol:* dx.doi.org/10.1021/tx100318m.

Ristimaki, A., Sivula, A., Lundin, J., Lundin, M., Salminen, T. & Haglund, C. (2002) Prognostic significance of elevated cyclooxygenase-2 expression in breast cancer, *Cancer Res* 62: 632–5.

Shao, Y.Y., Chen, C.C., Wang, H.Y., Chiu, H.L., Hseu, T.H. & Kuo, Y.H. (2008) Chemical constituents of Antrodia camphorata submerged whole broth *Nat Prod Res* 22:1151-7.

Sharma, R.A., Harris, A.L., Dalgleish, A.G., Steward, W.P. & O'Byrne, K.J. (2001) Angiogenesis as a biomarker and target in cancer chemoprevention, *Lancet Oncol* 2: 726–32.

Shibata, A., Nagaya, T., Imai, T., Funahashi, H., Nakao, A. & Seo1, H. (2002) Inhibition of NF-κB activity decreases the VEGF mRNA expression in MDA-MB-231 breast cancer cells, *Breast Cancer Res Treat* 73: 237–43.

Sliva, D. (2008) Suppression of cancer invasiveness by dietary compounds, *Nat Rev Cancer* 3:921-30.

Song, T.Y., Hsu, S.L. & Yen, G.C. (2005) Induction of apoptosis in human hepatoma cells by mycelia of *Antrodia camphorata* in submerged culture, *J Ethnopharmacol* 100: 158–67.

Soslow, R.A., Dannenberg, A.J., Rush, D., Woerner, B.M., Khan, K.N., Masferrer, J. & Koki, A.T. (2000) COX-2 is expressed in human pulmonary, colonic and mammary tumors, *Cancer* 89, 2637-2645.

Surh, Y.J. (2003) Cancer chemoprevention with dietary phytochemicals, *Nat Rev Cancer* 3:768-80.

Takeya, Y., Makino, H., Aoki, M., Miyake, T., Ozaki, K., Rakugi, H., Ogihara, T. & Morishita, R. (2008) *In vivo* evidence of enhancement of HGF-induced angiogenesis by fluvastatin, *Open genether J* 1: 1-6.

Talos, F. & Moll, U.M. (2010) Role of the p53 family in stabilizing the genome and preventing polyploidization, *Adv Exp Med Biol* 676:73-91.

Thomas, C.G., Vezyraki, P.E., Kalfakakou, V.P. & Evangelou, A.M. Vitamin C transiently arrests cancer cell cycle progression in S phase and G2/M boundary by modulating the kinetics of activation and the subcellular localization of Cdc25C phosphatase, *J Cell Physiol* 205:310-8.

Thu, Y.M. & Richmond, A. (2010) NF-κB inducing kinase: a key regulator in the immune system and in cancer, *Cytokine Growth Factor Rev* 21:213-26.

Verma, I.M. (2004) Nuclear factor (NF)-kappaB proteins: therapeutic targets, *Ann Rheum Dis* 63: ii57-61.

Wahl, G.M., Linke, S.P. & Paulson, T.G. (1997) Maintaining genetic stability through TP53 mediated checkpoint control, *Cancer Surv* 29:183-219.

Weng, C.J. & Yen, G.C. (2010) The in vitro and in vivo experimental evidences disclose the chemopreventive effects of *Ganoderma lucidum*on cancer invasion and metastasis, *Clin Exp Metastasis* 27: 361–9.

Westermarck, J., Li, S., Jaakkola, P., Kallunki, T., Grenman, R. & Kahari, V. M. (2000) Activation of fibroblast collagenase-1 expression by tumor cells of squamous cell carcinomas is mediated by p38 mitogen-activated protein kinase and c-Jun NH2-terminal kinase-2, *Cancer Res* 60, 7156-62.

Wu, S.H., Ryvarden, L. & Chang, T.T. (1997) *Antrodia camphorata* ("Niu-Chang-Chih"), new combination of a medicinal fungus in Taiwan. *Bot Bull Acad Sin* 38: 273-5.

Yang, C.M., Zhou, Y.J., Wang, R.J., Hu, M.L. (2009) Anti-angiogenic effects and mechanisms of polysaccharides from *Antrodia cinnamomea* with different molecular weights, *J Ethnopharmacol*123: 407–12.

Yang, H.L., Chen, C.S., Chang, W.H., Lu, F.J., Lai, Y.C., Chen, C.C., Hseu, T.H., Kuo, C.T., Hseu, Y.C. (2006) Growth inhibition and induction of apoptosis in MCF-7 breast cancer cells by *Antrodia camphorata*, *Cancer Lett* 231: 215–27.

Yang, H.L., Kuo, Y.H., Tsai, C.T., Huang, Y.T., Chen, S.C., Chang, H.W., Lin, E., Lin, W.H., Hseu, Y.C. (2011) Anti-metastatic activities of *Antrodia camphorata* against human breast cancer cells mediated through suppression of the MAPK signaling pathway, *Food Chem Toxicol* 49: 290–98.

Yeh, C.T., Rao, Y.K., Yao,C.J., Yeh,C.F., Li,C.H., Chuang, S.E., Luong, J.H.T., Lai, G.M., Tzeng,Y.M. (2009) Cytotoxic triterpenes from Antrodia camphorata and their mode of action in HT-29 human colon cancer cells, *Cancer Lett* 285: 73–79.

Zang, M. & Su, C.H. (1990) *Ganoderma comphoratum*, a new taxon in genus Ganoderma from Taiwan, China. *Acta Bot Yunnanical* 12: 395–396.